Applying Ethical Principles to Clinical Practice

Applying Ethical Principles to Clinical Practice provides a concise overview of bioethics, drawing especially on principlism, for all those who encounter moral dilemmas as part of their professional responsibilities to their patients.

Including an introductory chapter each on the principles of autonomy, beneficence, nonmaleficence, and justice, Glorioso then explores how these principles can apply in different clinical scenarios. The applied chapters look at end-of-life care, cancer care, intensive care, and the organization of health services. The book ends with chapters exploring how to establish healthcare ethics consultation services and develop your communication skills.

This guide is written in clear and accessible language and is designed for frontline healthcare professionals and their students.

Dominic Glorioso is the Associate Medical Director of Amedisys Hospice in Harrisburg, PA, USA. He is also an Assistant Clinical Professor of Internal Medicine at Duquesne University College of Osteopathic Medicine. In 2020, after many years as an internist and palliative care physician, Dr Glorioso decided to leave clinical practice and become a full-time student at Duquesne University in Pittsburgh, Pennsylvania. In 2023, he earned a PhD in clinical bioethics.

Applying Ethical Principles to Clinical Practice

DOMINIC GLORIOSO

Routledge
Taylor & Francis Group
LONDON AND NEW YORK

Designed cover image: Daniel Dinsmore

First published 2026
by Routledge
4 Park Square, Milton Park, Abingdon, Oxon OX14 4RN

and by Routledge
605 Third Avenue, New York, NY 10158

Routledge is an imprint of the Taylor & Francis Group, an informa business

British Library Cataloguing-in-Publication Data
A catalogue record for this book is available from the British Library

ISBN: 978-1-041-10241-0 (hbk)
ISBN: 978-1-041-10224-3 (pbk)
ISBN: 978-1-003-65412-4 (ebk)

DOI: 10.4324/9781003654124

Typeset in Vectora LH
by codeMantra

This book is dedicated to my wife, Barbara, who never wavered in her support for my decision to become a full-time student again, even after nearly 40 years in clinical practice.

Contents

Foreword

The author, Dr. Dominic Glorioso, and I have traveled a very similar path in the arena of palliative care and clinical ethics. Both disciplines are inextricably intertwined. Because of our close relationship that has developed over the years, I'm honored to write the foreword for this book, *Applying Ethical Principles to Clinical Practice*.

Dr. Glorioso brings principles alive through cases and his lived experience in the engagement of social and institutional contexts in which ethical dilemmas emerge.

This is not a passive text but a guide, a dialogue, and, at times, a direct challenge to our comfort as clinicians, administrators, and ethicists. The journey it offers is equal parts intellectual rigor, practical wisdom, and honest engagement with the limits of what ethical reasoning can achieve in the real world.

The principle of autonomy is laid bare in its complexity. The narrative repeatedly revisits real people. Beneficence and nonmalfeasance are unpacked as a source of much of modern medicine's anguish. Dr. Glorioso's reflection on human hope brings to life the very real trade-offs between technological possibility and the good life, between clinical optimism and the risk of paternalism. Justice never retreats to the background; it is present in every aspect of distributive resources and the often invisible bias that shapes who gets access to care. The text is explicit about the tough realities of who gets and who is denied or who is lost in the insurance labyrinth or abandoned due to administrative efficiency.

There is a persistent theme here: ethics is not just for ethicists. It is for every clinician, nurse, administrator, and family member faced with a choice that matters. The book's chapters on palliative care and patient-centered decision-making are particularly strong, offering practical frameworks for breaking bad news and the substituted judgment model for surrogate decision-making. These sections reinforce the idea that compassion and communication are skills that can and must be learned.

As someone who has spent years advising clinicians and organizations on ethical dilemmas, I found these pages both a comfort and a challenge. *Applying Ethical Principles to Clinical Practice* does not pretend that the right answer is always obvious or that there is a rulebook for the most difficult days in medicine. Instead, it offers what is perhaps most needed: A sense of company on the road, a reminder that wisdom is found as much in dialogue as in doctrine. For those new to bioethics, this book will serve as an invaluable guide. For the experienced practitioner, it serves as a mirror and a sounding board—a call to keep striving for honesty, justice, and empathy, even when the way forward is unclear.

I recommend Dr. Glorioso's book to anyone who understands that healthcare is, at its core, profoundly human—and therefore a profoundly ethical enterprise.

Rev. Dr. David Garvis, PhD
Adjunct Professor of Moral Theology, Ethicist
St. Mary's Seminary
Houston, TX

Introduction

Why I Wrote This Book

What a wonderful time to be working in healthcare! Recent medical breakthroughs have markedly enhanced how clinicians care for patients. Yet, with these advances come questions about the right thing to do. Do we need ethics? As the ethicist and physician Eric Cassell has stated, "To conceive of a physician practicing his profession without constant ethical decision-making is to conceive of a physician operating in a cultural vacuum and caring for a collection of static facts wrapped in human form."[1] Healthcare and ethics go hand in hand, and this book will attempt to show that for all practicing healthcare professionals.

At the beginning of life, new technologies have greatly improved the survival of infants that weigh less than two pounds at birth.[2] New advances have also made it possible to prolong life past anything previously imagined and to treat conditions considered to be untreatable. For example, we now have mRNA technology that can quickly produce highly effective and safe vaccines to diminish the effects of new organisms that could cause the next pandemic.[3] In addition, new targeted prostate and breast cancer treatments can significantly change how these common deadly diseases are treated.[4] Neural stimulation techniques can help those with paralysis to walk again. Artificial intelligence (AI) can do everything from sequencing genes to targeted cancer therapies to provide superior treatment protocols for sepsis.[5] Obesity, diabetes, and hyperlipidemia have all seen treatment advances that can reverse the adverse outcomes of these problems.[6] Machines can be substituted for failing human organs until they recover or can be replaced. No donor organs are available? No problem; soon, scientists can 3D print new organs for transplantation.[7] What if the patient dies in the hospital? Using extracorporeal membrane oxygenation (ECMO) with conventional cardiopulmonary resuscitation (CPR) called extracorporeal cardiopulmonary resuscitation (ECPR), we can cheat death by allowing time to fix the underlying etiology of the arrest.[8] All of the above technologies barely scratch the service of what is available in modern medicine.

DOI: 10.4324/9781003654124-1

However, these technologies have a negative side. They are expensive and do not always work in a way that provides a beneficial outcome. When this happens, ethical dilemmas occur. Very few problems in the hospital can match the chaos when these cases arise. Doctors, family members, friends, nurses, social workers, chaplains, lawyers, and even hospital administrators are often all painfully involved in resolving these quandaries. There may be many differing opinions on how to go ahead from all these people and disciplines.[9]

This book aims to help people deal with ethical dilemmas in healthcare. It will do so from a clinical point of view written by a physician with internal medicine and palliative care training and certification, who is also Catholic. My approach will be more clinical and practical rather than philosophical. That being said, the cases presented will require the reader to think!

Regarding being Catholic, that should not dissuade the reader who is not Catholic, Christian, or even religious from reading this book. When I was a hospital-based palliative care physician at an urban hospital, I had a considerable amount of house staff who were foreign medical graduates (FMGs). Several times, it occurred that one of the residents would come to me before graduation and state that they had just got a job at a Catholic hospital and they were concerned because they were Hindu, Islamic, Buddhist, or just non-Catholic. They were worried about what new rules they would need to know to work there. First, I told them, and you will see later in this chapter, that most secular healthcare ethics is surprisingly based on Catholic teaching. Second, most of what they learned from me (with few exceptions) about end-of-life care would be proper for Catholic hospitals. Artificial nutrition and hydration (ANH) would need further discussion, and medical assist in dying (MAID) would be forbidden. As new internists, they would not often be involved with beginning-of-life dilemmas; however, that will be covered in this book. When there is a difference between Catholic and secular bioethics, I will point that out.

One final reason why this book could be helpful to non-Catholics is that many medical issues have become political in the United States. Since the overturn of *Roe v. Wade*, it is now up to the individual states to legislate abortion policies. Some of the rhetoric on both sides can be difficult to grasp. The Catholic Church, by definition, places these dilemmas in the context of Christ's love and biblical teaching. Even if the reader disagrees with this position, understanding this view, which is not tainted by politics, should prove instructive.

Dealing with ethical dilemmas in healthcare is challenging. One concern is the different educational backgrounds of the professionals who face these problems. A clinical ethicist with a philosophical background will have developed considerable skills in their training.[10] However, these skills may leave the ethicist ill-prepared when faced with the challenges of helping patients, providers, and other parties resolve ethical concerns to help resolve uncertainties or conflicts between or among multiple parties in a timely fashion.[11] In addition, when faced with a clinical dilemma, philosophy-educated ethicists must avoid a lengthy search for truth and wisdom when a quick decision is needed.[12]

Physicians and nurses are at the other end of the spectrum. Although they are well-educated on clinical matters, they often have difficulty with different areas of learning. Even though Galen, the ancient Roman writer and physician, has said that anyone who claims to be a doctor must "know all parts of philosophy: the logical, the physical and the ethical,"[13] the need for this knowledge has been debated in present medical education.[14] For social workers, although there is a requirement for ethics education throughout their curriculum, it frequently does not specify what should be taught or how.[15] Finally, chaplains and social workers most likely do not have a philosophical or medical background yet are often involved with healthcare ethics.[16]

Not too long ago, healthcare was simple because treatment options were limited. Clinicians offered what they could, and most often, patients died regardless. Only in the last century have treatments for chronic illnesses been developed. Procedures were even designed to bring the dead back to life through resuscitation. The fact is that most often, patients are elderly and have multiple chronic illnesses. Treatment decisions, therefore, become more complex. For the first time, the question becomes, even though we can do something, should we? There are many examples of this dilemma, which will be explored later. Modern medicine can keep people alive for extended periods, but at what cost? Ventilators can keep people breathing when their lungs have failed. Likewise, left ventricular assist devices (LVADs) can support people with failing hearts and dialysis with those with failing kidneys. But what if the patients cannot come off these machines? Do we continue them, or do we stop them? Alternatively, maybe the decision is not to start them at all. By the way, who is going to make these decisions? Ideally, it would be the patient, but often, that person is too ill to make such a choice, or sometimes they choose not to make a choice. So then, who makes the choice: family, the physician, the hospital, the insurance company, the Church, the government?

THE RISE OF MEDICAL TECHNOLOGY AND REVOLUTIONARY IDEAS

Although positive, the increase in medical technology comes with a cost that has not previously been seen. For example, financial concerns now play a role in decision-making. Many of the innovative treatments now available are not covered by insurance. As a result, the choice to accept treatment can often lead to financial hardships and bankruptcy. The stress of these options can increase the risk of early death.[17] And what about quality of life? As before, who decides whether someone's life has quality? If it is the patient, many opt to forgo treatment if it negatively affects their lifestyle. Often, clinicians have problems with this situation. If only you would take one more pill or agree to one more treatment or surgery, you would be so much better (sic). On the other side of the spectrum are those (or their families) who want to avoid death, no matter the financial or personal cost. Moreover, what about the cost to the clinicians involved with the case; does that matter?[18]

One common ethical problem in hospitals involves families that cannot let go of their seriously ill loved one. It does not matter to them how old or sick their family member is or the almost zero chance for recovery; they still want everything done. By everything, they could mean CPR, life support, dialysis, surgery, the newest medications, and anything else they can find doing a Google search. So often, the clinical team, especially the nurses, feels that their actions are causing the patient to suffer. The physicians and other team members have to deal with the family that is begging, pleading, crying, praying, screaming, threatening, or whatever it takes to get the team to do every imaginable thing to keep the patient alive, no matter the cost, the pain or the chance of survival. Even if death can temporarily be postponed, what will be the quality of whatever amount of life that could be salvaged? Some will argue that this type of care should be considered futile, but even that term is controversial.[19] Does calling it medically ineffective care make it sound better?

Besides the difficulties caused by the exponential increase in science and technology, the number of people who make decisions has also changed. In the past, these decisions were made exclusively by physicians. It was felt that their education made them solely competent in deciding what was best for their patients. However, a new phenomenon occurred, and patient rights began to get national attention by the 1960s. In 1976, California was the first state to enact natural death legislation. The Natural Death Act allowed patients to refuse treatment even when their physicians decided it was best for them.[20] This law quickly became widespread, and by 1988, many states, including Arizona, Illinois, Kentucky, Maryland, Massachusetts, Michigan, Minnesota, New Hampshire, New York, Pennsylvania, Rhode Island, and Vermont, approved a patient's bill of rights by regulation or statute.

To further add to the complexity of medical decision-making, laws were placed to allow families and friends to make choices for their loved ones when they could no longer do so. As previously said, modern medical and technical procedures make extending human life beyond natural limits possible. Applying some of these procedures to an individual suffering an uncomfortable and challenging dying process may cause a loss of patient dignity and secure the extension of a precarious and burdensome life.[21] Therefore, legislation about advance care planning (ACP) was enacted by many states. The lawmakers said that the customary goal of ACP is to have patients make treatment choices in advance so that clinicians can provide care consistent with their wishes. Ideally, this conversation would occur with their clinicians and their chosen surrogates. The results are then written as a *living will.*[22] For many people, this process also included choosing a *healthcare power of attorney,* which involves preparing another trusted person to make medical decisions if the person can no longer make their own decisions.[23]

Besides the laws about healthcare decision-making, the 1970s had three medical events that forever influenced how medical technology has changed our values. The first event involved a remarkable beginning of life discovery, *in vitro* fertilization, or what was then called the first test tube baby. A baby girl named Louise Joy Brown was born by Cesarean section on July 25, 1978, in Oldham, a small town near Manchester, England. Her mother, Lesley, had been infertile for nine years and desperately wanted a baby. Her obstetrician, Patrick Christopher Steptoe, extracted the egg from the mother, and a physiologist, Robert Geoffrey Edwards, developed the method for the *in vitro* fertilization of the human ovum.[24] The ovum was reimplanted, and the pregnancy went ahead as usual. After the birth, there were questions about the morality of the procedure. The Catholic Church opposed it because the unused fertilized eggs were discarded. (Interestingly, this dilemma became relevant again in 2024 Alabama, where the disposal of frozen embryos became controversial.) However, beyond this singular opposition, more provocative questions arose about the "natural order of procreation" and "playing God" concerning reproduction.[25]

Another medical breakthrough during this time was the development of the artificial heart. This idea began in 1965, and in the summer of 1972, the National Heart and Lung Institute (NHLI) brought together a group of experts to discuss the development of a device that would be totally implantable in the chest or upper abdomen and have a similar cardiac output to a natural heart.[26] Even though this procedure's auspicious beginning raised numerous ethical questions, many praised this development as a step forward in treating people with end-stage heart disease. Institutional review boards (IRBs) were set up to discuss eligibility and consent policies.[27] However, others felt that the procedure was not likely to be of any benefit. Implanting an artificial heart was just too risky and expensive to help the common good. In contrast, others raised concerns about the psychological costs to recipients who would now become literally part man and part machine.[28]

The final point to be discussed was not a medical breakthrough but a tragic case that illustrates the burdens of technology and our right to refuse it. Twenty-one-year-old Karen Quinlan decided to meet her friends at a New Jersey bar for a night of partying on April 14, 1975. She was apparently trying to lose weight to fit into a dress and had been fasting for several days. Unfortunately, she overdid it by consuming a combination of alcohol and tranquilizers. [29] When she collapsed, her friends took her home, thinking she just needed to "sleep it off." However, she eventually stopped breathing, and they started CPR. At the hospital, it was revealed that she suffered extensive brain damage due to hypoxia (low levels of oxygen to the brain). Five months later, when it became clear that she would not recover, her family asked that she be removed from the ventilator. Fearing prosecution for homicide, her physicians refused, and after a prolonged legal battle, the NJ Supreme Court allowed her to be removed from life support in May 1976. However, maintained by a feeding tube, she lived for another nine years.[30] This decision had far-reaching consequences beyond this one case and set precedents for patients and their guardians, allowing them to refuse medical treatment based on the burden of the intervention and not prognosis, removing the long-held practice that only physicians could make this choice.[31] The Natural Death Act now had a face and a compelling story.

PHILOSOPHICAL FOUNDATIONS

The *Merriam-Webster Dictionary* describes ethics as "a set of moral principles." It often stands for the correct behavior or action when given a specific problem or set of circumstances. Moreover, bioethics refers to "a discipline dealing with the ethical implications of biological research and applications, especially in medicine."[32] As noted above, incidents that occurred in the 1970s seemed to spark an interest in bioethics. This movement developed its influence throughout Western countries in the 1980s and became a global effort in the 1990s. This initiative continues to the twenty-first century and will likely remain a medical discipline for a long time. Because of its longevity, Bioethics is now seen as "classic"—the opposite of pure "fashion."[33] However, 50 years seems minuscule compared to its ancient origins in philosophy.

Philosophy comes from the Greek word that means "love of wisdom,"[34] a simple definition but also a puzzling one. For neither word, love, nor wisdom, has a clear explanation. However, with this ambiguity, there is also beauty, and perhaps the reason why this field of study has persisted. Philosophy has the lengthiest ongoing record of argumentation and controversy in history. Other disciplines, such as medicine, law, and mathematics, are at least as old as philosophy (if not older).

Still, their teachers and students rarely consider what their ancestors created or understood. For example, medicine changes so rapidly that studies from only a decade ago may seem obsolete. However, from the beginning, philosophers have directed their insights toward opinions made by other philosophers, even going back to the ancient Greeks.[35] The allure of philosophy is that it allows teachers and learners to speak out constructively in response to challenges. Therefore, philosophy's value as a discipline exists in its tradition dedicated to examining, discovering, and meditating about life through dialogue, with a desire to question ways of thinking that challenge our mutual well-being.[36]

Socrates (469–399 BCE) is regarded as the originator of teaching through dialogue and discussions.[37] Healthcare professionals are familiar with this practice of education during teaching rounds in the hospital. The professor, physician, or instructor would ask their pupils questions about the patients they saw in front of the group. That unfortunate student would have to answer the query correctly or face further probing by the leader. Sometimes called "pimping" (especially by the humiliated learners), this style of teaching is more formally called the "Socratic method." The Roman statesman Cicero also credits Socrates as the first person to analyze ethics and who "brought down philosophy from the heavens, established it in cities, introduced it into families, and forced it to examine life, morals, and good and evil."[38] Unfortunately, Socrates was tried and convicted of being a "Sophist," a dangerous philosopher with destructive ideas. He was sentenced to death and drank the poison hemlock. Another famous philosopher, Plato (427–347 BCE), some forty years his junior, disputed this accusation and, through his writings, gave society much of what we know about Socrates' teachings since there is no recorded writing from Socrates.[39]

In his writings, Plato's student Aristotle (384–322 BCE) provided much of what we know about ancient ethics. First, he introduces the concept of virtue and describes it as something unique to humans and what separates us from animals. Then, as with Socrates and Plato before him, he insists that virtue is connected to human good at its best way—indeed, the only way—to secure what we most desire.[40] However, unlike many modern philosophers, Aristotle sees virtue as "a quality of individual human character, rather than embodied simply in terms of social behaviors."[41] By making virtue part of the human character and not just an action or behavior, Aristotle makes this idea a psychological characteristic with human reasoning as its primary focus. Just obeying laws is not enough. Something could be illegal and still virtuous and also legal and yet improper. As we will later see, rules take on a more significant stature when ethics is examined under religious and not philosophical concepts.[42]

A contemporary of Plato was Hippocrates (460–370 BCE), who wrote *Epidemics*; this text presented a series of clinical cases and a description of the climate and geography where the cases occurred. Amid this clinical reporting, the earliest warning about the practitioner's ethics appears perplexing. First, the author discusses the prognostic importance of "humors," bodily liquids that govern the individual's health.[43] Hippocrates conformed to the theory of four humors: blood, mucus (or phlegm), yellow bile, and black bile; an imbalance of these humors was essential in developing diseases.[44] Then, inexplicably, these words come out of context:

> *Declare the past, diagnose the present, foretell the future. As to diseases, make a habit of two things— to help and not harm. The art has three factors: the disease, the patient, and the physician. The physician is the servant of the art. The patient must work with the physician in combating the disease.*[45]

The text then returns to its clinical tone, discussing pain and fever. Nevertheless, this text clearly describes the connection between the patient, the physician, and the disease, which is far timelier than the discussion of "humors."

The next figure to be discussed is Galen (129–216 AD), a native of Pergamum who practiced in Rome. Among his numerous writings are many treatises and commentaries on ethics. In one short essay, "The Best Doctor Is Also a Philosopher," Galen contends that anyone who claims to be a doctor, a name made noble by Hippocrates, must "know all parts of philosophy: the logical, the physical and the ethical." He must be skilled at analyzing the problems presented to him and understanding the nature and function of the body within the physical world. A physician must also "practice temperance and despise money since all evil actions that men undertake are done either at the prompting of greed or under the spell of pleasure."[46] Galen's philosophical doctor is not merely a student of philosophical literature but also one whose life has been formed by fairness and temperance. He, therefore, will possess all other virtues since, according to Stoic doctrine, "all the virtues are connected as if by one string." Galen denounces physicians for avarice, contentiousness, and ignorance in his writings. He concludes that the ideal physician should be a student of all that affects health. A physician should also be fair-minded and live a modest, even austere life.[47]

The study of healthcare bioethics should focus on "ethical awareness" as it applies to everyday clinical dilemmas. For example, later in this book, there will be a discussion about futile care in the intensive care unit (ICU) setting. These decisions can be difficult and exhausting; ideally, a bioethics background should be helpful. Such education should be emotionally supportive as well. However, as it is taught, bioethics often falls short of this goal. As one author put it, "Current medical ethics teaching focuses largely on the cognitive realm with an emphasis on rational thinking and decision-making."[48] The knowledge of bioethics, especially from a philosophical background, will not readily say whether a decision is right or wrong. However, as Socrates, Plato, Aristotle, Cicero, and many others have said, it should help us ask the right questions.[49] Bioethics should continue examining, discovering, and meditating about life as the ancient Greek philosophers did so many years ago.

RELIGIOUS ROOTS

The earlier section explored philosophy as a "love of wisdom" as a foundation for modern ethics. Many scholars (but not all) also cite religion as essential for setting up contemporary bioethics.[50] Nevertheless, religion as an origin for ethics will be explored in this section. However, before that can be done, the origin of religion must be studied. Charles Darwin writes in his book *The Descent of Man*:

> *As soon as the important faculties of imagination, wonder, and curiosity, together with some power of reasoning, had become partially developed, man would naturally crave to understand what was passing around him, and would have vaguely speculated on his own existence.*[51]

So, how far back does religion go? In a 2009 article in *Science* by Elizabeth Culotta, she ponders how the archeological evidence can prove how long ago religion began. Burial sites in Africa and Israel dated to 100,000 years ago suggest that ancient peoples felt that something occurred when a person died more than just the body's death. Thirty thousand years ago, cave drawings in Europe also suggested that man perceived the world as more than physical. Eleven thousand years ago, evidence of temples and other possible religious structures was discovered in Turkey. These discoveries were suspect, however, since there was no recorded history to explain if these objects were religious in origin. Nevertheless, around 5000 years ago, religion could be confirmed because of the written language in Egypt and Mesopotamia.[52]

So now that the *where* and *when* have been discussed, a more complicated conversation should occur about *what* religion is. The dictionary defines religion as "a body of beliefs and practices regarding the supernatural and the worship of one or more deities."[53] However, the word's derivation is controversial. Cicero uses the term in his book *De Natura Deorum* (The Nature of Gods) to mean to "go through or read, over again speak or think over again," from the Latin word *relegere*.[54] However, most modern interpretations of the word state that it comes from the Latin word *religare*, meaning to bind or connect.[55] Nevertheless, even that interpretation is open to debate. The word "bind" (or tie down) seems negative and restrictive, while "connect" seems positive and unifying.

So, what makes up a religion? John Teehan is an Associate Professor of Philosophy at Hofstra University in New York. In his article "The Evolutionary Basis of Religious Ethics," he proposes three necessary aspects. The first is the presence of a supernatural agent. These could be "gods, ghosts, or spirits."[56] Although these agents in some religions could be animals, plants, places, weather phenomena (like thunder), or non-descript, they are often depicted as a person, such as Zeus, Athena, and other Greco-Roman gods.[57] The second part is rituals. These are frequently very elaborate and can evolve over time. One purpose of rituals is to connect or have a relationship with the supernatural agent. Another purpose is to group identity. (In the Catholic tradition, there is a hymn, "They Will Know We Are Christians by Our Love.") The third part is the establishment of rules.

This aspect is where there is much debate. For example, although a religion needs a set of laws or rules to define itself, does bioethics need religion? Father William E. Stempsey would be an excellent person to ask, having degrees in Medicine, Divinity, and Philosophy. In his article "*Homo Religiosus*: The Soul of Bioethics," he emphatically states that religion in bioethics is necessary since it deals with "the deepest mysteries of the human condition." [58] He further contends:

> *Although it is possible to be human and not to give a religious account of one's life, it seems difficult to be a thinking human being and not realize the depths of mystery in life, death, and suffering, the very core of bioethics. If these religious mysteries are the stuff of bioethics, bioethics must include religion.*[59]

Other scholars argue that religion is not necessary in bioethics, and its presence could be considered discriminatory. Because of the vast diversity seen in today's society, concerns exist that a religious approach could unjustly help some and not others. Timothy F. Murphy, in his article "In Defense of Irreligious Bioethics," states that bioethics "loses something important when it presumes in advance that religious views occupy any privileged status when it comes to theorizing decisions about health, health care, and biomedical innovation."[60] He further contends that not everyone is religious (he uses the term theist), and a nonreligious or irreligious view would have a more complete status in bioethics. He concludes that this approach would enable "the field to think more critically and independently than is otherwise possible and to work toward justice in bioethics without the expectation of a safety net of a life beyond this one."[61]

Lately, there has been a trend to secularize bioethics, that is, to remove any religious influence. Those who favor this approach would replace the religious aspects with scholasticism, natural law, and moral theology. Many would argue that this thinking aligns with the US's separation of Church and State.[62] However, Catholicism's influence on bioethics goes back centuries. For example, a Protestant professor of ethics, Joseph Fletcher from Harvard, saw that very few scholarly articles were written before 1960 by anyone other than Catholics.[63] Catholic teachings on ethics can be traced back to the fourth century with Saint Augustine and his writings on suicide.[64] In the thirteenth century, St. Thomas Aquinas introduced the Principle of Double Effect, which is still widely used in healthcare today.[65] The splendor and foundation of Catholic Bioethics is its unwavering belief in the sanctity of life. Thomas Huxley is reputed to have said, "Teach a child what is wise; that is morality. Teach him what is wise and beautiful; that is religion!" Since human life comes from God, who loves us, it has sacred value but is not absolute. The meaning and purpose of life are founded in the belief that Jesus Christ rose from the dead on Easter Sunday and that his followers can obtain everlasting life after death. These beliefs are still significant and create a background for bioethics in contemporary society.[66]

Catholic healthcare ethics, therefore, has a rich history and values that can be applied to contemporary medicine but is not without controversy. Despite its significant impact on bioethics, some aspects conflict with secular bioethics. For example, the Principle of Respect for Autonomy, described by the bioethicists Beauchamp and Childress, has some aspects contrary to Catholic teaching. This topic will be discussed in another chapter in detail. Still, they contend that Autonomy "encompasses, at a minimum, self-rule that is free from both controlling interference by others and from certain limitations such as an inadequate understanding that prevents meaningful choice. The autonomous individual acts freely per a self-chosen plan, analogous to how an independent government manages its territories and establishes its policies."[67]

In contrast, based on statements made by Pope John Paul II, Catholic theologian William E. May asserts that "When human autonomy is conceived as the creator and arbiter of good and evil, of right and wrong, we are no longer able to guide our choices by the truth but only by subjective and changing human opinions."[68] Other inconsistencies exist concerning reproductive rights and MAID, to name a few. Nevertheless, the influence of Catholic bioethics is still significant and cannot be ignored or replaced entirely by secular bioethics. Throughout this book, both sides will be explored in various clinical scenarios.

BIOETHICAL PRINCIPLES

> *In a word, it is incumbent on the physician that under all conditions, his bearing towards patients, the public, and fellow practitioners should be characterized by a gentlemanly deportment and that he constantly should behave toward others as he desires them to deal with him. Finally, these principles are primarily for the good of the public, and their enforcement should be conducted in such a manner as shall deserve and receive the endorsement of the community.*[69]

The above quote is taken from a 1945 article in the *Journal of Clinical Psychology* entitled "Principles of Medical Ethics." In an editor's note, D. Olin West, Secretary and General Manager of the American Medical Association (AMA), was acknowledged for providing this document to the journal so clinical psychologists could study a "working system of professional ethics" developing in the US.[70] A few points should be made about this position paper. First, it should not be dismissed for what now would be interpreted as being sexist or chauvinist. This article repeatedly refers to physicians as entirely masculine, although there were definitely women physicians at the time.[71] Second, although the article was about medical ethics, it focused almost exclusively on physicians. However, it does state that ethical principles for a "group or clinic" are the same as those for an individual. Much of the article deals with how physicians should behave and treat each other. Finally, about the treatment of patients, it says that "physicians should give timely notice of dangerous manifestations of the disease to the friends of the patient. He should neither exaggerate nor minimize the gravity of the patient's condition."[72] It is unclear why the AMA chose to tell the patient's friends to show critical medical information instead of the patients or their families. However, they comment on secrecy regarding infectious diseases and recommend that physicians treat others as they want to treat themselves or their families.

After World War II, there was a massive outburst of new medical technology aimed first at increasing military medicine but later at advancing medical treatments for all. Dr. Albert R. Jonsen, in his book *The Birth of Bioethics*, writes about how these medical discoveries, although in many ways miraculous, were also problematic: "The scientific training of which modern medicine was so proud seemed to transform the healer into the technician who was remote, difficult to see, and even more difficult to understand."[73] These so-called growing pains led to questions about how these new technologies could and should be used. In addition, these new treatments were expensive and also limited.

Of course, many people had something to say about these new medical discoveries. Initially, physicians tried to control these discoveries, but theologians and philosophers soon weighed in on how to ethically use these new technologies. Consequently, another problem that needed to be addressed was medical research. The Nazi atrocities in the postwar era were slowly being brought to light, and the results were horrifying. The Nuremberg Trials exposed how German physicians did medical experiments on non-German and vulnerable populations during the war. Besides condemning these barbaric procedures, actions were needed to define how medical experiments should be conducted. First, subjects for these experiments should do so voluntarily, and their safety should be a top priority. Second, the reasons for the experiments should be for the common good and not for financial gain. Third, these clinical trials should be transparent, and the results, good or bad, should be made known to the public. With technological advances, medical atrocities, and the need for ethical principles from physicians, theologians, philosophers, politicians, and others, a mandate ushered in a new era of bioethics.[74]

The work of two bioethicists, Tom L. Beauchamp and James F. Childress, will be introduced now and referenced frequently throughout this book. In their book *Principles of Biomedical Ethics*, in its multiple editions, a set of norms are set up that are basic for biomedical ethics. They contend that a "set of principles in a moral account should function as an analytical framework that expresses the general values underlying rules in the common morality. These principles can then function as guidelines for professional ethics."[75] The first edition of their book was published in 1979, and the ninth edition in 2019. Its persistence and durability speak for themselves. Their writings made famous the four bioethical principles of respect for autonomy, beneficence, nonmaleficence, and justice.

Autonomy refers to the moral principle of allowing individuals who can do so to make their own decisions. Beneficence refers to trying to do good for patients by considering risks, benefits, and costs with medical choices. In contrast, Nonmaleficence is the notion that we should avoid hurting or causing harm to patients. Finally, Justice refers to evenly distributing risks, benefits, and costs throughout the population.[76] This principle also deals with diverse topics, from vulnerable populations to sustainable healthcare systems. This book will start with a chapter for each principle, and the later chapters will explore these principles in specific clinical scenarios. The goal is to show how the contribution of principlism (using these ethical principles) can advance ethical and clinical collaboration when healthcare dilemmas need to be resolved.

NOTES

1 Eric Cassell, Hastings Center Report, 1973.
2 Amir M. Zayegh et al., "Trends in Survival, Perinatal Morbidities and Two-year Neurodevelopmental Outcomes in Extremely Low-birthweight Infants over Four Decades," *Paediatric and Perinatal Epidemiology* 36, no. 5 (September 2022): 594–602, https://doi.org/10.1111/ppe.12879.
3 "Cleveland Clinic Unveils Top 10 Medical Innovations for 2022—Cleveland Clinic Newsroom," accessed February 7, 2023, https://newsroom.clevelandclinic.org/2022/02/16/cleveland-clinic-unveils-top-10-medical-innovations-for-2022.
4 "Medical Science Breakthroughs of 2022: ALS, Diabetes, COVID," accessed February 7, 2023, www.usatoday.com/story/news/health/2022/12/19/medical-science-breakthroughs-2022/10858326002.
5 Matthieu Komorowski et al., "The Artificial Intelligence Clinician Learns Optimal Treatment Strategies for Sepsis in Intensive Care," *Nature Medicine* 24, no. 11 (November 2018): 1716–1720, https://doi.org/10.1038/s41591-018-0213-5.
6 "The Biggest Health and Biology Breakthroughs of 2022—Scientific American," accessed February 7, 2023, www.scientificamerican.com/article/the-biggest-health-and-biology-breakthroughs-of-2022.
7 "3D Bioprinting of Living Tissues," accessed February 7, 2023, https://wyss.harvard.edu/technology/3d-bioprinting.
8 Darryl Abrams et al., "Extracorporeal Cardiopulmonary Resuscitation in Adults: Evidence and Implications," *Intensive Care Medicine* 48, no. 1 (January 2022): 1–15, https://doi.org/10.1007/s00134-021-06514-y.
9 Leili Yekefallah et al., "Nurses' Experiences of Futile Care at Intensive Care Units: A Phenomenological Study," *Global Journal of Health Science* 7, no. 4 (January 14, 2015): 235–242, https://doi.org/10.5539/gjhs.v7n4p235.
10 Bjørn Hofmann, "The Role of Philosophy and Ethics at the Edges of Medicine," *Philosophy, Ethics, and Humanities in Medicine* 16, no. 1 (December 2021): 14, https://doi.org/10.1186/s13010-021-00114-w, page 1.
11 Kenneth Berkowitz et al., *Ethics Consultation: Responding to Ethics Questions in Health Care*, 2nd edition (New York: Springer, 2015), page vi.
12 Barbara Grondkowska, "Between Idle Chatter and the Pursuit of Wisdom. The Idea of Philosophy in the Thought of Nicholas of Cusa," *Entre La Charla Ociosa y La Búsqueda de La Sabiduría. La Idea de Fi Losofía En El Pensamiento de Nicolás de Cusa.* 54, no. 3 (September 2021): 475–500, page 477.
13 Albert R. Jonsen, *A Short History of Medical Ethics* (New York: Oxford University Press, 2000), page 10.
14 Laura L. Machin and Robin D. Proctor, "Engaging Tomorrow's Doctors in Clinical Ethics: Implications for Healthcare Organisations," *Health Care Analysis: An International Journal of Health, Philosophy and Policy* 29, no. 4 (December 1, 2021): 319–342, https://doi.org/10.1007/s10728-020-00403-z, page 321.
15 Greg L. Pugh, "A Model of Comparative Ethics Education for Social Workers," *Journal of Social Work Education* 53, no. 2 (April 3, 2017): 312–326, https://doi.org/10.1080/10437797.2016.1243497, pages 312–313.
16 "Chaplains Report Receiving No Ethics Education—ProQuest," accessed May 7, 2022, www-proquest-com.authenticate.library.duq.edu/docview/2544798116?accountid=10610.
17 Mary Kay Barton, "Bankruptcy Linked to Early Mortality in Patients with Cancer," *CA: A Cancer Journal for Clinicians* 66, no. 4 (July 2016): 267–268, https://doi.org/10.3322/caac.21305.
18 Betty R. Ferrell, "Understanding the Moral Distress of Nurses Witnessing Medically Futile Care," *Oncology Nursing Forum* 33, no. 5 (January 1, 2006): 922–930, https://doi.org/10.1188/06.ONF.922-930.
19 Dereddi Raja S. Reddy, John C. O'Horo, and Sumedh S. Hoskote, "Judgment of Futile Care in the ICU," *Critical Care Medicine* 43, no. 5 (May 2015): e151.

20 Diane Lynn Redleaf, Suzanne Baillie Schmitt and William Charles Thompson, "The California Natural Death Act: An Empirical Study of Physicians' Practices," *Stanford Law Review* 31, no. 5 (May 1979): 913–945, page 918.
21 "2006 Act 169" (Pennsylvania General Assembly, 2006), www.legis.state.pa.us/cfdocs/Legis/LI/uconsCheck.cfm?txtType=HTM&yr=2006&sessInd=0&smthLwInd=0&act=169.
22 Rebecca L. Sudore, "Redefining the 'Planning' in Advance Care Planning: Preparing for End-of-Life Decision Making," *Annals of Internal Medicine* 153, no. 4 (August 17, 2010): 256, https://doi.org/10.7326/0003–4819-153–4–201008170-00008.
23 Rebecca L. Sudore et al., "Defining Advance Care Planning for Adults: A Consensus Definition From a Multidisciplinary Delphi Panel," *Journal of Pain and Symptom Management* 53, no. 5 (May 2017): 821–832.e1, https://doi.org/10.1016/j.jpainsymman.2016.12.331.
24 Marc A. Shampo and Raymond A. Lee, "The World's First 'Test-Tube Baby'," *Journal of Pelvic Surgery* 8, no. 2 (April 3, 2002): 120–122.
25 John S. Feinberg, "A Baby at Any Cost and By Any Means? The Morality of In Vitro Fertilization and Frozen Embryos," *Trinity Journal* 14, no. 2 (1993): 143–173, pages 149–150.
26 Morris Bernard Kaplan, "The Case of the Artificial Heart Panel," *The Hastings Center Report* 5, no. 5 (October 1, 1975): 41–48, https://doi.org/10.2307/3561228.
27 F. R. Woolley, "Ethical Issues in the Implantation of the Total Artificial Heart," *The New England Journal of Medicine* 310, no. 5 (February 2, 1984): 292–296, https://doi.org/10.1056/NEJM198402023100505, pages 292–296.
28 Mary Jean Walker, "A Heart without Life: Artificial Organs and the Lived Body," *Hastings Center Report* 51, no. 1 (January 2021): 28–38, page 31.
29 Norman N. Cantor, "'In the Matter of Karen Quinlan': A Comment," *BioScience* 26, no. 4 (April 1, 1976): 257–259, https://doi.org/10.2307/1297348.
30 "How This Young Woman's Tragic Night out Changed Our View of Death," accessed February 20, 2023, https://nypost.com/2017/02/18/how-this-young-womans-tragic-night-out-changed-our-view-of-death/.
31 Robert M. Veatch, "Who Should Decide: The Case of Karen Quinlan," *Christianity and Crisis* 35, no. 22 (January 19, 1976): 329–331.
32 "Philosophy Definition & Meaning," accessed March 21, 2023, www.merriam-webster.com/dictionary/bioethics.
33 Diego Gracia, "Bioethics, from Stories to History," *Medicine, Health Care and Philosophy* 8, no. 1 (April 1, 2005): 119–122, page 119.
34 "Philosophy Definition & Meaning," accessed March 21, 2023, www.merriam-webster.com/dictionary/bioethics.
35 Fernando Leal and Hubert Marraud, "Argumentation in Philosophical Controversies," *Argumentation: An International Journal on Reasoning*, September 9, 2022, 1–25, https://doi.org/10.1007/s10503-022-09581-7, page 456.
36 Lynn Bowyer, "What Does Philosophy Do?," *Journal of Philosophy in Schools* 8, no. 1 (August 17, 2021): 71–103.
37 Noburu Notomi, "Socrates and the Sophists: Reconsidering the History of Criticisms of the Sophists," *Humanities* 11, no. 6 (December 7, 2022): 153, https://doi.org/10.3390/h11060153, page 1.
38 William Stull, "Reading the *Phaedo* in *Tusculan Disputations* 1," *Classical Philology* 107, no. 1 (January 2012): 38–52, https://doi.org/10.1086/663216.
39 Noburu Notomi, "Socrates and the Sophists: Reconsidering the History of Criticisms of the Sophists," *Humanities* 11, no. 6 (December 7, 2022): 153, https://doi.org/10.3390/h11060153, pages 2–5.
40 Nicholas D. Smith, "Some Thoughts about the Origin of Greek Ethics," *The Journal of Ethics* 5 (2001): 18–20.
41 Nicholas D. Smith, "Some Thoughts about the Origin of Greek Ethics," *The Journal of Ethics* 5 (2001): 18–20.
42 Nicholas D. Smith, "Some Thoughts about the Origin of Greek Ethics," *The Journal of Ethics* 5 (2001): 18–20, page 20.

43 Albert R. Jonsen, *A Short History of Medical Ethics* (New York: Oxford University Press, 2000).
44 Liddell, "Hippocrates of Cos (460–377 BC): RSM Symposium," *Clinical and Experimental Dermatology* 25, no. 1 (January 2000): 86–88, https://doi.org/10.1046/j.1365–2230.2000.0580d.x, page 86.
45 Albert R. Jonsen, *A Short History of Medical Ethics* (New York: Oxford University Press, 2000), page 2.
46 Albert R. Jonsen, *A Short History of Medical Ethics* (New York: Oxford University Press, 2000), page 10.
47 Albert R. Jonsen, *A Short History of Medical Ethics* (New York: Oxford University Press, 2000), page 10.
48 Paul Macneill, "Balancing Bioethics by Sensing the Aesthetic," *Bioethics* 31, no. 8 (October 2017): 631–643, page 632.
49 Jennifer Blumenthal-Barby et al., "The Place of Philosophy in Bioethics Today," *The American Journal of Bioethics* 22, no. 12 (December 2, 2022): 10–21, https://doi.org/10.1080/15265161.2021.1940355, page 14.
50 Timothy F. Murphy, "In Defense of Irreligious Bioethics," *The American Journal of Bioethics* 12, no. 12 (December 2012): 3–10, https://doi.org/10.1080/15265161.2012.719262, pages 3–10.
51 Culotta, Elizabeth, "On the Origin of Religion," *Science* 326, no. 5954 (November 6, 2009): 784–787.
52 Culotta, Elizabeth, "On the Origin of Religion," *Science* 326, no. 5954 (November 6, 2009): 784–787.
53 "43 Synonyms & Antonyms of Religion," accessed April 1, 2023, www.merriam-webster.com/thesaurus/religion.
54 Sarah F. Hoyt, "The Etymology of Religion," *Journal of the American Oriental Society* 32, no. 2 (1912): 126, https://doi.org/10.2307/3087765.
55 "Religion," accessed April 1, 2023, www.etymonline.com/word/religion.
56 John Teehan, "The Evolutionary Basis of Religious Ethics," *Zygon* 41, no. 3 (September 2006): 747–774, https://doi.org/10.1111/j.1467–9744.2005.00772.x, page 753.
57 John Teehan, "The Evolutionary Basis of Religious Ethics," *Zygon* 41, no. 3 (September 2006): 747–774, https://doi.org/10.1111/j.1467–9744.2005.00772.x, page 754.
58 William E. Stempsey, "Homo Religiosus: The Soul of Bioethics," *Journal of Medicine & Philosophy* 46, no. 2 (April 2021): 238–253, page 249.
59 William E. Stempsey, "Homo Religiosus: The Soul of Bioethics," *Journal of Medicine & Philosophy* 46, no. 2 (April 2021): 238–253, page 249.
60 Timothy F. Murphy, "In Defense of Irreligious Bioethics," *The American Journal of Bioethics* 12, no. 12 (December 2012): 3–10, https://doi.org/10.1080/15265161.2012.719262, page 3.
61 Timothy F. Murphy, "In Defense of Irreligious Bioethics," *The American Journal of Bioethics* 12, no. 12 (December 2012): 3–10, https://doi.org/10.1080/15265161.2012.719262, page 3.
62 Rev S Joseph Tham, "The Secularization of Bioethics," *The National Catholic Bioethics Quarterly*, 2008, 443–453.
63 Louise A. Mitchell, "A Brief History of Catholic Bioethic," *Ethics & Medics* 41, no. 7 (July): 3–4.
64 Hazel J. Markwell, "Bioethics for Clinicians: 27. Catholic Bioethics," *Canadian Medical Association Journal* 165, no. 2 (July 24, 2001): 189–192.
65 Daniel H .Weiss, "Aquinas's Opposition to Killing the Innocent and Its Distinctiveness Within the Christian Just War Tradition," *Journal of Religious Ethics* 45, no. 3 (September 2017): 481–509.
66 Hazel J. Markwell, "Bioethics for Clinicians: 27. Catholic Bioethics," *Canadian Medical Association Journal* 165, no. 2 (July 24, 2001): 189–192.
67 Tom L. Beauchamp and James F. Childress, *Principles of Biomedical Ethics*, eighth edition (New York: Oxford University Press, 2019), page 99.

68 Elliott Louis Bedford, "The Core Competencies: A Roman Catholic Critique," *HEC Forum* 23, no. 3 (September 2011): 147–169, https://doi.org/10.1007/s10730-011-9169-2, page 158
69 American Medical Association, "Principles of Medical Ethics," *Journal of Clinical Psychology* 1 (1945): 336–342, https://doi.org/10.1002/1097–4679(194510)1:4<336::AID-JCLP2270010417>3.0.CO;2-I, page 342
70 American Medical Association, "Principles of Medical Ethics," *Journal of Clinical Psychology* 1 (1945): 336–342, https://doi.org/10.1002/1097–4679(194510)1:4<336::AID-JCLP2270010417>3.0.CO;2-I, page 336.
71 "Graduates (1940s–1950s)," accessed April 18, 2023, https://onlineexhibits.library.yale.edu/s/100-years-women-ysm/page/women-medical-graduates-in-the.
72 American Medical Association, "Principles of Medical Ethics," *Journal of Clinical Psychology* 1 (1945): 336–342, https://doi.org/10.1002/1097–4679(194510)1:4<336::AID-JCLP2270010417>3.0.CO;2-I, page 336.
73 Albert R. Jonsen, *A Short History of Medical Ethics* (New York: Oxford University Press, 2000), page 12.
74 Albert R. Jonsen, *A Short History of Medical Ethics* (New York: Oxford University Press, 2000), pages 138–140.
75 Tom L. Beauchamp and James F. Childress, *Principles of Biomedical Ethics*, eighth edition (New York: Oxford University Press, 2019), page 12.
76 Tom L. Beauchamp and James F. Childress, *Principles of Biomedical Ethics*, eighth edition (New York: Oxford University Press, 2019), pages 12–13.

BIBLIOGRAPHY

Abrams, Darryl, Graeme MacLaren, Roberto Lorusso, Susanna Price, Demetris Yannopoulos, Leen Vercaemst, Jan Bělohlávek, et al. "Extracorporeal Cardiopulmonary Resuscitation in Adults: Evidence and Implications." *Intensive Care Medicine* 48, no. 1 (January 2022): 1–15. https://doi.org/10.1007/s00134-021-06514-y.

American Medical Association. "Principles of Medical Ethics." *Journal of Clinical Psychology* 1 (1945):336–342. https://doi.org/10.1002/1097-4679(194510)1:4<336::AID-JCLP2270010417>3.0.CO;2-I.

Barton, Mary Kay. "Bankruptcy Linked to Early Mortality in Patients with Cancer." *CA: A Cancer Journal for Clinicians* 66, no. 4 (July 2016): 267–268. https://doi.org/10.3322/caac.21305.

Beauchamp, Tom L., and James F. Childress. *Principles of Biomedical Ethics*. Eighth edition. New York: Oxford University Press, 2019.

Bedford, Elliott Louis. "The Core Competencies: A Roman Catholic Critique." *HEC Forum* 23, no. 3 (September 2011): 147–169. https://doi.org/10.1007/s10730-011-9169-2.

Berkowitz, Kenneth, et al. *Ethics Consultation: Responding to Ethics Questions in Health Care*. Second Edition. New York: Springer. 2015.

Blumenthal-Barby, Jennifer, Sean Aas, Dan Brudney, Jessica Flanigan, S. Matthew Liao, Alex London, Wayne Sumner, and Julian Savulescu. "The Place of Philosophy in Bioethics Today." *The American Journal of Bioethics* 22, no. 12 (December 2, 2022): 10–21. https://doi.org/10.1080/15265161.2021.1940355.

Bowyer, Lynn. "What Does Philosophy Do?" *Journal of Philosophy in Schools* 8, no. 1 (August 17, 2021): 71–103.

Cantor, Norman N. "'In the Matter of Karen Quinlan': A Comment." *BioScience* 26, no. 4 (April 1, 1976): 257–259. https://doi.org/10.2307/1297348.

Culotta, Elizabeth. "On the Origin of Religion." *Science* 326, no. 5954 (November 6, 2009): 784–87.

Feinberg, John S. "A Baby at Any Cost and By Any Means? The Morality of In Vitro Fertilization and Frozen Embryos." *Trinity Journal* 14, no. 2 (1993): 143–173.

Ferrell, Betty R. "Understanding the Moral Distress of Nurses Witnessing Medically Futile Care." *Oncology Nursing Forum* 33, no. 5 (January 1, 2006): 922–930. https://doi.org/10.1188/06.ONF.922-930.

Gracia, Diego. "Bioethics, from Stories to History." *Medicine, Health Care and Philosophy* 8, no. 1 (April 1, 2005): 119–122.

Grondkowska, Barbara. "Between Idle Chatter and the Pursuit of Wisdom. The Idea of Philosophy in the Thought of Nicholas of Cusa." *Entre La Charla Ociosa y La Búsqueda de La Sabiduría. La Idea de Fi* Losofía *En El Pensamiento de Nicolás de Cusa.* 54, no. 3 (September 2021): 475–500.

Hofmann, Bjørn. "The Role of Philosophy and Ethics at the Edges of Medicine." *Philosophy, Ethics, and Humanities in Medicine* 16, no. 1 (December 2021): 14. https://doi.org/10.1186/s13010-021-00114-w.

Hoyt, Sarah F. "The Etymology of Religion." *Journal of the American Oriental Society* 32, no. 2 (1912): 126. https://doi.org/10.2307/3087765.

Jonsen, Albert R. *A Short History of Medical Ethics*. New York: Oxford University Press, 2000.

Kaplan, Morris Bernard. "The Case of the Artificial Heart Panel." *The Hastings Center Report* 5, no. 5 (October 1, 1975): 41–48. https://doi.org/10.2307/3561228.

Komorowski, Matthieu, Leo A. Celi, Omar Badawi, Anthony C. Gordon, and A. Aldo Faisal. "The Artificial Intelligence Clinician Learns Optimal Treatment Strategies for Sepsis in Intensive Care." *Nature Medicine* 24, no. 11 (November 2018): 1716–1720. https://doi.org/10.1038/s41591-018-0213-5.

Leal, Fernando, and Hubert Marraud. "Argumentation in Philosophical Controversies." *Argumentation: An International Journal on Reasoning*, September 9, 2022, 1–25. https://doi.org/10.1007/s10503-022-09581-7.

Liddell. "Hippocrates of Cos (460–377 BC): RSM Symposium." *Clinical and Experimental Dermatology* 25, no. 1 (January 2000): 86–88. https://doi.org/10.1046/j.1365-2230.2000.0580d.x.

Machin, Laura L., and Robin D. Proctor. "Engaging Tomorrow's Doctors in Clinical Ethics: Implications for Healthcare Organisations." *Health Care Analysis: An International Journal of Health, Philosophy and Policy* 29, no. 4 (December 1, 2021): 319–342. https://doi.org/10.1007/s10728-020-00403-z.

Macneill, Paul. "Balancing Bioethics by Sensing the Aesthetic." *Bioethics* 31, no. 8 (October 2017): 631–643.

Markwell, Hazel J. "Bioethics for Clinicians: 27. Catholic Bioethics." *Canadian Medical Association Journal* 165, no. 2 (July 24, 2001): 189–192.

Mitchell, Louise A. "A Brief History of Catholic Bioethic." *Ethics & Medics* 41, no. 7 (July): 3–4.

Murphy, Timothy F. "In Defense of Irreligious Bioethics." *The American Journal of Bioethics* 12, no. 12 (December 2012): 3–10. https://doi.org/10.1080/15265161.2012.719262.

Notomi, Noburu. "Socrates and the Sophists: Reconsidering the History of Criticisms of the Sophists." *Humanities* 11, no. 6 (December 7, 2022): 153. https://doi.org/10.3390/h11060153.

Pugh, Greg L. "A Model of Comparative Ethics Education for Social Workers." *Journal of Social Work Education* 53, no. 2 (April 3, 2017): 312–326. https://doi.org/10.1080/10437797.2016.1243497.

Reddy, Dereddi Raja S., John C. O'Horo, and Sumedh S. Hoskote. "Judgment of Futile Care in the ICU." *Critical Care Medicine* 43, no. 5 (May 2015): e151.

Redleaf, Diane Lynn, Suzanne Baillie Schmitt and William Charles Thompson. "The California Natural Death Act: An Empirical Study of Physicians' Practices." *Stanford Law Review* 31, no. 5 (May 1979): 913–945.

Shampo, Marc A., and Raymond A. Lee. "The World's First 'Test-Tube Baby'." *Journal of Pelvic Surgery* 8, no. 2 (April 3, 2002): 120–122.

Smith, Nicholas D. "Some Thoughts about the Origin of Greek Ethics." *The Journal of Ethics* 5 (2001): 18–20.

Stempsey, William E. "Homo Religiosus: The Soul of Bioethics." *Journal of Medicine & Philosophy* 46, no. 2 (April 2021): 238–253.

Stull, William. "Reading the *Phaedo* in *Tusculan Disputations* 1." *Classical Philology* 107, no. 1 (January 2012): 38–52. https://doi.org/10.1086/663216.

Sudore, Rebecca L. "Redefining the 'Planning' in Advance Care Planning: Preparing for End-of-Life Decision Making." *Annals of Internal Medicine* 153, no. 4 (August 17, 2010): 256. https://doi.org/10.7326/0003-4819-153-4-201008170-00008.

Sudore, Rebecca L., et al. "Defining Advance Care Planning for Adults: A Consensus Definition From a Multidisciplinary Delphi Panel." *Journal of Pain and Symptom Management* 53, no. 5 (May 2017): 821–832.e1. https://doi.org/10.1016/j.jpainsymman.2016.12.331.

Teehan, John. "The Evolutionary Basis of Religious Ethics." *Zygon* 41, no. 3 (September 2006): 747–774. https://doi.org/10.1111/j.1467-9744.2005.00772.x.

Tham, Rev S. Joseph. "The Secularization of Bioethics." *The National Catholic Bioethics Quarterly*, 2008, 443–453.

Veatch, Robert M. "Who Should Decide: The Case of Karen Quinlan." *Christianity and Crisis* 35, no. 22 (January 19, 1976): 329–331.

Walker, Mary Jean. "A Heart without Life: Artificial Organs and the Lived Body." *Hastings Center Report* 51, no. 1 (January 2021): 28–38.

Weiss, Daniel H. "Aquinas's Opposition to Killing the Innocent and Its Distinctiveness Within the Christian Just War Tradition." *Journal of Religious Ethics* 45, no. 3 (September 2017): 481–509.

Woolley, F. R. "Ethical Issues in the Implantation of the Total Artificial Heart." *The New England Journal of Medicine* 310, no. 5 (February 2, 1984): 292–296. https://doi.org/10.1056/NEJM198402023100505.

Yekefallah, Leili, Tahereh Ashktorab, Houman Manoochehri, and Alavi Majd Hamid. "Nurses' Experiences of Futile Care at Intensive Care Units: A Phenomenological Study." *Global Journal of Health Science* 7, no. 4 (January 14, 2015): 235–242. https://doi.org/10.5539/gjhs.v7n4p235.

Zayegh, Amir M., et al. "Trends in Survival, Perinatal Morbidities and Two-year Neurodevelopmental Outcomes in Extremely Low-birthweight Infants over Four Decades." *Paediatric and Perinatal* Epidemiology 36, no. 5 (September 2022): 594–602. https://doi.org/10.1111/ppe.12879.

Chapter 1
The Ethical Principle of Autonomy

INTRODUCTION

In the United States, the concept of "freedom of choice "is vital to the idea of Constitutionally protected rights. Indeed, our heritage is based on freedom. Therefore, the ethical concept of autonomy is crucial and troublesome when placed in the medical arena. People can choose or refuse medical treatments without exception, right? What if the choice is based on wrong information or is harmful to the person? What if that medical decision could cause harm to others? So, should there be exceptions to autonomy?

The word autonomy comes from the Greek *autos* ("self ") and *nomos* ("rule," "governance," or "law"), initially referred to as the self-rule or self-governance of independent territories. However, autonomy has since been used for individuals and has acquired meanings as distinct as self-governance, liberty rights, privacy, individual choice, and free will. Clearly, autonomy is not a univocal concept in either ordinary English or contemporary philosophy. It needs to be refined in light of particular objectives, specifically healthcare.[1]

Autonomy, therefore, means self-rule free from controlling interference. When a patient has capacity, they have the right to make their own medical choices and take responsibility for the consequences of these decisions. Healthcare ethics has spent much time and energy delving into one aspect of self-rule: the right to decline medical treatment. It is easy to see how the right to refuse care is essential to medical autonomy. If we are to be self-governing agents, no other person should have the authority to force us to receive medical treatment. If another person did have this authority, the person who received the unchosen medical treatment would not be free to govern oneself; the *governor* would rather be the authority figure who used force or coercion to treat the patient against the patient's will.[2] Therefore, according to a self-chosen plan, the

DOI: 10.4324/9781003654124-2

autonomous individual acts freely, which is analogous to how an independent government manages its territories and sets its policies.[3] While this sounds good, in reality, especially in healthcare, this is not always the case. Many patients do not have the above-mentioned "self-chosen plan "and may not be interested in making one. Carl Schneider writes, "While patients largely wish to be informed about their medical circumstances, a substantial number of them (especially the elderly and the very sick) do not want to make their own medical decisions, or perhaps even to participate in those decisions in any very significant way."[4]

Along with the problem of autonomous individuals not wanting to make decisions, there is a problem with these people making what many would call "bad" decisions. In the mid-1980s, several papers on the impact of motorcycle helmet laws were published. The advocates of personal choice in wearing or not wearing helmets then and now use an autonomy-based argument that riders have the right to feel "the wind in their hair." However, the critics of the unabashed autonomy view noted that we all pay the price of peeling such "free riders" off the pavement. Therefore, such a personal choice has an actual cost, which can be expressed in dollars. Several writers were sympathetic to this latter position.

Further, they contended that economic considerations alone could not provide an adequate moral response to the autonomy-based right-of-riders-to-feel-wind-in-their-hair argument. Instead, they claimed that there is a social, moral obligation to be concerned about the safety of riders along with the economic cost of motorcycle accidents to society. Therefore, they advanced an ethical argument for the interests of the "commons," a distinct minority approach in mainstream bioethics, then and now.[5]

Whether a person decides to wear a motorcycle helmet will most likely have little effect on most other people except for a rise in their automobile insurance. One can choose not to be a passenger on a motorcycle when the driver is not wearing a helmet. However, some health choices can affect others more directly, which is a significant dilemma. For example, this country is currently experiencing the COVID-19 pandemic. As of July 2021, the CDC had reported over 600,000 deaths in the United States. Fortunately, several highly effective vaccines became available, yet many refused to get vaccinated. This problem brought the concept of autonomy to the forefront. Young people especially have been resistant to getting vaccinated, arguing that studies have shown a tiny percentage of severe illnesses from COVID-19 in this population. However, vaccinating this group could slow down the spread of this virus to more vulnerable populations. Does autonomy justify this refusal? This debate will be further discussed in a later section.

AUTONOMY PART 1—PATIENT HAS CAPACITY

As Tom L. Beauchamp and James F. Childress stated in their book Principles of Biomedical Ethics, "The autonomous individual acts freely in accordance with a self-chosen plan, analogous to how an independent government manages its territories and sets its policies. A person of diminished autonomy, by contrast, is in some way under the control of others and cannot consider or act on their desires and plans."[6] The authors further explain that prisoners and mentally retarded individuals often have diminished autonomy. To have autonomy, an individual should have both the freedom and the mental ability to make decisions on their behalf. They call these two conditions: (1) liberty (independence from controlling influences) and (2) agency (capacity for intentional action). So basically, a sane person not in prison should be able to make decisions. Unfortunately, even in the United States, that is not always the case.

Born on December 2, 1981, Britney Jean Spears is an American singer and songwriter. She is recognized for shaping the resurgence of teen pop through the late 1990s and early 2000s. As a result, she is referred to as the "Princess of Pop." With popular songs such as "... Baby One More Time," she quickly rose in the charts, and her first four albums sold an astonishing 30 million copies. Unfortunately, Ms. Spears encountered the pressures created by sudden fame and wealth, like other child stars before her.

Moreover, she had a chaotic private life, culminating in a very public breakup with her lover, Justin Timberlake, in 2002. To complicate things further, she married a childhood friend from Louisiana in Las Vegas in 2004, which lasted a mere 55 hours. Then, only nine months later, she married a local backup dancer, Kevin Federline. After the birth of their second son in November 2006, she again filed for divorce.[7] Britney was "bad" in the Fall of 2007: she was on drugs, she drank until she was sick, she was an unfit mother and ex-wife, she avoided the gym, and she had inappropriate sexual relations. Her hair was messy. She ate junk food. She was angry. Britney no longer embodied the all-American girl.

Then, the tangible shift happened over December 2007 and early January 2008: that shift from "bad" to "mad." She had post-partum depression and bipolar disease, and was perceived to be out of control. On the night of January 3, 2008, Britney was involuntarily held at Cedars-Sinai Medical Centre. Images were captured of her being carted out of her home, and "despite being strapped to a gurney, Spears is smiling and laughing as she is put in an ambulance."[8] Because of her erratic behavior, Britney's parents, Jamie and Lynn Spears, filed for conservatorship in 2008.

Spears, who is now in her forties, spent thirteen years living under a conservatorship, a legal structure in which a person's personal, economic, and legal decision-making power is ceded to others. Conservatorship (called guardianship in most states) is intended for people who cannot care for themselves. During the period of Spears's conservatorship (2008–2021), she released four albums, headlined a global tour that grossed one hundred and thirty-one million dollars, and had a successful four-year show in Las Vegas. However, her conservators, who include her father, Jamie Spears, controlled her spending, communications, and personal decisions.[9] This agreement is typically used to protect the old, people with mental disabilities, or the extremely ill. Ms. Spears was unable to make critical (or even trivial) personal or financial decisions without the consent of her father, Jamie Spears, and a lawyer, Andrew M. Wallet. From a drink at Starbucks to a song on iTunes, her most everyday purchases are recorded in court documents as part of the arrangement to protect the great fortune she has earned but does not ultimately control.[10]

The conservatorship control over Britney even had control over her medical issues. For example, she stated that she was given pills daily and had no control over that. She also stated that she could not get married or have children: "I have an IUD inside myself right now, so I don't get pregnant. I wanted to take the IUD out so I could start trying to have another baby, but the so-called team won't let me go to the doctor to take it out because they don't want me to have any more children."[11]

Driven by growing popular demand over Britney Spears's conservatorship, a bill proposed by two House of Representatives members would allow Ms. Spears (and other individuals) to petition a judge to change their personal guardian or conservator. This bill, the Freedom and Right to Emancipate from Exploitation Act or the FREE Act, was presented by its co-sponsors Representative Nancy Mace, Republican of South Carolina, and Representative Charlie Crist, Democrat of Florida. The bill allows individuals to have the right to ask that their private guardian or conservator be changed to either a family member, a private individual, or a public guardian employed by the State. The bill argues that this would provide more accountability for the current guardianship system. For a guardian to be replaced, individuals must prove that abuse or fraud has occurred in Court. The legislation could also provide insight into guardianships and conservatorships in the United

States.[12] This case illustrates that autonomy should not be taken for granted in the United States and needs to be further explored.

Informed Consent

Informed consent plays a fundamental part in the modern healthcare delivery system. Completing a consent form for procedures, transfusions, and other activities is commonplace in inpatient and outpatient medical settings. The form, intended to be written proof of the discussion between a healthcare provider and the patient, has become a medicolegal necessity. Moreover, informed consent is the core of what autonomy means in healthcare. The provider gives patients important information, and they then have the right to consent or refuse.

Virtually all top medical and research codes and institutional rules of ethics now hold that physicians and investigators must obtain the informed consent of patients and subjects before any substantial intervention. Throughout the early history of concern about research subjects, consent requirements appeared primarily to minimize potential harm. Reducing risk and avoiding unfairness and exploitation are reasons for many professional, regulatory, and institutional controls. However, since the mid-1970s, the primary justification for informed consent requirements has been to protect autonomous choice, a loosely defined goal often buried in broad discussions of protecting the rights of patients and research subjects. Historically, we can claim little beyond that a general, amorphous societal demand has emerged to protect patients' and subjects' rights, particularly their autonomy rights.[13] However, what defines informed consent?

One cannot make decisions about oneself without the correct information. In a perfect world, informed consent is a process of education—a conversation between a healthcare provider and a patient or their family that helps them to make the best possible decision regarding care.[14] This need for accurate information is the foundation of one of the most discussed bioethical issues in the contemporary era. Even the name informed consent implies that one should be informed before consenting.[15] Autonomy requires, then, not only the right to make self-governing choices but also the tools (such as information) that aid one in the process.[16]

The information component refers to the disclosure of information and comprehension of what is disclosed. The consent component refers to both a voluntary decision and an authorization to proceed. Legal, regulatory, philosophical, medical, and psychological pieces of literature tend to favor the following elements as the components of informed consent: "(1) competence, (2) disclosure, (3) understanding, (4) voluntariness, and (5) consent."[17] Some writers present these elements as the building blocks for a definition of informed consent: One gives informed consent to an intervention if (and perhaps only if) one is competent to act, receives a thorough disclosure, comprehends the disclosure, acts voluntarily, and consents to the intervention. This application works well when the patient agrees with the healthcare team, but that does not necessarily guarantee informed consent.

For example, a patient may have already decided what they want in an informed manner before seeing a health professional. Consequently, it is crucial to distinguish informational exchanges through which patients elect medical interventions from acts of approving and authorizing those interventions. In other words, is the patient agreeing with the physician because they have already made their own decision based on their own research? In an article entitled "Introduction: Autonomy in Healthcare" by James Stacey Taylor, he discusses the issue with patients who have made up their minds about a diagnosis or a treatment plan before meeting with their clinicians having "investigated" independently their medical condition. He contends that these patients are not truly competent—and so their decisions should not provide the buffer against interference competent choices should be held to—for they are not deliberating well when they make medical decisions before seeing a healthcare professional.

Moreover, he argues that such patients are also not truly informed, for they cannot accurately determine which sources of medical information they should trust. They might fail to believe the information their healthcare team provides them.[18] Thus, shared decision-making is a worthy medical ideal, but it neither defines nor displaces informed consent.[19] Moreover, this situation can worsen when the patient disagrees with the healthcare team.

Basil Varkey gave this example in an article titled "Principles of Clinical Ethics and Their Application to Practice," the following case was presented. A 56 year-old attorney and current pack-a-day cigarette smoker for more than 30 years were found to have a five-centimeter solitary right upper lobe pulmonary mass on a chest radiograph done during an insurance application. He is asymptomatic, and his examination is normal. If this is lung cancer, which is the probable and most significant diagnosis to consider, early surgical resection provides the best prospects for a cure. Therefore, his physician recommended a bronchoscopic biopsy and subsequent resection in consultation with a chest surgeon. Although the patient understands the treatment plan and the significance of not delaying the treatment, he refuses this plan. He states that he does not think he has cancer. He also fears the surgery will kill him, and even when told of the low mortality of surgery and the importance of removing the mass before it spreads, he refuses treatment.[20] Should the patient be allowed to make this decision?

Clinicians need to be aware of the significance of informed consent. Informed consent must not be seen merely as a legal procedure but as a device to educate their patients and increase their participation in decision-making. The scope of informed consent involves more than just surgical procedures. It adds a whole new dimension to medicine by allowing patients to question their treatment options. Adding a medical social worker to the consent process may be explored to ease the burden on the doctors and could be less intimidating. Also, modifying the informed consent form may be considered to include all the required information in simple, patient-friendly language.[21] Next, in a world where patients and families do their research at "Google University," agreeing with a procedure may not be enough to fulfill the requirements for informed consent. Finally, there will be times when a patient is genuinely informed about a procedure and still disagrees with the healthcare team. This conundrum will be discussed in a later section.

Capacity Defined

> *Amen, amen, I say to you, when you were younger, you used to dress yourself and go where you wanted; but when you grow old, you will stretch out your hands, and someone else will dress you and lead you where you do not want to go.*
>
> —John 21:18 (New American Bible)

Usually, when decisions have to be made in medical practice, there is a consultation between the patient and the clinicians involved. The physician's job with the patient is to provide information and help the patient with decision-making. Treatment can proceed if the patient and the clinical team agree on a course of action. However, there may be uncertainty and even disagreement when the patient is presented with therapeutic options. Suppose the patient is elderly or has been very ill. In that case, there may be a question as to whether or not the patient has the ability or capacity to make medical decisions. Thus, formal accounts of autonomy share a somewhat speculative focus, including some requirements describing the necessary characteristics or capacities for decision-making.[22] Many patients and potential subjects are not competent to give valid consent. Questions about competence focus on whether patients are capable, psychologically or legally, of adequate decision-making. Competence in decision-making is closely connected to autonomous decision-making, as well as to the validity of consent.[23] Capacity refers to the functional determination of whether an individual patient can adequately make a specific decision, such as financial decisions, or perform a particular task, such as driving.

In contrast, competency is the legal determination of whether an impaired mental capacity limits a patient's ability to make a legally relevant decision or action. Physicians play an essential role in this process: in most cases, capacity determinations are made in the clinic without adjudication, and even in cases that progress to legal hearings to determine competency, evidence from clinicians is often crucial. Importantly, capacity is context and decision-specific: a patient may retain the capacity for some decisions, even if other types of decisions are lost.[24] However, when clinicians determine that a patient lacks decision-making capacity, the outcome may be the same as those attending a legal determination of incompetence.[25]

Competence judgments serve a gatekeeping role in healthcare by recognizing persons whose decisions should be sought or accepted from persons whose decisions need not or should not be sought or accepted. For example, health professionals' judgments of a person's lack of capacity may lead them to overrule that person's decisions, turn to informal surrogates for decision-making, or even ask the Court to appoint a guardian to protect their interests if no family members can fill this role.[26] The healthcare team routinely makes this determination with virtually every patient encounter where treatment options are presented. To obtain informed consent, a patient must demonstrate four abilities: to understand the information presented, appreciate how it relates to their situation, rationally use it to make a decision and maintain a consistent choice over time.[27] Although obvious, other authors would add a fifth condition, the ability to communicate that choice.[28] This determination is time and question-sensitive. For example, although a patient may be able to answer a question now, they may lose that ability later if their medical condition worsens.

Moreover, a person may be able to make some decisions, such as I do not want you to attempt resuscitation if I die, but not others, such as financial determinations.[29] As with all medical decisions, clinicians can make false-positive and false-negative errors. A false-positive error would determine that a patient lacks capacity when to make decisions. Such a determination deprives a person of their autonomy. However, a false-negative error is also problematic, as it allows a patient who lacks the capacity to make decisions that could be detrimental to their health.[30] From an ethical standpoint, this is challenging, and there are no easy solutions as often these determinations are subjective and time-consuming. In addition, there are no imaging studies that can determine capacity.[31] Surrogate decision-making will be discussed later, especially in the context of the frail elderly. However, some capacity determinations can be particularly challenging.[32]

A psychiatrist at an eating disorder facility once commented that the patients he saw were the most brilliant, educated, and articulate people he had ever met.[33] Nevertheless, these patients were killing themselves because they felt they were overweight or that food was toxic. These patients can often demonstrate the four capacities stated above, but do they genuinely have the ability to make medical decisions about themselves? Anorexia Nervosa is an eating disorder where the individual has an intense fear of gaining weight despite abnormally low body weight. Persons with this disorder strongly value managing their weight and shape, using extreme efforts often significantly affecting their lives.[34]

In cases where a refusal to eat has led to possible death by starvation, the legal and ethical situation is complicated. Unlike many other potentially fatal illnesses, treating anorexia can prevent death by using nasogastric feeding (a tube that goes into the nose and stomach) to restore weight. However, an unwilling patient can remove a nasogastric tube, so for it to be effective, the patient may have to be chemically or physically restrained during feeding; that is, they must be force-fed. Force-feeding is a controversial medical procedure described as "inhuman and degrading treatment."[35]

Treating anorexic patients with a feeding tube can sometimes be justified when they are acutely ill. Many of these patients, especially women, can develop hypophosphatemia. This condition can cause delirium (an altered mental status), worsening anorexia, and, under extreme conditions, even death. Giving these patients a feeding tube until this electrolyte imbalance is treated may correct the mental status changes and allow the patient to make healthier decisions.[36] However, a nasogastric tube is only a short-term treatment for an acute problem, not a long-term solution for anorexia nervosa.

A difficult balancing act must be performed in treating anorexia patients; pragmatism and compassion must be considered. Offering palliative care to the patient to alleviate the physical suffering caused by malnutrition is not just about respecting their refusals. It is also not about acting in their best interests and is even not, strictly speaking, discontinuing ineffective treatment. Long-term tube feeding by sedating or physically restraining the patient is clearly not an ethical or realistic option. Ultimately, compassion and respecting the patient's dignity and integrity from their perspective may be the best and only conclusion.[37] Gender-affirming treatment is another topic to be addressed when discussing autonomy. This particular item has become a recurrent topic in our society. It has surfaced in many issues, including women's sports, beer commercials, school curriculum, and parent's rights, to name just a few. For simplicity, this discussion will not include the rare condition where children are born with "ambiguous genitalia," where surgery and other treatments are often used to help them live an ordinary life. This section will look at people born with one sex who wish to be another.

People who wish to change their sex are often diagnosed with gender dysphoria. The most recent DSM-5 classification for gender dysphoria, published in 2013, can be problematic, to say the least. Opponents state that including this diagnosis in the DSM implies that a person having a transgender identity has a mental health problem, even though the DSM is clear that only people in distress or impaired would meet the diagnostic criteria. This scenario presents a Catch-22: unless a person has a mental disorder, they cannot get treatment, but if they have a mental disorder, how can they consent to treatment?[38] Treatment for gender dysphoria can vary widely. Psychological support ranges from assisting with exploring gender identity to helping with making the social transition to living as one's affirmed gender. Medical interventions include affirmation of the patient's gender identity through hormone treatment and often gender-affirming surgery.[39]

The results of medical and surgical treatments are substantial depending on the transition and often include preventing puberty, sterilization, double mastectomies, and orchiectomies (removing the testicles). These circumstances propose an obvious problem: do patients with a mental disorder have autonomy? Other questions arise, such as whether minors can decide to seek treatment and whether parents should be excluded from decision-making if they disagree with their child. Finally, since many of these procedures are irreversible, should less aggressive treatments be explored with children who, by definition, have psychiatric issues? There are no clear answers to these questions. The Catholic Church does not have any specific directives regarding transgender interventions. Still, since they often involve sterilization, clearly, the Church would be against them.

Additionally, an ethicist at the National Catholic Bioethics Center, John A. Di Camillo, states, "In the end, there is no authentic transition either anthropologically or biologically—just mutilation."[40] Others, however, will argue that gender is not a fixed entity and that an autonomous patient with capacity can make this choice. Although I have provided some definitions and concerns, some of these debates are far from settled.

Autonomy versus Beneficence

The ethical principle of beneficence is a group of norms for providing and balancing benefits against risks and costs.[41] With medicine, we should always strive to do what is best for the patient. However, we should also respect patients' choices, especially if they have autonomy. As John Stuart Mill states, "Autonomous actions should not be subjected to controlling constraints by others." This principle of respect for autonomy needs specification in particular contexts to become a practical guide to conduct, and appropriate specification will, in due course, incorporate valid exceptions. Autonomy is often considered the highest principle in contemporary medical ethics. However, a closer analysis of autonomy shows that it is a flawed entity upon which to base medical decisions.[42]

One of the more baffling moral dilemmas in medicine occurs when the ethical obligation to protect a patient's welfare conflicts with the duty to protect the patient's rights.[43] For instance, pain management must look at the person's desire to be comfortable and the person's safety. Clinicians should follow the principles of beneficence and nonmaleficence and provide effective pain management while avoiding opioid overprescribing. These responsibilities are simultaneously balanced with respecting patient autonomy.[44]

What if respect for patient autonomy correlates with higher satisfaction scores? A nationally representative study determined that higher patient satisfaction was associated with lower emergency department utilization, higher inpatient utilization, more significant total healthcare expenditures, and higher expenditures on prescription drugs. The most satisfied patients also had a statistically significantly higher mortality risk than the least satisfied patients.[45] It is often difficult to decide what is best for patients with autonomy; perhaps it is worse when they do not.

In the US, reforms for laws regarding patients with mental illness were based on contemporary thoughts of constitutional limitations on state power and requirements for due process. Globally, these considerations have been framed by intrinsic human rights to liberty and autonomy. Current commitment laws typically involve periodic reviews of the committed patients' condition, which focuses on whether commitment criteria continue to be met and places that determination in the hands of individuals acting almost as judges. It is clear that contemporary civil commitment processes aim to protect the basic rights of liberty, even in the danger of less effective treatment, more rapid decompensation, and higher re-hospitalization rates. In these processes, rights precede treatment considerations: beneficence is less needed than autonomy.[46]

Although it seems autonomy takes precedence over other ethical principles, it is not absolute. This principle of respect for autonomy needs specification in particular contexts to become a practical guide to conduct, and appropriate specification will incorporate valid exceptions.[47] To illustrate this, what if an individual's decision has the potential to harm themselves or others? The former dilemma has been discussed for both laws to allow for physician-assisted suicide and justification for aggressive care at the end of life.

A significant problem with treating dying patients is the promotion of autonomy in living, which wrongfully prioritizes life's sanctity over its dignity. This practice is recognized when aggressive medical efforts are misused. Unfortunately, these attempts at prolonging life can quickly turn into dragging out an inevitable death. When death seems the alternative, enormous amounts of money and resources are often used to buy time for the patient or their loved ones at the end of life.[48] Sometimes, the patient has asked for this type of treatment, but their family often states that their loved one would have wanted this. Ultimately, the medical team is sometimes forced to choose between what the patient wants (autonomy) and appropriate treatment (beneficence.)

The other problem is when we overprioritize dignity over sanctity. The Oregon Death with Dignity Act is a crucial example of a legal policy implemented to guarantee that a dying patient has autonomy. The act originated as a quest for patient empowerment in end-of-life situations. However, it soon dissolved into an attempt to end suffering quickly and allow patient choices that could lead to immediate death. This bill, entitled Measure 16, was eventually seen as an affirmation "of the ideology of patient control and self-determination."[49] Heart-wrenching stories from dying patients were used to convince people that this legislation needed to be passed. The impact of Measure 16 in Oregon, even though limited in actual practice, will most likely, in the future, have ethical ramifications that will indeed not be limited to Oregon and a handful of other states. This obvious stand-off between autonomy and beneficence will continue as other states adopt similar legislation.

Finally, what happens when an autonomous person's decision about their health adversely affects others? Since the inception of this book, COVID-19 has become a vital part of the discussion regarding autonomy. In the middle of 2022, there were 66,992 new cases diagnosed in the US, and over 80% were from the delta variant. When many Americans felt that the worst of the pandemic was behind them, the emergence of COVID variants raised the possibility of a resurgence, which could lead to more mask mandates, lockdowns, and even more deaths. Confronted with a steep decline in vaccination rates, President Biden said that his administration would direct agents door to door, set up workplace clinics, and recommend employers provide paid time off as a part of a plan to reach tens of millions of unvaccinated Americans.[50] At what point does the autonomy to get vaccinated or not clash with the beneficence of mandating vaccinations?

Decades before the COVID-19 pandemic, Beauchamps and Childress, in their book *Principles of Biomedical Ethics*, stated:

> *The requirement to benefit may be overridden if we can produce a major benefit by causing a minor harm, or a major benefit for many people while causing a minor harm for only a few. Thus, for example, many public health programs, such as vaccinations, could cause harm to a certain percentage of the population while providing a major benefit to other parts of the population.*[51]

The argument for autonomy that an adult might invoke weakens as the risk to others by their non-participatory conduct increases: it is more justified to limit autonomy when its use harms others. COVID-19 is more contagious and more lethal than influenza, though the risk of death and hospitalization increases with age. The delta variant of COVID-19 appears to be more infectious than the initial strain, but not more deadly. Thus, the risk of this virus to healthy children seems minimal. However, healthy, unvaccinated children who do not receive the vaccine can get—and transmit—the virus to those vulnerable. This group could include classmates with medical conditions that put them at high risk if they get COVID-19. It could also include high-risk school employees such as teachers, administrators, or janitors over 60 years old, with weak immune systems, or conditions like diabetes or heart disease.[52]

The vaccines appear safe and effective, although the Johnson and Johnson vaccine has reported thrombosis (blood clots)[53] and heart muscle inflammation with the Pfizer and Moderna products.[54] Although the vaccines have been effective in preventing deaths, vaccinated people can still get sick and transmit COVID. These unfortunate effects have caused some people to question the usefulness of vaccinating. Vaccine reluctance is an old phenomenon that represents a severe threat to global health, as shown by the return of some childhood infections (e.g., outbreaks of measles and pertussis.) The gigantic leaps in developing efficacious and safe COVID-19 vaccines within a short period were unprecedented.

Nevertheless, COVID-19 vaccine hesitancy can limit global efforts to control the pandemic's destructive health and socio-economic effects.[55] Considering the perceived (and actual) risks from the available COVID-19 vaccines and their confirmed weaknesses, introducing a mandatory policy would be practically and ethically debatable. Risk communication aims to shape decision-making by complying with individual choices, but COVID-19 mandates significantly disregard personal autonomy.[56]

To get more people vaccinated, paying individuals to get the shot against COVID-19 may seem an adequate scheme, but such an approach is expensive and challenging. Further research should consider implementing COVID-19 mandates with groups that do not endorse vaccination on a large scale.[57] However, private companies, schools, health systems, and airlines may impose mandatory vaccine protocols, even when government agencies can or will not. Whether this approach will be enough to get to the threshold needed for herd immunity is unknown, and at least for now, a government mandate is unlikely to occur unless conditions get a lot worse.[58]

AUTONOMY PART 2—PATIENT DOES NOT HAVE CAPACITY

This section will examine patients' challenges when they cannot make healthcare decisions themselves. Most patients cannot make decisions for themselves when they are very ill. So, how do healthcare professionals decide on their course of action? If the patient had written out directions on how to proceed in various scenarios, that would be helpful, but does such a document cover all possible scenarios? What about family; can they make decisions regarding their loved ones that respect that person's autonomy? What if family members cannot agree? Finally, why not allow the healthcare team to do what they think is best? After all, is that not their area of expertise? Historically, several cases have occurred that can illustrate this dilemma. Both cases involve young women who suffered devastating injuries that prevented them from making medical decisions, forcing the family, the healthcare team, and, ultimately, the State to decide.

In an old car without seat belts, Nancy Cruzan was driving home from work in the early morning of January 11, 1983. She swerved on an icy, deserted Missouri country road, and her car flipped and crashed. The 25-year-old woman tumbled out and landed facedown in a water-filled ditch.[59] Massive injuries resulted in her falling unconscious and unresponsive to outside stimuli. Doctors estimated that Nancy's brain had been without oxygen for at least fourteen minutes before she was found, which, along with multiple cerebral contusions, caused severe brain damage.[60] Later that morning, Nancy's father received the phone call in the night that all parents fear, the one telling him that his daughter had been in a severe car accident and might not survive. Nancy's family spent the next several days in the hospital waiting room, not wanting to risk going home to shower, hoping and praying for good news.[61] On February 7, almost a month after his daughter was admitted to the hospital, Joe Cruzan finally signed a piece of paper titled "Hospital Consent to Operation, Anesthesia, and Other Services, to consent to surgery." This document allowed the hospital to place a gastrostomy feeding tube and a surgically placed hose in her stomach to enable her to receive nutrition.[62]

About seven years later, on February 25, 1990, Terri Schiavo suffered cardiac arrest, apparently caused by a potassium imbalance that led to a severe hypoxic brain injury. She was taken to the Humana Northside Hospital. She later was also given a percutaneous endoscopic gastrostomy (PEG) to provide nutrition and hydration.[63] On June 18, 1990, the Court appointed her husband, Michael, as guardian; her parents did not object.[64] What happens to Ms. Cruzan and Ms. Schaivo? Questions arose about what is considered good ethical treatment when the person can no longer make decisions. Both families had to resort to legal means to decide whether the PEG tube should remain or be removed.

When it became clear that Ms. Cruzan had virtually no chance of waking up, her parents asked that the Missouri State Hospital terminate the artificial hydration and nutrition provided by the PEG tube. However, the healthcare team refused to do so without court approval. The parents were subsequently successfully authorized to end treatment by a state trial court, which found that someone in Ms. Cruzan's situation had a fundamental constitutional right to refuse treatment and direct the withdrawal of "death-prolonging procedures." On appeal, however, the Missouri Supreme Court reversed the decision. The Court recognized that the common-law doctrine of informed consent included a right to refuse treatment but did not consider it applicable here. In addition, the Court declined to interpret the state constitution as giving a right of privacy so broad as to support an unrestricted right to refuse treatment. Finally, the Court rejected the argument that Ms. Cruzan's parents could order an end to treatment by concluding that no one could make that choice for an incompetent person absent the formalities required by the State's living-will statute or when clear and convincing documentation of the person's wishes are absent.[65]

The case then went to the US Supreme Court, which upheld the State Court's decision. The decision distinguished the rights of competent persons—who, the Court assumed, have a constitutionally protected right to refuse hydration and nutrition—from those of incompetent persons. However, in late 1990, Ms. Cruzan's parents were granted a second hearing in state court, which the State of Missouri did not oppose. Her parents presented new evidence that convinced a judge that Ms. Cruzan would not have wanted to live in PVS. He ordered the feeding tube removed. Although anti-euthanasia groups unsuccessfully sought to intervene. Nancy Cruzan died a few days later.

Terri Schiavo's case was even more gruesome regarding the ultimate removal of her tube feedings. Her husband, Michael, and her parents, the Schindlers, had a "falling out" regarding her care. Michael wanted the feedings to cease her tube feedings, stating that she would never have wanted to live this way. Her parents opposed this, saying that they felt that she would choose life. In May of 1998, Michael Schiavo petitioned the Court to allow the removal of Ms. Schiavo's feeding tube; the Schindlers opposed it, saying that she would want to remain alive.[66] This legal battle went on for over seven years. It involved then-Florida Governor Jeb Bush, who tried to use his authority to prevent the feeding tube's removal. The Florida House of Representatives even passed a bill, "Terri's Law," that allowed the governor to issue a "one-time stay in certain cases."[67]

On March 2, 2004, Pope John Paul II addressed the World Federation of Catholic Medical Associations and the Pontifical Academy for Life Congress on "Life-Sustaining Treatments and Vegetative State: Scientific Advances and Ethical Dilemmas." His remarks spark even more widespread interest and controversy in an already horrific case.[68] Another year of legal battles ensued; however, the Supreme Court refused to hear the case. The Peg tube was removed on March 18, 2005, and Terri Schiavo died on March 31, 2005.[69]

The complete ethical ramifications of the above two cases are beyond the scope of this chapter. However, these cases do illustrate the problems with surrogate decision-making. Neither Terri nor Nancy could say what they would want under the tragic circumstances they found they faced. There is no evidence to suggest that their parents felt nothing but love for their daughters and wanted the best for them. However, the Cruzans fought hard to have the feeding tube removed from their daughter, while the Schindlers fought hard to keep it in. Again, two loving families with two completely different decisions. As was discussed in the previous section, there sometimes is a conflict between dignity and sanctity.[70] The dignity paradigm would argue to remove the tube, while the sanctity paradigm would keep the feeding going to preserve life. The problem is, what would the patient want if they could wake up and tell us?

Surrogate Decision Making

As previously mentioned, most patients cannot decide for themselves when critically ill.[71] Often, family members are asked to help with the decision-making process. Ideally, these family members would know the patient well enough to be able to make choices based on their loved one's values with some degree of certainty. Their confidence would also be centered on written documentation from their ill loved ones stating their choices in various medical circumstances. Armed with this information, the surrogates would meet with the healthcare team, knowing that their decisions would respect the patient's autonomy and values. Unfortunately, this is often not the case.[72] Meaningful discussions between patients and their surrogates about risks and benefits, complex trade-offs, and preferences are usually deferred until more emergent occasions, making it more challenging, if not impossible, for those discussions to be thoughtful and well-grounded.[73] Despite these obstacles, decisions have to be made by someone.

Unless the patient has assigned in writing a decision-maker to be utilized when they can no longer make decisions, the healthcare team will look to the "next-of-kin" to help with decision-making. However, every State has its own statutes regarding who that person is and how much authority they have. For example, the "next-of-kin" is the healthcare representative in Pennsylvania. The spouse and children of a previous relationship are the first to be called, followed by current children, parents, and siblings (in that order). The healthcare representative can only make decisions regarding life-sustaining treatments if the patient has "an end-stage medical condition or is permanently unconscious."[74] Otherwise, it is assumed that the patient would want these treatments. The two apparent problems with this method are evident: the person designated as the decision-maker may not be the person that the patient wants, and secondly, that person may lack the authority (based on state law) to make the most critical decisions regarding life support and feeding tubes. If the patient had designated in writing a decision-maker, that person (called the *healthcare agent* or *healthcare power of attorney*) would have the same authority as the patient to make treatment decisions, including life support and feeding tubes.[75]

Jurisdictions base their next of kin rules on the alleged closeness to the individual. Such relationships are prioritized partly because a spouse, child, or sibling is likely to be reachable and willing to decide. Also, there is a premise that this person will likely have relevant information that the medical team lacks. It is not that the spouse, child, or sibling has a special moral right to decide for their relative. Instead, the thought is that this person possesses knowledge that makes them more likely than anyone else to make an appropriate decision.[76] This premise, however, is not always accurate, and the surrogate designated by state law may have difficulty making these decisions. Multiple studies indicate that this can be problematic.[77]

Surrogates vary in how they accurately predict patients' preferences for medical treatment. Their predictive accuracy most often falls between chance (50%)

and high (close to 100%) levels, yet factors contributing to this large variability have yet to be identified. However, patient–surrogate disagreement may arise because surrogates simply do not know patients' preferences.[78] For example, higher rates of life-sustaining treatments are observed when children are the sole decision-makers than when the spouse is involved.[79] This discrepancy could be because the spouse knows their partner's preferences better. Alternatively, spouses and children may have different views about whether life-sustaining treatments are beneficial or consistent with the patient's wishes. This dilemma requires patients to prepare their surrogate decision-makers with information about the type of care they would want to receive in various hypothetical situations while still cognitively normal.[80] When this type of information is lacking and the predictive accuracy is low, best-interest standards are often utilized.

Substituted Judgment versus Best Interest Standard

The substituted judgment standard (SJS) was initially described in several nineteenth-century English court judgments, including *Ex Parte Whitbread* (1815), *In Re Blair* (1836), and *In Re Earl of Carysfort* (1840). At the time, English courts were allowed to give away incompetent adults' property only in ways that aided the person. This principle stopped courts from giving away the property of incompetent adults in ways that did not benefit the individual, even if the individual would have endorsed this decision. In the *Whitbread* case, this principle prevented the courts from distributing money to close needy families, even when it was evident that the person would have wanted to help their families. However, the courts permitted the SJS to address this concern, which allowed them to consider how the incompetent individuals would have wanted their money used.[81]

Similarly, we can look at this standard today regarding healthcare decisions. Like the nineteenth-century British judges, are we limiting decisions regarding incompetent patients to judgments that benefit the individual (best interest) or to a decision based on what we think the individual would have wanted (substituted judgment)? Is one of these standards superior to the other?

The best interest standard for surrogate decision-making requires the establishment of objective criteria based on community norms. Therefore, developing best interest standards necessitates public discussion about end-of-life care and consensus regarding the specific situations in which surrogates have decision-making authority. This standard is incomplete since it fails to consider the individual patient's values and relationships.[82] However, as we saw in the Schiavo and Cruzan cases, knowing a patient's values can be elusive.

Best interest standard (BIS) makes sense when dealing with patients with preferences that cannot be known, such as infants and those born with cognitive disabilities. The BIS requires the surrogate(s) to assess the benefits and risks of treatment alternatives, including quality-of-life (QOL) considerations. Parents are the natural surrogates for children, so their interpretation of the best interest and healthcare decision-making should be supported. Exceptions to this may arise when parents demand ongoing treatment found futile by the medical team or when refusal of necessary treatment is considered medically neglectful. When the benefits of treatment are evident, or when further care is pointless, the BIS can be straightforwardly applied, but in circumstances of uncertain prognosis, the child's best interests may not be apparent; in these "gray zones," QOL considerations predominate, and the BIS empowers parents to make these difficult decisions.[83]

If the values of a formally competent but now incompetent patient are not written down or known to the surrogates, the BIS is also often employed. Under the BIS, a surrogate decision-maker must determine the highest net benefit among the available options, assigning different weights to the patient's interests in each option and discounting or subtracting inherent risks or costs. Thus, the term *best* is used because the surrogate must maximize benefit through a comparative assessment establishing the highest net benefit. In addition, the best interests standard protects another's well-being by assessing the risks and benefits of various treatments and alternatives to treatment, considering pain and suffering, and evaluating restoration or loss of functioning. It is, therefore, inescapably a quality-of-life judgment.[84] That is a difficult decision for a surrogate, especially if there is no document or conversation to rely on, and often there is not.

Some authors have used the term *substituted interest* as a way to help surrogates make decisions when the patient's preferences have not been made clear. When families are asked to make medical decisions for an incompetent patient, the substituted interests model would have clinicians guide them by emphasizing an individualized and patient-centered approach.[85] Moreover, clinicians would combine these principles with empirical evidence about what individuals value and how they make decisions. This model emphasizes authenticity (i.e., a decision valid to who the person really is) rather than the autonomy the patient cannot exercise.[86]

The substituted interests model reframes surrogate decision-making as an approach that promotes the patient as a unique person in the context of their relationships, applying the patient's authentic values, wishes, and real interests as best they can be known. To accomplish this, the clinician asks the family a series of questions in a way that helps them formulate their thoughts. Knowing your loved one, the clinician may ask what you think would be most essential for them right now. This model seems to respect patient rights and to serve each patient's unique cultural, spiritual, familial, psychological, and clinical circumstances—what clinicians want to do for all patients, those who can speak for themselves and those who cannot.[87]

Advance Care Planning

The customary objective of advance care planning has been to have patients make treatment decisions in advance so clinicians can attempt to provide care consistent with their wishes. Ideally, this conversation occurs with their clinicians and surrogates. The results are written as a *living will* and a *healthcare power of attorney*.[88] Unfortunately, these forms are rarely completed; when they are, they often do not have the needed conversations.[89] Advance care planning intends to help ensure that people receive care that reflects their values, goals, and preferences during severe and chronic illnesses. For many people, this process may include choosing and preparing another trusted person to make medical decisions if the person can no longer make their own decisions.[90] Therefore, an advance directive serves as a guide, providing critical information and stating whether patients intend their preferences to be followed strictly or loosely and who should be involved in making decisions. Most importantly, encouraging discussions about decision-making with loved ones becomes central to advance care planning.[91]

At best, however, advance directives are still a form of substituted judgment. Decisions are based on what a person says in the past regarding a future condition. Using the substituted judgment standard, is what a person desires now the same as what they would want in the future? One author states that a "major determinant of changing preferences is adaptability. For example, patients often cannot envision coping with disability and report the desire to forgo aggressive treatments in such states. However, once patients experience those health states, they are often more willing to accept even invasive treatments with limited benefits. On the other hand, some patients may shift their goals from life prolongation to comfort."[92] While it is not unusual for patients to change their minds as their illness progresses, it remains vital that a patient with capacity be allowed to make these decisions.[93]

A living will does not trump an autonomous patient, and most laws state that a living will only has power when a patient lacks capacity.[94] However, what if the loss of capacity is not permanent? In this case, the goal should be to get the patient to a point, if possible, to make decisions for themselves if they so choose. However, surrogates are often used to make decisions when a seriously ill patient's capacity is unlikely to return. Therefore, selecting an appropriate decision-maker is critical. Unfortunately, allowing this decision to be made by a state's "next-of-kin" legislature may not place the most suitable person in charge.[95] The agent or proxy in a durable power of attorney (DPOA) should know the patient's values intimately and can respond to unexpected events. In addition, the agent can ask questions, assess risks and costs, speak to relatives and friends of the patient, consider a variety of therapeutic options, seek the opinions of other physicians, and evaluate the patient's condition and prospects of recovery in short, engage in the same complex decision-making process that the patient would undertake if able to do so.[96]

Therefore, patients are encouraged to complete a DPOA form and prepare family and friends so that the person they choose to make medical decisions can be flexible.[97] Even if the living will is completed, goals and values change, and only a surrogate close to the patient can act as a valid surrogate during challenging times.[98]

Will their wishes be supported if a patient has completed a living will and a healthcare power of attorney and then loses capacity? The answer is maybe. It depends on the interpretation of the terms used. For instance, the standard terminology to describe when a living will is valid is when the patient has an "end-stage condition." This phrase assists a practitioner in feeling more comfortable with a decision that a disease has reached a final point. Determining that a patient has an end-stage condition no longer needs to be documented by two practitioners by law, even though this may be required in a person's advance directive.[99] However, even with this description, physicians and families sometimes do not recognize that the patient's condition is end-stage and that the living will demands should apply. Advance directives are usually insufficient to prevent the feared outcome of loss of personhood and dignity in advanced dementia.[100] As previously discussed, sanctity often overcomes dignity in these decisions.[101]

Advance directives can effectively identify decision-makers and outline patient healthcare wishes and priorities. However, converting advance directives into operational care plans for seriously ill patients at a high risk of facing a health crisis can be challenging for providers. For care plans to be effective, they must be translated into medical orders, which drive actions in medical settings. Without medical orders to the contrary, standardized medical protocols such as cardiopulmonary resuscitation (CPR) usually take over when an emergency occurs.[102] Healthcare innovators in Oregon, in 1991, began to articulate a process that looked at the disconnect between existing advance directives and the increasing need for clear, convincing, and actionable medical orders for severely ill or frail patients where death within the next year would not be surprising.

The physician order for life-sustaining treatment (POLST) was developed to bridge this gap.[103] POLST is a conversation tool that plainly addresses the type of medical treatment you would want at the end of life; it allows seriously ill patients to have more autonomy with their treatment decisions and helps patients discuss their choices with their healthcare team and loved ones. In addition, POLST can reduce patient and family suffering and ensure patient wishes are known and honored. The POLST process starts with discussing the treating clinician and the patient with severe illness or frailty (or the patient's authorized surrogate) to understand their current health status and medical decision options. Step two interprets those choices and goals into medical language, precisely with a set of medical orders that address likely critical decisions, for instance, cardiopulmonary resuscitation (CPR), the level of medical intervention desired in the event of an emergency, decisions regarding the level of comfort desired, decisions regarding further hospitalizations, whether to use artificial nutrition and hydration (ANH) and, in some states, the use of ventilators and antibiotics. The final steps in completing the POLST involve having clinicians confirm that POLST will follow the patient across all care settings, be honored, and be reviewed.[104]

Opponents of the POLST program have concerns regarding the value of seriously ill patients' choices and what happens if patients change their minds once the POLST is completed. Furthermore, critics often cite the inherent power imbalance between patients and their clinicians, stating that POLST is not "protective enough" and is "more about withholding treatment" than patient Autonomy.[105] For instance, the United States Conference of Catholic Bishops (USCCB) has stated that the POLST does not require the patient to sign the document as currently utilized. Additionally, once signed by the physician, it becomes an order to the medical staff and may override the patient's own past advance directives and even the patient's appointment with a healthcare agent. Furthermore, it may be applied to patients not in a terminal situation who only need antibiotics, nutrition, hydration, or other proportionate nonaggressive care.[106] Therefore, the POLST paradigm is often banned in Catholic hospitals.[107]

However, these concerns are not unique to POLST, as similar arguments have been made regarding advance directives.[108] In fact, other Catholic authors have stated that the POLST paradigm supports care in the context of the *Ethical and Religious Directives for Catholic Health Care Services* (ERDs). They state that POLST is a patient-centered process, respecting human dignity while acknowledging that death is an inevitable part of life. POLST forms complement advance directives by converting an individual's wishes regarding medical treatment into a medical order and guiding surrogate decision-makers.[109] For a POLST to be valid, an ongoing conversation must occur between healthcare providers, patients, and families. A form is just a piece of paper. It carries no weight if the necessary concentration is not given to the critical conversation and the professional duty placed upon healthcare providers to honor the requests from that conversation. Only then can the POLST become actionable, resulting in the kind of tender care that seriously ill patients deserve. POLST, when done well, can help preserve human dignity during life's final transition.[110]

Catholic versus Secular Autonomy

In the previous section we introduced the ERDs and how there are times when they differ from secular laws. So now, let us discuss the topic of autonomy as it relates to Catholic teaching. ERDs, first published in 1948 and with the sixth and most recent editions published in 2018, are "theological principles that guide the Church's vision of healthcare."[111] The United States Conference of Catholic Bishops (USCCB) defines the services Catholic Hospitals can provide and sets healthcare guidelines for Catholics involved in these services. These directives deserve further discussion.

There has always been a strong connection between the Church and treating the sick. Even a cursory reading of the Gospels will show multiple examples where Jesus healed people from numerous diseases, including blindness, leprosy, lameness, bleeding, being mute, and mental disorders, to name just a few. This tradition between healthcare and the Catholic Church goes back centuries and reflects a common goal: caring for the sick is rooted in the spirit of Christ and His love for us. From ancient times, there was an association between hospices that assist weary travelers and the development of early hospitals to treat the infirm. There are similarities between the Church and the practice of medicine as both strive to help the sick. However, the teachings of the Church are more comprehensive and deal with Catholic society as a whole. In contrast, medicine tends to be more specific, as it looks to treat individual patients. Therefore, the relationship between these communities has to be defined every so often.[112]

As early as the sixteenth century, theologians and medical professionals began working together to define medical and patient care norms.[113] Fast forward to the nineteenth and twentieth centuries in the United States, where Catholic medical institutions grew and developed (under the jurisdiction of the diocesan bishops) in much the same way Church-based hospices formed in the Middle Ages. So, in 1915, the Catholic Health Association was founded to improve the quality of medical care and ethical concerns of the time. The first written directives of ethical norms were compiled in 1921 in Detroit by Rev. Michael Burke and were just one page long. Essentially, it was a list of "do's and don'ts."[114] These rules were often displayed in the operating rooms of Catholic Hospitals in the US and Canada, much like the rules one would see when you enter a park: "No open fires," "No dogs without a leash," "No alcoholic beverages," and so on. As can be imagined, this brief document lacked any scriptural or biblical content.

First published in 1947, the ERDs were created by theologians and healthcare professionals from the United States and Canada based on Catholic teaching. Initially, it was up to the local bishops to accept these directives for their diocese. Not all dioceses accepted these directives for various reasons, so the National Conference of Catholic Bishops, now called the USCCB, was requested to revise and approve a new set of ERDs. The revised directives were completed in 1971 and were more universally adopted. Nevertheless, the ERDs still came across as a list of "do's and don'ts," not unlike its predecessors. It took another 23 years for the modifications to be published.

In 1994, a new version was issued with significant changes. The ERDs now focused on human dignity, social justice, and the Church's moral doctrine. This revision vow framed the "do's and don'ts" in terms that expressed the sanctity of life and God's love for us. Along a similar line, a year later, Pope John Paul II issued the *Evangelium Vitae* (The Gospel of Life) to "reiterate the view of the Roman Catholic Church on the value of life and to warn against violating the sanctity of life." Both of these documents convey the Catholic Church's stance on abortion, euthanasia, and birth control, as well as other concerns like the invitro fertilization method of conception. John Paul II and the Church voiced worries that these actions added to a growing "culture of death." Therefore, the Church needed to advocate for a "culture of life" by explaining why human life has worth and dignity.

Simply put, God loves and created us in His image and likeness. He sent Jesus, his only begotten son, so that all people could saved and experience eternal life. In the decades that have followed since the late pontiff issued EV, his message has extended to denouncing terrorist attacks, wars, increases in suicides, school shootings, and human trafficking, as well as easier access to abortions, and controversies and opinions surrounding global healthcare as these events have added to a devaluing of human life.[115] Every innocent human being, therefore, is unconditionally equal to all others. Thus, the EV, along with the ERDs, clearly define moral norms against the direct taking of the life of an innocent human being and other violations with no privileges or exceptions for anyone. All human beings are precious in His sight. The ERDs then became more than just a set of rules; they were now a moral and biblical explanation of how healthcare should be practiced in the US. (The word *love* is mentioned a dozen times in the ERDs, reinforcing the idea of its divine origin.) Finally, ERDs were subdivided into six sections, and these changes have persisted in subsequent editions released in 2001, 2009, and the most recent 2018 version.[116]

So, it is easy to appreciate why the ERDs would be against physician-assisted suicide, abortion, and euthanasia, as these procedures represent acts of "extreme autonomy" and would be contrary to a culture of life proposed by Pope John Paul II. Sadly, some, if not all, of these actions are considered healthcare practices in the US and other countries. This book will critically examine these clinical items to discuss the ethics involved. As a Catholic physician, however, there are times when my conscience struggles with Catholic teachings as well. This dilemma occurs when there is an emphasis on ERDs as absolute laws that must always be obeyed versus what is often referred to as "best practices" in medicine. Catholic healthcare workers, at times, have to choose between two courses of action, one recommended by the medical profession and the other as directed by the ERDs. In a later chapter on nonmaleficence, this question will be discussed regarding concerns about the beginning and end of life. But for now, let us look at an issue with Catholic hospitals regarding the sterilization of women.

According to Directive 53 of ERDs:

> *Direct sterilization of either men or women, whether permanent or temporary, is not permitted in a Catholic health care institution. Procedures that induce sterility are permitted when their direct effect is the cure or alleviation of a present and serious pathology, and a simpler treatment is unavailable.*[117]

Direct sterilizations, such as tubal ligations, if performed to prevent future pregnancies, are prohibited, even if the procedure is done to avoid a medical problem that may arise in a future pregnancy. However, medically necessary procedures to treat "a present and serious pathology" like cancer of the uterus, a tubal pregnancy, or a damaged uterus are allowed and are considered "indirect sterilization" even if the procedure causes sterility. This distinction between direct and indirect sterilization has been a contentious point for many years, despite repeated revision of the ERDs by the bishops, as well as Vatican efforts to clarify the teaching, and can cause some ethical dilemmas.[118]

Suppose a woman has serious health concerns such as heart disease or asthma where pregnancy would likely cause death. Situations such as these place Catholic health providers in the predicament of having to choose between Church teaching and what is widely considered "good medicine. Additionally, if the woman has a uterus that was damaged by a C-section, where another pregnancy would be dangerous, the Church would allow a hysterectomy but not a tubal ligation, even though the latter is less invasive and would essentially have the same clinical outcome. The Church's official stance is that women could still use natural family planning (with a failure rate of 24%, according to the CDC). From a medical standpoint, tubal ligation would be the most successful and least invasive way to save a woman from a perilous situation. One could argue that an even less invasive procedure of all would be to have the husband get a vasectomy; the procedure is less invasive than tubal ligation, and the husband most likely does not have the medical issues that the wife does that make pregnancy perilous for her. Of course, this procedure is prohibited for men, as well. Why, then, should medical professionals allow a woman to be placed in such a predicament?

The general introduction of the ERDs states:

> *The dialogue between medical science and Christian faith has for its primary purpose the common good of all human persons. It presupposes that science and faith do not contradict each other. Both are grounded in respect for truth and freedom. Allowing direct sterilizations under these specific circumstances could help settle an issue that can cause conflict with women, Catholic institutions, and healthcare workers who are trying to do the right thing on the deepest level.*[119]

This narrative is not meant to disrespect the Catholic tradition but to encourage healthcare professionals to remain ever-vigilant in ethical treatments for our patients. Suppose you are a medical professional working at a Catholic institution. In that case, the ethics committee and other structures will assist you in your decision-making. However, as we will see later in the chapter on nonmaleficence, this method is not foolproof, and problems can still occur. One extreme would be to take a purely "deontological" view, encouraging a strict "letter of the law" approach with the involved ERDs. Another way would be a "consequentialist" approach focusing on the best or the least harmful result. However, this approach often ignores the act itself. As with most extreme approaches, the truth usually lies somewhere in the middle.

The task is even more daunting for Catholic professionals working at a secular hospital. But what do you do if your patient insists on a procedure such as direct sterilization? Most Catholic hospitals see patients who are not Catholic, and many are located in rural areas where a secular hospital is not nearby. One choice would be to refer the patient to a colleague willing to do what the patient requests.

However, some would question abandonment problems with this decision. Additionally, referring the woman to another hospital can also be seen as illicit under Directives 70 and others of the ERDs.[120]

Dealing with this ethical dilemma can be troubling for Catholic health professionals and their patients. Prayer and consultation with a Catholic Chaplain or pastor are strongly recommended when faced with these dilemmas. It should be noted that ERDs are not the same as the Code of Canon Law of the Catholic Church (usually called "the Code"). The Code applies to the entire Western Church, and the Pope establishes it. In contrast, the ERDs are instituted by the US Conference of Catholic Bishops and are concerned only with Catholic healthcare services in the United States. The rules may differ if you are in a medical practice outside the US. In the end, the final decision should be based on moral decision-making. Perhaps the best advice for Catholics comes directly from the ERDs: "As new knowledge and new technologies expand, each person must form a correct conscience based on the moral norms for proper health care."[121]

CONCLUSION

A patient's rights, including freedom of choice, are essential to healthcare, reflected in the ethical principle of autonomy. Nevertheless, with this right comes a responsibility from the healthcare team to ensure that the patient's choice is indeed valid. The first section of this chapter looked at autonomy, which is when the patient can make informed decisions regarding their own body. We then looked at a patient's capacity regarding their intellectual ability to make choices. Next, we looked at the clinician's responsibility to genuinely inform patients of their choices. Finally, we discussed incidences where the patient's choice might conflict with what is best for them or others.

The second part of this chapter deals with decision-making when patients cannot make these determinations for themselves. First, we looked at the various kinds of surrogate decision-makers and their responsibility to the patient. Next, we looked at best interest versus substituted judgment concepts and how both models are potentially flawed. Advance care planning and POLST were discussed, along with the Catholic Church's issues with POLST, to illustrate the potential flaws in this paradigm. The POLST, when used correctly, can be a force to increase patient autonomy. Nevertheless, when misused, considerable threats to patient autonomy are likely. Healthcare professionals must diligently monitor these risks to patient autonomy. Finally, we discussed the difference between secular and Catholic autonomy.

TAKE-HOME POINTS

- Autonomy refers to the right of individuals to make their own decisions regarding medical treatment.
- Informed consent is a process of education—a conversation between a healthcare provider and a patient or their family that helps them to make the best possible decision regarding care.
- Capacity refers to the functional determination of whether an individual patient can adequately make a specific decision, such as a medical decision, or perform a particular task, such as driving.
- The healthcare team most often determines whether a patient has capacity, and psychiatry is usually unnecessary.
- When a patient does not have capacity, another mechanism must be utilized for decision-making regarding healthcare.
- Surrogate decision-making allows another person to make decisions for the patient. Although it would be ideal for this person to be named in writing by the patient, often it is done by "next-of-kin" rules as determined by local jurisdictions.
- Surrogates have the task of making decisions for the patient based on their knowledge of the patient and what the patient would decide to do if they could.
- The best interest standard requires the surrogate(s) to assess the benefits and risks of treatment alternatives, including quality-of-life (QOL) considerations.
- Advance care planning allows patients to make treatment decisions in advance and put them in writing so clinicians can attempt to provide care consistent with their wishes.
- Catholic autonomy involves bringing Catholic teachings and values into the decision-making process.

NOTES

1 Tom L. Beauchamp and James F. Childress, *Principles of Biomedical Ethics*, eighth edition (New York: Oxford University Press, 2019), page 99.

2 Maura Priest, "Autonomy-Centered Healthcare," *HEC Forum : An Interdisciplinary Journal on Hospitals' Ethical and Legal Issues* 30, no. 3 (September 2018): 297–318, https://doi.org/10.1007/s10730-018-9355–6, page 300.

3 Tom L. Beauchamp and James F. Childress, *Principles of Biomedical Ethics*, eighth edition (New York: Oxford University Press, 2019), page 99.

4 Carl Schneider, *The Practice of Autonomy : Patients, Doctors, and Medical Decisions* (Oxford University Press, 1998).

5 Jonathan D. Moreno, "The Triumph of Autonomy in Bioethics and Commercialism in American Healthcare," *Cambridge Quarterly of Healthcare Ethics* 16, no. 4 (October 2007): https://doi.org/10.1017/S096318010707051X, page 417.

6 Tom L. Beauchamp and James F. Childress, *Principles of Biomedical Ethics*, eighth edition (New York: Oxford University Press, 2019), page 99.
7 Serge F. Kovaleski and Joe Coscarelli, "Is Britney Spears Ready to Stand on Her Own?," *New York Times*, May 4, 2016.
8 Voronka, Jijian, "Making Bipolar Britney: Proliferating Psychiatric Diagnoses through Tabloid Media," *Radical Psychology* 7, no. 2 (n.d.): 1–21.
9 Ronan Farrow and Jia Tolentino, "Britney Spears's Conservatorship Nightmare," *The New Yorker*, July 3, 2021, www.newyorker.com/news/american-chronicles/britney-spears-conservatorship-nightmare.
10 Serge F. Kovaleski and Joe Coscarelli, "Is Britney Spears Ready to Stand on Her Own?," *New York Times*, May 4, 2016.
11 Ronan Farrow and Jia Tolentino, "Britney Spears's Conservatorship Nightmare," *The New Yorker*, July 3, 2021, www.newyorker.com/news/american-chronicles/britney-spears-conservatorship-nightmare.
12 Aishvarya Kavi, "A Bipartisan Bill Seeks to 'Free Britney' and Others Who Ask a Judge to Replace Their Guardian or Conservator," *The New York Times*, July 20, 2021.
13 Tom L. Beauchamp and James F. Childress, *Principles of Biomedical Ethics*, eighth edition (New York: Oxford University Press, 2019), page 118.
14 H. Vikas et al., "How Informed Is the Informed Consent?," *Journal of Family Medicine and Primary Care* 10, no. 6 (2021): 2299, https://doi.org/10.4103/jfmpc.jfmpc_2393_20.
15 Maura Priest, "Autonomy-Centered Healthcare," *HEC Forum : An Interdisciplinary Journal on Hospitals' Ethical and Legal Issues* 30, no. 3 (September 2018): 297–318, https://doi.org/10.1007/s10730-018-9355-6, page 300.
16 Maura Priest, "Autonomy-Centered Healthcare," *HEC Forum : An Interdisciplinary Journal on Hospitals' Ethical and Legal Issues* 30, no. 3 (September 2018): 297–318, https://doi.org/10.1007/s10730-018-9355-6, page 301.
17 Tom L. Beauchamp and James F. Childress, *Principles of Biomedical Ethics*, eighth edition (New York: Oxford University Press, 2019), page 122.
18 James Stacey Taylor, "Introduction: Autonomy in Healthcare," *HEC Forum* 30, no. 3 (September 2018): 187–189, https://doi.org/10.1007/s10730-018-9360-9, page 189
19 Tom L. Beauchamp and James F. Childress, *Principles of Biomedical Ethics*, eighth edition (New York: Oxford University Press, 2019), page 120.
20 Basil Varkey, "Principles of Clinical Ethics and Their Application to Practice," *Medical Principles and Practice* 30, no. 1 (February 1, 2021): 17, https://doi.org/10.1159/000509119, page 23
21 H. Vikas et al., "How Informed Is the Informed Consent?," *Journal of Family Medicine and Primary Care* 10, no. 6 (2021): 2299, https://doi.org/10.4103/jfmpc.jfmpc_2393_20.
22 A. P. Schwab, "Formal and Effective Autonomy in Healthcare," *Journal of Medical Ethics* 32, no. 10 (October 1, 2006): 575–579, https://doi.org/10.1136/jme.2005.013391, page 576
23 Tom L. Beauchamp and James F. Childress, *Principles of Biomedical Ethics*, eighth edition (New York: Oxford University Press, 2019), page 112.
24 R. Ryan Darby and Bradford C. Dickerson, "Dementia, Decision Making, and Capacity," *Harvard Review of Psychiatry* 25, no. 6 (November 2017): 270–278, https://doi.org/10.1097/HRP.0000000000000163.
25 Tom L. Beauchamp and James F. Childress, *Principles of Biomedical Ethics*, eighth edition (New York: Oxford University Press, 2019), page 112.
26 Tom L. Beauchamp and James F. Childress, *Principles of Biomedical Ethics*, eighth edition (New York: Oxford University Press, 2019), page 112.
27 R. Ryan Darby and Bradford C. Dickerson, "Dementia, Decision Making, and Capacity," *Harvard Review of Psychiatry* 25, no. 6 (November 2017): 270–278, https://doi.org/10.1097/HRP.0000000000000163.
28 Christine K. Cassel, ed., *Geriatric Medicine: An Evidence-Based Approach*, 4th ed (New York: Springer, 2003), page 1235.

29 R. Ryan Darby and Bradford C. Dickerson, "Dementia, Decision Making, and Capacity," *Harvard Review of Psychiatry* 25, no. 6 (November 2017): 270–278, https://doi.org/10.1097/HRP.0000000000000163.
30 Christine K. Cassel, ed., *Geriatric Medicine: An Evidence-Based Approach*, 4th ed (New York: Springer, 2003), page 1237.
31 R. Ryan Darby and Bradford C. Dickerson, "Dementia, Decision Making, and Capacity," *Harvard Review of Psychiatry* 25, no. 6 (November 2017): 270–278, https://doi.org/10.1097/HRP.0000000000000163.
32 Ryan, C., and Callaghan, S, "Treatment Refusal in Anorexia Nervosa: The Hardest of Cases," *Journal of Bioethical Inquiry* 11, no. 1 (2014): 43–45.
33 Steve Karp, personal communication, July 29, 2021.
34 Mayo Clinic Staff, "Anorexia Nervosa," www.mayoclinic.org/diseases-conditions/anorexia-nervosa/symptoms-causes/syc-20353591.
35 Sam Boyle, "How Should the Law Determine Capacity to Refuse Treatment for Anorexia?," *International Journal of Law and Psychiatry* 64 (May 2019): 250–259, https://doi.org/10.1016/j.ijlp.2019.05.001.
36 L. Haglin, "Hypophosphataemia in Anorexia Nervosa," *Postgraduate Medical Journal* 77, no. 907 (May 1, 2001): 305–311, https://doi.org/10.1136/pmj.77.907.305.
37 Simona Giordano, "Anorexia Nervosa: A Case for Exceptionalism in Ethical Decision Making," *Philosophy, Psychiatry, & Psychology* 26, no. 4 (2019): 315–331, https://doi.org/10.1353/ppp.2019.0047.
38 Kate Cooper et al., "The Phenomenology of Gender Dysphoria in Adults: A Systematic Review and Meta-Synthesis," *Clinical Psychology Review* 80 (August 2020): 101875, https://doi.org/10.1016/j.cpr.2020.101875.
39 Kate Cooper et al., "The Phenomenology of Gender Dysphoria in Adults: A Systematic Review and Meta-Synthesis," *Clinical Psychology Review* 80 (August 2020): 101875, https://doi.org/10.1016/j.cpr.2020.101875.
40 Eric Plemons, "Not Here: Catholic Hospital Systems and the Restriction Against Transgender Healthcare," *CrossCurrents* 68, no. 4 (December 2018): 533–549, https://doi.org/10.1111/cros.12341.
41 Tom L. Beauchamp and James F. Childress, *Principles of Biomedical Ethics*, eighth edition (New York: Oxford University Press, 2019), page 220.
42 Hannah B. Martin and Daryl F. Sas, "Autonomy vs. Selflessness at the End of Life," *Ethics & Medicine: An International Journal of Bioethics* 31, no. 2 (June 22, 2015): 109.
43 Marcia Abramson, "Autonomy vs. Paternalistic Beneficence: Practice Strategies," *Social Casework: The Journal of Contemporary Social Work* 70, no. 2 (February 1, 1989): 101.
44 Beth D. Darnall and Michael E. Schatman, "Autonomy vs Paternalism in the Emergency Department: The Potential Deleterious Impact of Patient Satisfaction Surveys," *Pain Medicine* 14, no. 7 (July 2013): 968.
45 Joshua J. Fenton, "The Cost of Satisfaction: A National Study of Patient Satisfaction, Health Care Utilization, Expenditures, and Mortality," *Archives of Internal Medicine* 172, no. 5 (March 12, 2012), https://doi.org/10.1001/archinternmed.2011.1662, page 409.
46 Abhishek Jain and Paul S. Appelbaum, "Balancing Autonomy and Beneficence at the Time of Psychiatric Discharge," *Israel Journal of Health Policy Research* 7, no. 1 (January 2, 2018), https://doi.org/10.1186/s13584-017-0201-0, page 2.
47 Tom L. Beauchamp and James F. Childress, *Principles of Biomedical Ethics*, eighth edition (New York: Oxford University Press, 2019), page 105; John Stuart Mill, *Utilitarianism*, in vol. 10 of the *Collected Works of John Stuart Mill* (Toronto: University of Toronto Press, 1969), ch. 1, p. 207; ch. 2, pp. 210, 214; ch. 4, pp. 234–35.
48 Hannah B. Martin and Daryl F. Sas, "Autonomy vs. Selflessness at the End of Life," *Ethics & Medicine: An International Journal of Bioethics* 31, no. 2 (June 22, 2015): 109.
49 Hannah B. Martin and Daryl F. Sas, "Autonomy vs. Selflessness at the End of Life," *Ethics & Medicine: An International Journal of Bioethics* 31, no. 2 (June 22, 2015): 109.

50 Michael D. Shear and Noah Weiland, "Biden Calls for Door-to-Door Vaccine Push; Experts Say More Is Needed," *New York Times*, August 2, 2001.
51 Tom L. Beauchamp and James F. Childress, *Principles of Biomedical Ethics*, eighth edition (New York: Oxford University Press, 2019), page 412.
52 Dorit R. Reiss and Arthur L. Caplan, "Considerations in Mandating a New Covid-19 Vaccine in the USA for Children and Adults," *Journal of Law and the Biosciences* 7 (2020): 1–9.
53 Jessica R. MacNeil et al., "Updated Recommendations from the Advisory Committee on Immunization Practices for Use of the Janssen (Johnson & Johnson) COVID-19 Vaccine After Reports of Thrombosis with Thrombocytopenia Syndrome Among Vaccine Recipients—United States, April 2021," *MMWR. Morbidity and Mortality Weekly Report* 70, no. 17 (April 30, 2021): 651–656, https://doi.org/10.15585/mmwr.mm7017e4.
54 Ann Marie Navar et al., "Temporal Associations Between Immunization With the COVID-19 mRNA Vaccines and Myocarditis: The Vaccine Safety Surveillance System Is Working," *JAMA Cardiology*, June 29, 2021, https://doi.org/10.1001/jamacardio.2021.2853.
55 Malik Sallam, "COVID-19 Vaccine Hesitancy Worldwide: A Concise Systematic Review of Vaccine Acceptance Rates," *Vaccines* 9, no. 2 (February 16, 2021): 160, https://doi.org/10.3390/vaccines9020160.
56 Kathryn Buckner, "Would It Be Ethically Problematic to Introduce Mandatory Vaccination for COVID-19?," *Linguistic & Philosophical Investigations*, no. 20 (January 2021): 55–64.
57 Kathryn Buckner, "Would It Be Ethically Problematic to Introduce Mandatory Vaccination for COVID-19?," *Linguistic & Philosophical Investigations*, no. 20 (January 2021): 55–64.
58 Michael D. Shear and Noah Weiland, "Biden Calls for Door-to-Door Vaccine Push; Experts Say More Is Needed," *New York Times*, August 2, 2001.
59 Alain L. Sanders, "Ethics: Whose Right to Die? The Supreme Court Will Finally Wrestle with the Ultimate Question," *Time*, December 11, 1989.
60 Kurt Darr, "After Cruzan, Hospitals and the Right to Die," *Hospital Topics* 69, no. 4 (1991): 4.
61 William H. Colby, "Nancy Cruzan and the Withhold Versus Withdraw Dilemma," *The American Journal of Bioethics: AJOB* 19, no. 3 (March 2019): 1–2, https://doi.org/10.1080/15265161.2019.1580964.
62 William H. Colby, "Nancy Cruzan and the Withhold Versus Withdraw Dilemma," *The American Journal of Bioethics: AJOB* 19, no. 3 (March 2019): 1–2, https://doi.org/10.1080/15265161.2019.1580964.
63 Kenneth W. Goodman, ed., *The Case of Terri Schiavo: Ethics, Politics, and Death in the 21st Century* (Oxford ; New York: Oxford University Press, 2010), page 225.
64 Kenneth W. Goodman, ed., *The Case of Terri Schiavo: Ethics, Politics, and Death in the 21st Century* (Oxford ; New York: Oxford University Press, 2010), page 226.
65 Kurt Darr, "After Cruzan, Hospitals and the Right to Die," *Hospital Topics* 69, no. 4 (1991): 4.
66 Kenneth W. Goodman, ed., *The Case of Terri Schiavo: Ethics, Politics, and Death in the 21st Century* (Oxford ; New York: Oxford University Press, 2010), page 227.
67 Kenneth W. Goodman, ed., *The Case of Terri Schiavo: Ethics, Politics, and Death in the 21st Century* (Oxford ; New York: Oxford University Press, 2010), page 233.
68 Kenneth W. Goodman, ed., *The Case of Terri Schiavo: Ethics, Politics, and Death in the 21st Century* (Oxford ; New York: Oxford University Press, 2010), page 236.
69 Kenneth W. Goodman, ed., *The Case of Terri Schiavo: Ethics, Politics, and Death in the 21st Century* (Oxford ; New York: Oxford University Press, 2010), page 247.
70 Hannah B. Martin and Daryl F. Sas, "Autonomy vs. Selflessness at the End of Life," *Ethics & Medicine: An International Journal of Bioethics* 31, no. 2 (June 22, 2015): 109.
71 E. E. Frezza, D. M. Squillario, and T. J. Smith, "The Ethical Challenge and the Futile Treatment in the Older Population Admitted to the Intensive Care Unit," *American Journal of Medical Quality : The Official Journal of the American College of Medical Quality* 13, no. 3 (1998): 121–126.
72 Krishnaswamy Sundararajan et al., "Posttraumatic Stress Disorder in Close Relatives of Intensive Care Unit Patients' Evaluation (PRICE) Study," *Australian Critical Care* 27, no. 4 (November 1, 2014): 183–187.

73 Rebecca M. Crimmins, Lydia Elliott, and Darren T. Absher, "Palliative Care in a Death-Denying Culture: Exploring Barriers to Timely Palliative Efforts for Heart Failure Patients in the Primary Care Setting," *American Journal of Hospice and Palliative Medicine* 38, no. 1 (January 2021): 77–83, https://doi.org/10.1177/1049909120920545.

74 M. Lowenthal, "Act 169: Pennsylvania's New Advance Directive Law: Implications for Health Care Providers," *Pennsylvania Nurse* 62, no. 4 (December 2007): 22–23.

75 M. Lowenthal, "Act 169: Pennsylvania's New Advance Directive Law: Implications for Health Care Providers," *Pennsylvania Nurse* 62, no. 4 (December 2007): 22–23.

76 Daniel Brudney, "The Different Moral Bases of Patient and Surrogate Decision-Making," *Hastings Center Report* 48, no. 1 (February 1, 2018): 37–41.

77 Micah Y. Baum et al., "Does It Matter Who Decides? Outcomes of Surrogate Decision-Making for Community-Dwelling, Cognitively Impaired Older Adults Near the End of Life," *Journal of Pain and Symptom Management*, January 1, 2021.

78 Rachael Spalding, "Accuracy in Surrogate End-of-Life Medical Decision-Making: A Critical Review," *Applied Psychology: Health and Well-Being* 13, no. 1 (February 1, 2021): 3, https://doi.org/10.1111/aphw.12221.

79 Micah Y. Baum et al., "Does It Matter Who Decides? Outcomes of Surrogate Decision-Making for Community-Dwelling, Cognitively Impaired Older Adults Near the End of Life," *Journal of Pain and Symptom Management*, January 1, 2021.

80 Micah Y. Baum et al., "Does It Matter Who Decides? Outcomes of Surrogate Decision-Making for Community-Dwelling, Cognitively Impaired Older Adults Near the End of Life," *Journal of Pain and Symptom Management*, January 1, 2021.

81 John Phillips and David Wendler, "Clarifying Substituted Judgement: The Endorsed Life Approach: Table 1," *Journal of Medical Ethics* 41, no. 9 (September 2015): 723–730, https://doi.org/10.1136/medethics-2013–101852.

82 Rachael Spalding, "Accuracy in Surrogate End-of-Life Medical Decision-Making: A Critical Review," *Applied Psychology: Health and Well-Being* 13, no. 1 (February 1, 2021): 3, https://doi.org/10.1111/aphw.12221, page 4

83 Naomi Laventhal and Melissa Constantine, "The Harms of a Duty: Misapplication of the Best Interest Standard," *American Journal of Bioethics* 12, no. 4 (2012): 17–19, page 17

84 Tom L. Beauchamp and James F. Childress, *Principles of Biomedical Ethics*, eighth edition (New York: Oxford University Press, 2019), page 141.

85 Daniel P. Sulmasy and Lois Snyder, "Substituted Interests and Best Judgments: An Integrated Model of Surrogate Decision Making," *JAMA* 304, no. 17 (November 3, 2010): 1946, https://doi.org/10.1001/jama.2010.1595.

86 Brudney Daniel, "Choosing for Another: Beyond Autonomy and Best Interests," *The Hastings Center Report* 39, no. 2 (March 1, 2009): 31–37.

87 Daniel P. Sulmasy and Lois Snyder, "Substituted Interests and Best Judgments: An Integrated Model of Surrogate Decision Making," *JAMA* 304, no. 17 (November 3, 2010): 1946, https://doi.org/10.1001/jama.2010.1595.

88 Rebecca L. Sudore, "Redefining the 'Planning' in Advance Care Planning: Preparing for End-of-Life Decision Making," *Annals of Internal Medicine* 153, no. 4 (August 17, 2010): 256, https://doi.org/10.7326/0003–4819-153–4–201008170-00008.

89 Rebecca L. Sudore, "Redefining the 'Planning' in Advance Care Planning: Preparing for End-of-Life Decision Making," *Annals of Internal Medicine* 153, no. 4 (August 17, 2010): 256, https://doi.org/10.7326/0003–4819-153–4–201008170-00008.

90 Rebecca L. Sudore et al., "Defining Advance Care Planning for Adults: A Consensus Definition From a Multidisciplinary Delphi Panel," *Journal of Pain and Symptom Management* 53, no. 5 (May 2017): 821–832.e1, https://doi.org/10.1016/j.jpainsymman.2016.12.331.

91 Daniel P. Sulmasy and Lois Snyder, "Substituted Interests and Best Judgments: An Integrated Model of Surrogate Decision Making," *JAMA* 304, no. 17 (November 3, 2010): 1946, https://doi.org/10.1001/jama.2010.1595.

92 Rebecca L. Sudore, "Redefining the 'Planning' in Advance Care Planning: Preparing for End-of-Life Decision Making," *Annals of Internal Medicine* 153, no. 4 (August 17, 2010): 256, https://doi.org/10.7326/0003-4819-153-4-201008170-00008.
93 Marianna Chaves, "Advance Directives: The Consecration of Autonomy and Dignity of the Human Being," *Medicine and Law* 32, no. 4 (2013): 515–524, page 519.
94 M. Lowenthal, "Act 169: Pennsylvania's New Advance Directive Law: Implications for Health Care Providers," *Pennsylvania Nurse* 62, no. 4 (December 2007): 22–23.
95 M. Lowenthal, "Act 169: Pennsylvania's New Advance Directive Law: Implications for Health Care Providers," *Pennsylvania Nurse* 62, no. 4 (December 2007): 22–23.
96 Thaddeus A. Hoffmeister, "The Growing Importance of Advance Medical Directives," *Military Law Review* 177 (2003): 110–132, page 122.
97 Rebecca L. Sudore, "Redefining the 'Planning' in Advance Care Planning: Preparing for End-of-Life Decision Making," *Annals of Internal Medicine* 153, no. 4 (August 17, 2010): 256, https://doi.org/10.7326/0003-4819-153-4-201008170-00008.
98 Thaddeus A. Hoffmeister, "The Growing Importance of Advance Medical Directives," *Military Law Review* 177 (2003): 110–132, page 117.
99 M. Lowenthal, "Act 169: Pennsylvania's New Advance Directive Law: Implications for Health Care Providers," *Pennsylvania Nurse* 62, no. 4 (December 2007): 22–23, page 22.
100 Donald O. Kollisch, Robert B. Santulli, and James L. Bernat, "The Limits of Advance Directives in Maintaining Autonomy in Patients with Advanced Dementia," *The American Journal of Medicine*, January 1, 2021.
101 Lindy Willmott, "Advance Directives Refusing Treatment as an Expression of Autonomy: Do the Courts Practise What They Preach?," *Common Law World Review* 38, no. 4 (December 2009): 295–341, https://doi.org/10.1350/clwr.2009.38.4.0198, page 40.
102 Judy Thomas and Charles Sabatino, "Patient Preferences, Policy, and POLST," *Generations* 41, no. 1 (2017): 102–109, page 103.
103 In the US, this program goes by different names according to the state, such as Medical Order for Life-Sustaining Treatment (MOLST), Physician Order for Scope of Treatment (POST), Pennsylvania Order For Life-Sustaining Treatment (POLST), etc.
104 Judy Thomas and Charles Sabatino, "Patient Preferences, Policy, and POLST," *Generations* 41, no. 1 (2017): 102–109, page 104.
105 Sebastian Agredo, "POLST," *Voices in Bioethics* 1 (2014).
106 "Advance Medical Directives: Planning for Your Future," *United States Conference of Catholic Bishops*, n.d.
107 Judie Brown, "Lives 'Unworthy of Being Lived' and POLST," *Catholic Lane*, August 2, 2012.
108 Sebastian Agredo, "POLST," *Voices in Bioethics* 1 (2014).
109 Gerald D Coleman and Margaret R McLean, "POLST Supports Care in Context of ERDs," *Health Progress* 93, no. 6 (November 2012): 58–65, Page 62
110 Sebastian Agredo, "POLST," *Voices in Bioethics* 1 (2014).
111 Eric Plemons, "Not Here: Catholic Hospital Systems and the Restriction Against Transgender Healthcare," *CrossCurrents* 68, no. 4 (December 2018): 533–549, https://doi.org/10.1111/cros.12341.
112 Daniel M. Cowdin, "Sterilization, Catholic Health Care, and the Legitimate Autonomy of Culture," *Christian Bioethics* 4, no. 1 (1998): 14–44.
113 Kevin D. O'Rourke, "A Brief History," *Health Progress*, December 2001.
114 Kevin D. O'Rourke, "A Brief History," *Health Progress*, December 2001.
115 Ashley L. Allen, "The Sacredness Of Life In A Culture Of Death," *Southwestern Journal of Theology* 64, no. 2 (2022): 85–97.
116 Richard S. Myers, "Evangelium Vitae and Constitutional Law," *Life and Learning* 30 (2020): 65–87.
117 United States Conference of Catholic Bishops, *Ethical and Religious Directives for Catholic Health Care Services*, sixth edition (Washington, DC: United States Conference of Catholic Bishops, June 2018).

118 Ann Carey, "Texas Hospital Challenges Bishop on Sterilizations," *Our Sunday Visitor*, December 28, 2008.
119 Daniel M. Cowdin, "Sterilization, Catholic Health Care, and the Legitimate Autonomy of Culture," *Christian Bioethics* 4, no. 1 (1998): 14–44.
120 United States Conference of Catholic Bishops, *Ethical and Religious Directives for Catholic Health Care Services*, sixth edition (Washington, DC: United States Conference of Catholic Bishops, June 2018).
121 United States Conference of Catholic Bishops, *Ethical and Religious Directives for Catholic Health Care Services*, sixth edition (Washington, DC: United States Conference of Catholic Bishops, June 2018).

BIBLIOGRAPHY

Abramson, Marcia. "Autonomy versus Paternalistic Beneficence: Practice Strategies." *Social Casework: The Journal of Contemporary Social Work* 70, no. 2 (February 1, 1989): 101.

Agredo, Sebastian. "POLST." *Voices in Bioethics* 1 (2014).

Allen, Ashley L. "The Sacredness Of Life In A Culture Of Death." *Southwestern Journal of Theology* 64, no. 2 (2022): 85–97.

Baum, Micah Y., Joseph J. Gallo, Marie T. Nolan, Kenneth M. Langa, Scott D. Halpern, Mario Macis, and Lauren Hersch Nicholas. "Does It Matter Who Decides? Outcomes of Surrogate Decision-Making for Community-Dwelling, Cognitively Impaired Older Adults Near the End of Life." *Journal of Pain and Symptom Management*, January 1, 2021.

Beauchamp, Tom L., and James F. Childress. *Principles of Biomedical Ethics*. Eighth edition. New York: Oxford University Press, 2019.

Boyle, Sam. "How Should the Law Determine Capacity to Refuse Treatment for Anorexia?" *International Journal of Law and Psychiatry* 64 (May 2019): 250–259. https://doi.org/10.1016/j.ijlp.2019.05.001.

Brown, Judie. "Lives 'Unworthy of Being Lived' and POLST." *Catholic Lane*, August 2, 2012.

Brudney Daniel. "Choosing for Another: Beyond Autonomy and Best Interests." *The Hastings Center Report* 39, no. 2 (March 1, 2009): 31–37.

Brudney, Daniel. "The Different Moral Bases of Patient and Surrogate Decision-Making." *Hastings Center Report* 48, no. 1 (February 1, 2018): 37–41.

Buckner, Kathryn. "Would It Be Ethically Problematic to Introduce Mandatory Vaccination for COVID-19?" *Linguistic & Philosophical Investigations*, no. 20 (January 2021): 55–64.

Carey, Ann. "Texas Hospital Challenges Bishop on Sterilizations," *Our Sunday Visitor*, December 28, 2008.

Cassel, Christine K., ed. *Geriatric Medicine: An Evidence-Based Approach*. 4th edition. New York: Springer, 2003.

Chaves, Marianna. "Advance Directives: The Consecration of Autonomy and Dignity of the Human Being." *Medicine and Law* 32, no. 4 (2013): 515–524.

Colby, William H. "Nancy Cruzan and the Withhold Versus Withdraw Dilemma." *The American Journal of Bioethics: AJOB* 19, no. 3 (March 2019): 1–2. https://doi.org/10.1080/15265161.2019.1580964.

Coleman, Gerald D, and Margaret R McLean. "POLST Supports Care in Context of ERDs." *Health Progress* 93, no. 6 (November 2012): 58–65.

Cooper, Kate, Ailsa Russell, William Mandy, and Catherine Butler. "The Phenomenology of Gender Dysphoria in Adults: A Systematic Review and Meta-Synthesis." *Clinical Psychology Review* 80 (August 2020): 101875. https://doi.org/10.1016/j.cpr.2020.101875.

Cowdin, Daniel M. "Sterilization, Catholic Health Care, and the Legitimate Autonomy of Culture." *Christian Bioethics* 4, no. 1 (1998): 14–44.

Crimmins, Rebecca M., Lydia Elliott, and Darren T. Absher. "Palliative Care in a Death-Denying Culture: Exploring Barriers to Timely Palliative Efforts for Heart Failure Patients in the Primary Care Setting." *American Journal of Hospice and Palliative Medicine* 38, no. 1 (January 2021): 77–83. https://doi.org/10.1177/1049909120920545.

Darby, R. Ryan, and Bradford C. Dickerson. "Dementia, Decision Making, and Capacity." *Harvard Review of Psychiatry* 25, no. 6 (November 2017): 270–278. https://doi.org/10.1097/HRP.0000000000000163.

Darnall, Beth D., and Michael E. Schatman. "Autonomy vs Paternalism in the Emergency Department: The Potential Deleterious Impact of Patient Satisfaction Surveys." *Pain Medicine* 14, no. 7 (July 2013): 968.

Darr, Kurt. "After Cruzan, Hospitals and the Right to Die." *Hospital Topics* 69, no. 4 (1991): 4.

Farrow, Ronan, and Jia Tolentino. "Britney Spears's Conservatorship Nightmare." *The New Yorker*, July 3, 2021, www.newyorker.com/news/american-chronicles/britney-spears-conservatorship-nightmare.

Fenton, Joshua J. "The Cost of Satisfaction: A National Study of Patient Satisfaction, Health Care Utilization, Expenditures, and Mortality." *Archives of Internal Medicine* 172, no. 5 (March 12, 2012): 405. https://doi.org/10.1001/archinternmed.2011.1662.

Frezza, E. E., D. M. Squillario, and T. J. Smith. "The Ethical Challenge and the Futile Treatment in the Older Population Admitted to the Intensive Care Unit." *American Journal of Medical Quality : The Official Journal of the American College of Medical Quality* 13, no. 3 (1998): 121–126.

Giordano, Simona. "Anorexia Nervosa: A Case for Exceptionalism in Ethical Decision Making." *Philosophy, Psychiatry, & Psychology* 26, no. 4 (2019): 315–331. https://doi.org/10.1353/ppp.2019.0047.

Goodman, Kenneth W., ed. *The Case of Terri Schiavo: Ethics, Politics, and Death in the 21st Century*. Oxford: Oxford University Press, 2010.

Haglin, L. "Hypophosphataemia in Anorexia Nervosa." *Postgraduate Medical Journal* 77, no. 907 (May 1, 2001): 305–311. https://doi.org/10.1136/pmj.77.907.305.

Hoffmeister, Thaddeus A. "The Growing Importance of Advance Medical Directives." *Military Law Review* 177 (2003): 110–132.

Jain, Abhishek, and Paul S. Appelbaum. "Balancing Autonomy and Beneficence at the Time of Psychiatric Discharge." *Israel Journal of Health Policy Research* 7, no. 1 (January 2, 2018). https://doi.org/10.1186/s13584-017-0201-0.

Kavi, Aishvarya. "A Bipartisan Bill Seeks to 'Free Britney' and Others Who Ask a Judge to Replace Their Guardian or Conservator." *The New York Times*, July 20, 2021.

Kollisch, Donald O., Robert B. Santulli, and James L. Bernat. "The Limits of Advance Directives in Maintaining Autonomy in Patients with Advanced Dementia." *The American Journal of Medicine*, January 1, 2021.

Kovaleski, Serge F., and Joe Coscarelli. "Is Britney Spears Ready to Stand on Her Own?" *New York Times*, May 4, 2016.

Laventhal, Naomi, and Melissa Constantine. "The Harms of a Duty: Misapplication of the Best Interest Standard." *American Journal of Bioethics* 12, no. 4 (2012): 17–19.

Lowenthal, M. "Act 169: Pennsylvania's New Advance Directive Law: Implications for Health Care Providers." *Pennsylvania Nurse* 62, no. 4 (December 2007): 22–23.

MacNeil, Jessica R., et al. "Updated Recommendations from the Advisory Committee on Immunization Practices for Use of the Janssen (Johnson & Johnson) COVID-19 Vaccine After Reports of Thrombosis with Thrombocytopenia Syndrome Among Vaccine Recipients—United States, April 2021." *MMWR. Morbidity and Mortality Weekly Report* 70, no. 17 (April 30, 2021): 651–656. https://doi.org/10.15585/mmwr.mm7017e4.

Martin, Hannah B., and Daryl F. Sas. "Autonomy vs. Selflessness at the End of Life." *Ethics & Medicine: An International Journal of Bioethics* 31, no. 2 (June 22, 2015): 109.

Moreno, Jonathan D. "The Triumph of Autonomy in Bioethics and Commercialism in American Healthcare." *Cambridge Quarterly of Healthcare Ethics* 16, no. 04 (October 2007): 415. https://doi.org/10.1017/S096318010707051X.

Myers, Richard S. "Evangelium Vitae and Constitutional Law." *Life and Learning* 30 (2020): 65–87. https://search.ebscohost.com/login.aspx?direct=true&AuthType=sso&db=rfh&AN=ATLAi9KZ210208000790&site=eds-live&scope=site&custid=s9004660.

Navar, Ann Marie, Elizabeth McNally, Clyde W. Yancy, Patrick T. O'Gara, and Robert O. Bonow. "Temporal Associations Between Immunization With the COVID-19 mRNA Vaccines and Myocarditis: The Vaccine Safety Surveillance System Is Working." *JAMA Cardiology*, June 29, 2021. https://doi.org/10.1001/jamacardio.2021.2853.

O'Rourke, Kevin D. "A Brief History." *Health Progress*, December 2001.

Phillips, John, and David Wendler. "Clarifying Substituted Judgement: The Endorsed Life Approach: Table 1." *Journal of Medical Ethics* 41, no. 9 (September 2015): 723–730. https://doi.org/10.1136/medethics-2013-101852.

Plemons, Eric. "Not Here: Catholic Hospital Systems and the Restriction Against Transgender Healthcare." *CrossCurrents* 68, no. 4 (December 2018): 533–549. https://doi.org/10.1111/cros.12341.

Priest, Maura. "Autonomy-Centered Healthcare." *HEC Forum : An Interdisciplinary Journal on Hospitals' Ethical and Legal Issues* 30, no. 3 (September 2018): 297–318. https://doi.org/10.1007/s10730-018-9355-6.

Reiss, Dorit R., and Arthur L. Caplan. "Considerations in Mandating a New Covid-19 Vaccine in the USA for Children and Adults." *Journal of Law and the Biosciences* 7 (2020): 1–9.

Ryan, C., & Callaghan, S. "Treatment Refusal in Anorexia Nervosa: The Hardest of Cases." *Journal of Bioethical Inquiry* 11, no. 1 (2014): 43–45.

Sallam, Malik. "COVID-19 Vaccine Hesitancy Worldwide: A Concise Systematic Review of Vaccine Acceptance Rates." *Vaccines* 9, no. 2 (February 16, 2021): 160. https://doi.org/10.3390/vaccines9020160.

Sanders, Alain L. "Ethics: Whose Right to Die? The Supreme Court Will Finally Wrestle with the Ultimate Question." *Time*, December 11, 1989.

Schneider, Carl. *The Practice of Autonomy : Patients, Doctors, and Medical Decisions.* Oxford University Press, 1998.

Schwab, A. P. "Formal and Effective Autonomy in Healthcare." *Journal of Medical Ethics* 32, no. 10 (October 1, 2006): 575–579. https://doi.org/10.1136/jme.2005.013391.

Shear, Michael D and Weiland, Noah. "Biden Calls for Door-to-Door Vaccine Push; Experts Say More Is Needed." *New York Times*, August 2, 2001.

Spalding, Rachael. "Accuracy in Surrogate End-of-Life Medical Decision-Making: A Critical Review." *Applied Psychology: Health and Well-Being* 13, no. 1 (February 1, 2021): 3. https://doi.org/10.1111/aphw.12221.

Sudore, Rebecca L. "Redefining the 'Planning' in Advance Care Planning: Preparing for End-of-Life Decision Making." *Annals of Internal Medicine* 153, no. 4 (August 17, 2010): 256. https://doi.org/10.7326/0003-4819-153-4-201008170-00008.

Sudore, Rebecca L., Hillary D. Lum, John J. You, Laura C. Hanson, Diane E. Meier, Steven Z. Pantilat, Daniel D. Matlock, et al. "Defining Advance Care Planning for Adults: A Consensus Definition From a Multidisciplinary Delphi Panel." *Journal of Pain and Symptom Management* 53, no. 5 (May 2017): 821–832.e1. https://doi.org/10.1016/j.jpainsymman.2016.12.331.

Sulmasy, Daniel P., and Lois Snyder. "Substituted Interests and Best Judgments: An Integrated Model of Surrogate Decision Making." *JAMA* 304, no. 17 (November 3, 2010): 1946. https://doi.org/10.1001/jama.2010.1595.

Sundararajan, Krishnaswamy, Michelle Martin, Srinivas Rajagopala, and Marianne J. Chapman. "Posttraumatic Stress Disorder in Close Relatives of Intensive Care Unit Patients' Evaluation (PRICE) Study." *Australian Critical Care* 27, no. 4 (November 1, 2014): 183–187.

Taylor, James Stacey. "Introduction: Autonomy in Healthcare." *HEC Forum* 30, no. 3 (September 2018): 187–189. https://doi.org/10.1007/s10730-018-9360-9.

Thomas, Judy, and Charles Sabatino. "Patient Preferences, Policy, and POLST." *Generations* 41, no. 1 (2017): 102–109.

United States Conference of Catholic Bishops. *Ethical and Religious Directives for Catholic Health Care Services*. Washington, DC: United States Conference of Catholic Bishops. Sixth Edition. June 2018.

Varkey, Basil. "Principles of Clinical Ethics and Their Application to Practice." *Medical Principles and Practice* 30, no. 1 (February 1, 2021): 17. https://doi.org/10.1159/000509119.

Vikas, H., Ananth Kini, Nishant Sharma, Naveen R. Gowda, and Anant Gupta. "How Informed Is the Informed Consent?" *Journal of Family Medicine and Primary Care* 10, no. 6 (2021): 2299. https://doi.org/10.4103/jfmpc.jfmpc_2393_20.

Voronka, Jijian. "Making Bipolar Britney: Proliferating Psychiatric Diagnoses through Tabloid Media." *Radical Psychology* 7, no. 2 (n.d.): 1–21.

Willmott, Lindy. "Advance Directives Refusing Treatment as an Expression of Autonomy: Do the Courts Practise What They Preach?" *Common Law World Review* 38, no. 4 (December 2009): 295–341. https://doi.org/10.1350/clwr.2009.38.4.0198.

Chapter 2
The Ethical Principle of Beneficence

INTRODUCTION

In this chapter, the principle of beneficence, as stated by Beauchamp and Childress, will be explored. When describing beneficence, the authors state that healthcare providers' activities toward their patients should "contribute to their welfare."[1] The *Merriam-Webster Dictionary* states that beneficence comes from the Latin *beneficus*, which in turn comes from *bene*, meaning *good*, and *facere*, meaning *to do*.[2] Simply put, what is done to the patient by the provider should benefit the patient. Or, as the Dalai Lama said, "It is not enough to be compassionate—you must act."

Working for the patient's benefit is a fundamental ethical value in medical practice. Some have described beneficence as the foundational commitment of medicine, which is that medicine predominantly exists to benefit patients and society.[3] Healthcare companies, therefore, try to emphasize this idea in their marketing. For example, some of the slogans used to promote their organizations seem to define beneficence: "Empowering people to improve their lives," "Keeping you well," "We're here for you," "Get better here," "A better place to get better," "Well-being for life," "Bringing loving care to health care," "Helping people feel better," "Caring people … caring for people," and finally, "Bringing loving care to health care." These concepts tend to define the very purpose or mission of healthcare systems. In the following pages, the perceptions of beneficence will be explored within the confines of healthcare. The first section will define beneficence as an ethical principle and a practical guide for medical decision-making. The second section will look at some controversies dealing with beneficence, especially in the setting of the other ethical principles.

DOI: 10.4324/9781003654124-3

UNDERSTANDING BENEFICENCE

Healthcare is here to do good; that is the easy part. Taking a patient who is ill and helping them become well sounds simple. However, many cases in medicine are not that simple. Often, patients are already chronically ill and become even sicker. Getting them disease-free or well is not an option; many will not survive this new sickness. Then, the tricky part is defining what good is. In these cases, do we do everything possible knowing that, most likely, the treatment will be unsuccessful? Studies have shown that providing ongoing care to patients without the possibility of any meaningful chance for recovery is costly and can be directly detrimental to other patients' care.[4] Also, how do we define success? How clinicians define success may differ from how patients and families define it.[5]

Beneficence Described in Non-principlism Ethical Theories

Beauchamp and Childress use a set of principles that include beneficence as an analytical framework that expresses the general values underlying rules in common morality. Beneficence, however, can be looked at through other ethical theories besides principlism, and in this way, the concept of what is good for the patient can be further examined. This section will examine beneficence through casuistry, deontology, and consequentialism theories. This section is not meant to be an expert analysis of these different philosophies but rather a brief survey of these ideas. It is intended to show how this topic has been debated. The hope is that this will stimulate the reader to contemplate what doing good for a patient means.

The first theory is casuistry, which is the philosophy of resolving moral dilemmas by carefully evaluating the *cases* to which these rules apply. Indeed, the word casuistry comes from the Latin word *casus,* meaning case. Therefore, casuistry interprets and resolves moral problems by focusing on specific cases rather than applying ethical theories and principles.[6] This approach compares a given case with the clearcut paradigmatic case.[7] The critical issue is whether the given case so closely resembles a paradigmatic case that it should be resolved in a similar matter or whether it should be separated and treated differently.

In some cases, the application of ethical realities will be clear-cut. In more complex cases, it might be unclear whether the guidelines apply or whether different guidelines might provide opposing opinions.[8] This theory concludes that no ethical problem is totally unique, and regardless of how novel, it bears some resemblance to more familiar problems. The more typical ones will often be ones for which decisions have been offered and sometimes accepted. Therefore, one compares the new case with the more familiar one. Occasionally, in the more unusual cases, one will recognize that the issues under which the moral discussion proceeds are inadequate because the circumstances have distinctly or even subtly changed. In this opinion, ethical reasoning is primarily reasoning by comparison, seeking to identify cases similar to the one under examination and discern whether the changed situations justify a different judgment in the new case than in the former.[9] The casuistic method offers an in-depth way to learn healthcare bioethics. It teaches how to break an ethical dilemma into its parts and compare them with other cases to determine an appropriate resolution.[10]

The trouble with a casuistry approach to beneficence is that it is sometimes difficult to conclude that the present case is the same as the paradigm case. Based solely on paradigmatic cases, can one assume that one patient's good is good for others? Indeed, it is possible that the given case is not equivalent and raises genuine ethical uncertainty. Moreover, there could be other ethical principles involved. In other words, more than one concern may exist that cannot be resolved based on the comparison with a paradigmatic case. The challenge is to identify, weigh, and balance the demands of the particular case and determine a unique course of action. Whereas studying cases may be a way to help learn about clinical ethics, this method may fall short when resolving specific situations. Cases and their related ethical problems should not be looked at from the position of a moral critic (top-down reasoning) but rather from the perspective of the one facing the problem (bottom-up reasoning).[11] Each situation is unique and must be appreciated for its individual circumstances. Furthermore, deciding what is good for a patient should be precise and deeply personal.

The next approach is the deontological approach. The dictionary definition of *deontology* is the theory or study of moral obligation.[12] The term is derived from the Greek *deon*, meaning "that which is binding, needful, right, proper."[13] Often called deontological (i.e., a theory that some features of actions other than or in addition to consequences make actions right or wrong), this type of theory is now increasingly called Kantian, because the ethical thought of Immanuel Kant (1724–1804) has most deeply shaped its formulations.[14]

Deontology is similar to casuistry in that it is a top-down approach. This theory begins with basic concepts of right and wrong and then examines the case. However, this philosophy is similar to how casuistry tries to link a specific case with a standard paradigmatic one. This theory also tends to be absolute because the rules applied have few exceptions.[15] For example, Kant famously denounced lying, even if it would save someone's life.[16] Lying is wrong and never acceptable in deontological theory, where rules are more important than outcomes.[17]

Kant does believe that beneficence toward those in need is a universal duty of human beings. In Kantian ethics, the duty of beneficence is a categorical imperative that must be universally applicable to all rational beings. Although his theory is based on rules, Kant believed in treating humanity as an end, never merely as a means. Treating humanity as an end is acknowledging the non-comparable worth of every human, regardless of race, religion, or nationality, making one another's equals. When human beings are considered as ends in themselves, they must actively fulfill their needs and potential.[18] Therefore, for Kant, the idea of humanity captures inclusive beneficence: as (in his own words) "a lawgiving reason, which includes the whole species (and so myself as well) in its idea of humanity as such, includes me as giving universal law along with all others in the duty of mutual benevolence, following the principle of equality."[19]

The book that Kant's above quote was taken from is entitled *Practical Philosophy*. Nevertheless, one could question how practical his philosophy is when dealing with actual patients. Moreover, because deontological theory deals with absolutes,[20] its practicality is questionable. Childress states that principles and rules are used through "application and balancing."[21] For example, in Kantian theory, lying, and killing are both considered entirely immoral.

Nevertheless, suppose you are a physician caring for a dying patient who promised to do all you can to keep them comfortable. However, keeping the patient comfortable could include potent analgesic medications that could ultimately kill the patient. Preventing suffering could also involve removing the patient from life support, which would almost certainly result in the patient's death. So, no solution for the physician would be appropriate according to deontological theory. The physician cannot fulfill the promise to make the patient comfortable without actions that could kill the patient. Because moral rules are unconditional for Kant, he seems to say that we are obligated to both actions, which is impossible. The physician would have to accept a system with only one absolute rule, like not lying or giving up absolutes.[22] Following this theory would not allow the physician to treat the patient correctly and would go against the principle of beneficence. Using deontology alone would put rules and obligations over the physician's personal relationship and obligation to the patient.

The final ethical theory to discuss is consequentialism. Compared to casuistry and deontology, the derivation and meaning of this term are more fundamental; the moral value of an action should be determined by the value of its results.[23] This theory proposes that the "ends justify the means." It states that the correct act in any situation is the one that generates the best overall result, as determined from an impersonal perspective that gives equal weight to the interests of each affected party[24] (or parties.) This theory is often divided into egoistic consequentialism and universal consequentialism, sometimes called Utilitarianism. The former states that the act should benefit the individual, whereas the latter proposes that the result should benefit the whole and not just the individual.[25] Compared to casuistry and deontology, consequentialism uses a more bottom-up approach; it looks at the actions and draws conclusions based on the results.[26]

Therefore, the principal consequentialist structure of utilitarianism is that whether an act can be considered virtuous is defined in terms of the good it produces and that rightness depends only on the results of the act itself.[27] On the surface, utilitarianism seems reasonable. For example, who would deny that we should minimize evil in healthcare and increase positive value? The theory is pragmatic in that we all often engage in a utilitarian method of calculating what should be done by balancing goals and resources and considering the needs of everyone affected.[28] For healthcare professionals, outcomes are critical. Most clinicians are familiar with the triple and quadruple aims of healthcare. The triple aim looks at improving the individual care experience, improving populations' health, and reducing the per capita care costs for populations. The quadruple aim adds preventing provider burnout as a goal.[29] Therefore, it is easy to conclude that a theory based on outcomes would be familiar and attractive to healthcare professionals.

However, consequentialism has problems that need to be considered. Some authors feel that it is not an entirely adequate moral theory. They argue that if the action is immoral, the consequences should not matter.[30] For example, looking at the triple aim goals stated above, suppose the action to improve patient experience and decrease cost was to allow patients to have any medication they want without the inconvenience and expense of seeing a clinician. The decline in population health that this would cause could be offset by removing the minority of patients who are very ill and tend to pull down the other two goals as well. But, of course, these actions would be considered absurd, no matter the result of the triple aim goals. Therefore, a dilemma is created if consequentialism is looked at simply as a numbers game.

Nevertheless, other philosophers use consequentialism to apply an approach that considers immediate and easy quantifiable consequences as well as intrinsic and less easily measurable effects.[31] Nonmeasurable items, especially intention, play an essential role in this method. When intentionality plays a vital role in consequentialism, it becomes similar to proportionality. In this concept, any action may result in a bad outcome in some situations, and the choice becomes which outcome is the least harmful. In this sense, it is not what the consequences of the action are alone, but also what was the intention of the act that was done. Hence, this approach is sometimes called intrinsic consequentialism. The term intrinsic is used to determine whether the "human person was adequately considered."[32]

Another way to consider consequentialism in a clinical context is to look at antibiotic stewardship programs (ASP) in nursing homes (NH). Antibiotic use is pervasive in NH settings. Over 70% of NH residents may receive at least one course of antibiotics annually, with 40% to 75% of prescriptions deemed inappropriate or inconsistent with guidelines.[33] Efforts to decrease the improper use of antibiotics have resulted in institutions enacting ASP. The reasons given for this application would be cutting costs, reducing the development of antibiotic-resistant bacterial strains, and preventing antibiotic side effects.[34] The most common justification for antibiotic use in this population is urinary tract infections (UTIs.) However, the error rate in diagnosing UTIs is high. Signs and symptoms can be subtle and may include the absence or reduced intensity of fever or unspecific, such as a sudden change in mental or functional status in this group than in younger people. Older adults also less often show common signs of a UTI, such as frequency and dysuria.[35] There are valid reasons for not treating suspected UTIs in elderly patients without reasonable diagnostic criteria; however, there are also problems with not treating suspected UTIs as well. A study showed a significant increase in the risk of bloodstream infection and all-cause death rate, and hospital admission rate associated with no antibiotics and deferred antibiotics contrasted with immediate antibiotics in the elderly with a diagnosis of UTI. The study suggested that the early initiation of antibiotics for UTIs in older high-risk groups (especially men aged over 85 years) should be proposed to prevent serious complications.[36]

Therefore, whether to treat a suspected UTI in an elderly patient can be problematic from a consequentialist perspective. Should the decision be made because of ASP guidelines or to prevent hospitalizations and deaths in this cohort? Perhaps this question cannot be answered by this approach. Diagnostic excellence in the care of older adults requires awareness of the risks of errors of commission, inappropriate antibiotic use, and the risks of omission, not using an antibiotic. A personalized approach to setting care goals is essential for all patients and older adults. Evaluating older patients with multiple chronic conditions requires a balance of finding a diagnosis while supporting the patient's physical and cognitive function. Personalizing care includes aggressively seeking a diagnosis and treatment if the patient wants to engage in the process and understands the potential risks of the interventions.[37]

So, in conclusion, consequentialism sounds like an appealing way to look at beneficence in that outcomes define it. In contrast to the other two theories discussed, casuistry and deontology, it offers some semblance of logic in that it focuses on results rather than what was done in previous similar cases or the rules. It fails, however, in that it does not consider the act itself or the intention of the act. It also can fail to consider how an action affects an individual in deference to how it affects the whole's greater good.

The Concept of Well-being

> *Medicine should be about healing people and making them happy.*
>
> —Deepak Chopra[38]

This quote gets to the very heart of this section as it looks at the duality of healthcare. There are physical challenges, such as healing the body, and intellectual challenges, such as making people happy. On the surface, The principle of beneficence appears straightforward: do the right thing. However, as the saying goes, "The devil is in the details." In healthcare, the actions taken have to do more than just not hurt the patient; they should strive to provide a positive outcome.[39] Indeed, there would be little argument if it was as simple as curing diseases and making patients well. The debate occurs with defining the right thing and who should define it. Patients and physicians often do not agree with the proposed course of treatment, which can cause moral distress. One study found that a likely reason for concern is feeling like the physician's care plan includes more aggressive life-sustaining treatment than they believe appropriate. The clinician may feel conflicted about whether to honor a surrogate's request for a particular care plan, even when they feel it is inappropriate. Doing what the family or surrogate wants may be an ethically correct approach since guidelines for surrogate decision-making give surrogates the authority to speak for the patient. However, many feel that physicians should protect patients from medically ineffective care, even if a surrogate chooses them. Resolving these conflicting goals can often lead to moral distress.

Nevertheless, other studies have shown that doing just what a patient wants is also problematic. For example, in a study examining emergency department patients, those with higher satisfaction scores had poorer outcomes. The researchers found that higher patient satisfaction results were associated with some adverse consequences, including greater inpatient use, higher overall healthcare and prescription drug expenditures, and increased mortality in a nationally representative sample. When patients see their healthcare clinicians, they often bring a set of requests, and their satisfaction correlates with how well the clinician fulfills patient desires. Patient requests can also affect how the physician prescribes medications for the patient.[40] So often, physicians are put in a position of doing things that, at the very least, are not beneficial to the patient.[41]

Therefore, conflict occurs when physicians try to do what a patient wants (Autonomy) versus what they think is suitable for the patient (Beneficence). Johan Christiaan Bester (director of bioethics for UNLV) has written extensively about well-being. He states that the interests of a patient are not only related to known clinical data about health but also to what the patient thinks is good for them. Acting in a patient's best interests requires considering both elements: those scientifically known to be correct and those associated with the patient's goals, values, and wishes.[42] Therefore, he tries to put this conflict in perspective by stating that beneficence should make patients better off by attempting to advance their interests. Interests are a vital part of well-being, so to say that "clinicians make patients better off (or advance the interests of patients) is the same thing as saying that clinicians advance the well-being of patients."[43]

Consequently, within the well-being theory, the first idea is subjective and is generally referred to as desire-fulfillment (i.e., how well someone is doing is based on the extent to which their desires are fulfilled). What is good for a person is derived from their view of what is good for them. This unique and personal view of the good is derived from a set of values and goals from that person's life. Since interests are a vital component of well-being, interests, therefore, must be determined by the individual in this view.[44] The patient or their surrogates decide what is best for the patient. When a patient's life is examined, how well they do on each item on the list of interests, goals, and desires describes their well-being.[45]

On the contrary, the objective theory formulates different factors that define a patient's well-being. With this theory, none of the decisions are exclusively derived from the person's desires or view of the good. In this view, well-being is an objective construct. Others, especially clinicians, can see someone and determine whether they are doing well or not, are healthy, and are doing well or poorly, independently of what the patient thinks. According to this view, interests are objective and not determined by the person's thoughts.[46]

Not all ethicists agree with Bester's well-being approach to beneficence. Laurence B. McCullough (Distinguished Emeritus Professor Baylor College of Medicine) states that Bester makes two assertions: beneficence-based ethical obligations "work for the patient's good," and that good is explicated as well-being.[47] He then goes on to say that this concept differs from Beauchamp and Childress's textbook, the *Principles of Bioethics*. The authors state, "The principle of beneficence refers to a statement of moral obligation to act for the benefit of others." They then characterize beneficence in healthcare as originating in "a health professional's assumption of obligations through entering a profession and taking on professional obligations."[48] McCullough then points out that no appeal to well-being is made in their account of beneficence's general and specific principles. He then concludes that Bester's proposal to deploy a "hybrid conception of well-being for medical practice" does not succeed because no appeal to well-being is required to understand the meaning and clinical application of the ethical principle of beneficence in bioethics or professional ethics in medicine.[49] This conclusion proposes that the physician has a professional obligation to do what is best for the patient irrespective of the patient's view of the good, which is essential in the well-being concept of Bester. Is that what Beauchamp and Childress are saying?

In a final article on this topic by Norah Jacobson (Department of Psychiatry, University of Toronto) and Diego S. Silva (Centre for Bioethics, University of Toronto) entitled *Dignity Promotion and Beneficence*, the authors challenge this rather one-sided view of beneficence. They introduce the concept of Dignity Promotion. If the primary goal of beneficence is doing good for the patient, then Dignity Promotion complements these processes by addressing how care is provided.[50] This approach addresses well-being, emphasizing that what is good for the individual is derived from the patient's view of the good. The authors also state that this approach is consistent with Beauchamp and Childress's definition of beneficence. The beneficent act always involves a healthcare provider and a patient. Beneficence in a healthcare context is based on relationships, not because the idea of being relational is fundamental to beneficence; you show beneficence to someone, but also because there is no healthcare provider without a patient and no patient without a healthcare provider.[51]

In conclusion, the concept of well-being takes in the duality of beneficence. It involves doing what is physically best for the patient, i.e., diagnosis, treatment, and rehabilitation. It also considers the goals, values, and beliefs of the patient. In healthcare, this is sometimes referred to as the patient-centered model instead of the disease-centered model. This approach involves communication skills needed to understand the patient's perspective. It requires exploring the patient's feelings, ideas, concerns, and experiences regarding the impact of the illness and what the patient expects from the physician.[52] It also involves treating the patient with dignity.

CONCERNS WITH BENEFICENCE

This section will discuss two clinical issues under Beneficence: Paternalism and Futile care. Clinicians are often faced with the problem of patients not agreeing with the proposed course of treatment. As stated in the first section, beneficence does not just mean acting based on clinical grounds alone. Instead, it needs to look at the person and not just as a patient with a disease. Eric Cassell puts it best in his groundbreaking book *The Nature of Suffering*:

> *In the light of the present intense and growing interest in medical ethics, it may be surprising that there is no logical reason why a medicine directed primarily at diseases should also encompass ethical problems. To be concerned with moral problems is to be concerned with persons. Where medicine is focused on diseases, the sick person as person is not central, and consequently, neither are decisions that arise from the moral nature of the person. Indeed, clashes between technological and moral imperatives are currently a commonplace in medical practice. Few guidelines exist for resolving the conflict between the demands of the disease and the other needs of a sick person, which suggests the possibility that something might be considered appropriate treatment even if it were, at the same time, unreasonable or inappropriate in terms of the patient.*[53]

As a palliative care physician, I had a patient who described her visit with her oncologist as similar to taking her daughter to her pediatrician. As her daughter was the focus of the pediatrician, her cancer was the focus of her oncologist—she was only there to provide transportation and pay the bill.

Paternalism

A family arrives by multiple ambulances at your emergency department after their minivan was involved in an accident. The family consists of two parents, an elderly grandmother, a 16-year-old daughter, and an eight-year-old son. All of them have multiple lacerations, blunt force trauma, and internal bleeding. They are all in serious condition and will need surgery. The team attempts to stabilize them and types and crosses them for blood. As they try to get consent filled out for blood transfusions from the adults who are still conscious, you find out that everyone in the family is a Jehovah's Witness. You feel that all five of them will need to be transfused to survive but are told by the father that none of them wants to receive blood. Do you transfuse them anyway because it will save their lives?

Jehovah's Witnesses is a religion that began in the US in the nineteenth century. Followers believe in the infallibility of the Bible and claim to practice the proper form of the Christian faith. Healthcare workers must understand that witnesses refuse any medical treatment involving blood use, such as transfusions, based on multiple Biblical references. Although this directive is not considered absolute, those in violation are asked to leave the church in front of the congregation. This process is called disfellowship and is believed necessary to keep the congregation pure. This ostracization continues until the person has demonstrated that they are worthy of re-entering the church, and could last from a few months to a year.[54]

Jehovah's Witnesses often carry a card, a type of advance directive, stating they do not want to be transfused. Believers feel that even severe anemia can be tolerated and that alternative treatments are available.[55] However, it is unclear if the witness understands the limits that a body can tolerate severe anemia, specifically when other comorbidities exist.[56] This situation presents a problem for the emergency staff, who feel duty-bound to save the lives of this family. For the adult family members who are awake and can answer questions, the emergency team will follow their wishes and keep an open dialog with the patient as their condition progresses. However, the minor children would most likely be transfused despite protests from the parents. Sometimes, a court order is required, and usually, the result is to transfuse when the child's life is at stake.[57] Some cases have made exceptions for "mature teenagers" when the transfusion is for a chronic situation, not an emergency.[58] For adult family members who do not have capacity but have either the "no blood" card or a valid healthcare power of attorney, substituted judgment procedures are followed just as they would be for other life-sustaining treatments. Courts will sometimes, but not always, be sympathetic to healthcare professionals who decide to transfuse the patient in an emergency when there is a question of the validity of the advance directive or the proxy decision maker.[59]

In the above scenario, the moral dilemma of deciding between autonomy and beneficence becomes apparent for the healthcare professional in this unenviable position of caring for multiple Jehovah's Witness patients after an automobile accident. Other clinical situations are also challenging, and clinicians often lament that their patients would do much better if they only listened to them. Of course, they want what is best for their patients, and who better to know what is best than the physician?

In a *Journal of the American Medical Association* article from 1914, the author writes about the "standardization of a surgeon" in towering terms. He states that medicine is "a profession ennobled by men actuated solely by their desire to devote their time and their talents to the relief of suffering humanity, willing, yes, glad at any time if need be to lay down their own lives for those of their fellow men."[60] How could you doubt someone with that kind of enthusiasm? Clinicians can get very upset when they feel patients are not making correct choices, which usually means agreeing with them. Moral distress can occur when a clinician is restrained from acting on deeply held beliefs, compromising their professional integrity. Although it was first noted in the nursing literature, there is evidence that moral distress is a common problem, regardless of the profession, and has damaging effects even for physicians. Traumatic stress disorder, burnout, quitting your job, and depression have all been recognized as the results of this problem.[61]

However, it was not always like this; in the past, patients usually agreed with their physicians and followed their orders. Patient rights began to get national attention by the 1960s, and in 1976, California became the first state to enact natural death legislation. The Natural Death Act allowed patients to refuse treatment even when it went against their physician's demands.[62] This law quickly became popular, and by 1988, many states, including Arizona, Illinois, Kentucky, Maryland, Massachusetts, Michigan, Minnesota, New Hampshire, New York, Pennsylvania, Rhode Island, and Vermont, adopted a patients' bill of rights by regulation or statute.

However, the American Medical Association (AMA) delayed adopting its version of the Patient's Bill of Rights until 1989, primarily because it did not take it seriously. Five of the provisions enacted, including patients' rights to access medical record information and make treatment decisions and the rights to respect, confidentiality, and continuity of care, seem to have been directly taken from the state bills. Finally, in 1990, the Patient Self-Determination Act was passed, allowing patients to choose their treatment, including withholding life-sustaining treatments.[63] Why the AMA took 14 years from the California Natural Death Act to take a stand can most likely be attributed to paternalism.

The *Oxford English Dictionary* defines paternalism as "the principle and practice of paternal administration, government as by a father. The father analogy presumes two features of the paternal role: that the father acts thoughtfully following his idea of the interests of his children and that he makes all or at least some of the decisions relating to his children's welfare rather than letting them make those decisions. Commonly, a father will tell a child; you will do as I say if you know what is good for you. Suppose the child asks why, and the father will answer because I said so. In healthcare relationships, the analogy extends further: The clinician is the expert and is in an authoritative position to determine the patient's best interests. From this perspective, a healthcare professional is like a loving parent with dependent, often ignorant, and fearful children. Paternalism always involves some form of interference with or refusal to conform to another person's preferences regarding their own welfare.[64]

This interference between the patient's preferences and welfare is a cause for concern. Autonomy usually wins out in contemporary Western bioethics when dealing with competent patients. However, beneficence typically wins when dealing with incompetent patients, although autonomy must be considered. The following sections will explore three aspects of paternalism: paternalism regarding competent patients, paternalism regarding incompetent patients with surrogates, and paternalism regarding incompetent patients without surrogates.

One interpretation of paternalistic behavior is the deliberate interference with a patient's freedom of choice, without their consent, to benefit or prevent harm to them.[65] This action can occur when the patient disagrees with the physician. Therefore, medical paternalism occurs when a physician determines that a patient does not understand the necessity of an offered treatment, and the patient declines and then makes the decisions on behalf of the patient. If the patient is genuinely competent, the action is called *hard paternalism*. Moreover, if a patient is considered not fully competent at the time of the encounter, the physician in such a situation may make decisions in the patient's best interest; this is called *soft paternalism*.[66]

What happens if a competent patient refuses possibly lifesaving therapies the physician offers? If a physician finds that a patient's preference conflicts with the physician's beliefs about what is harmful, then the physician might try to persuade the patient to change their mind. The physician might attempt to inform the patient so that he agrees with the proposed treatment, as stated in the film *The Godfather*, and he will "make him an offer he cannot refuse."[67] Sometimes, this coercion by the physician is given the euphemism of nudging. The doctor might use different strategies, from soft nudges to decisions based on hard paternalism. Nudging is used all the time in clinical situations. Often, there is no neutral way of informing patients about their treatment choices. A surgeon may tell a patient they will die without this operation. Patients who do not have preexisting preferences concerning their treatment choices will most likely agree to the recommendations. Therefore, nudging is acceptable, and nudges must be done to promote choices as endorsed by the "best interest standard."[68] Those with preexisting preferences can easily resist nudging and ask for options.[69] Even though the physician often knows and understands more than the patient about medical matters, this does not imply that they always know what is in their best interest. However, after adequate information about the consequences of different treatment options has been acquired to prevent misunderstandings, the physician must respect a competent patient's values and preferences.[70]

Therefore, the goal is to decide based on adequate information given by the physician to a competent patient. This objective is often called shared decision-making. When a shared decision cannot be reached in contemporary medical ethics, respect for patient autonomy is frequently considered the primary principle to follow. At the same time, paternalism is seen as less favorable. Nevertheless, there is sometimes a need for physician-driven decision-making, and it is far more common than many physicians care to admit. Unfortunately, the subtleties of medical decision-making are complex, and standards delineating a balance between patient autonomy and medical paternalism remain undefined. Moreover, the unique nature of patient-specific values and preferences often undermines efforts to generate decision-making guidelines. This variability leaves physicians to interpret situation-dependent conditions without explicit instructions.[71]

Indeed, patient autonomy needs to be respected; nevertheless, autonomy should not be invoked as an excuse for abandoning professional responsibility or justification for unjust, futile use of resources. It is too easy to justify poor decisions by stating that the clinician just did what the patient or family wanted. Physicians need to be both cautious and conscientious regarding paternalistic decision-making. They should be transparent about how decisions are made and promote shared decision-making fervently. However, physicians also need to balance this with the responsibility to ensure the highest standards of ethical practice are enacted and embrace those decisions in patients' best interest to ensure that beneficence is also acknowledged.[72]

For patients who lack competency, the burden of decision-making now requires the involvement of surrogates. Much of what was said about autonomy and paternalism with competent patients must apply to the surrogate. The best interest principle states that a surrogate chooses what will best serve the patient's interests, in other words, maximally promoting the patient's good."[73] The power of a surrogate to predict what their loved one would want in certain situations can be challenging. Several studies have measured the ability of family members to predict patients' choices about their treatment. One published study revealed that surrogates predict ICU patients' treatment preferences with only 68% accuracy. Also, even when the patient designated a surrogate or had a prior surrogate-patient discussion, it often failed to improve the accuracy of the surrogate decision.[74] Besides this uncertainty, the emotional impact on family members is also burdensome. Families are typically very anxious when a loved one is admitted to an ICU. Many family members also report depression, sleep disturbances, and symptoms of post-traumatic stress disorder (not unlike the moral distress that clinicians can sometimes feel with challenging cases).[75] These challenges are accelerated when decisions have to be made, and physicians often need to take a more paternalistic approach while respecting the autonomy of the patient and their families.[76]

The final category is decision-making for incompetent patients with no advance directive or surrogate. These patients are variously termed the "unbefriended," "unrepresented," or "patients without proxies." Their numbers are significant. In 2003, an American Bar Association report estimated that 4% of individuals in nursing homes lacked family to serve as surrogate decision-makers. In 2006, another study found that 16% of incapacitated ICU patients lacked surrogates for seven months, and 5.5% of deaths were incapacitated patients who lacked surrogates.[77] This group of patients is challenging and often requires clinicians to make decisions with little if any, knowledge of the patient's preferences. When no surrogate is identified, healthcare professionals usually find contrasting legal requirements that vary by jurisdiction. In some states, treating clinicians may accept the power to make decisions for their unrepresented patients, but other states expressly forbid this practice.[78] Ideally, a decision-making process for unrepresented patients would include diverse opinions from persons who recognize the regional culture and state laws, such as social workers, attorneys, or chaplains. Additionally, choices should be made free of financial stakes or other personal conflicts.

Unfortunately, this rarely occurs, and one study showed that 81% of critical decisions for hospitalized patients without a surrogate were made by the treating team alone or in consultation with only one other physician, ostensibly disregarding the above recommendations.[79] Beneficence for this cohort requires efforts to prevent paternalism, even if single clinician decision-making is done merely out of necessity. Healthcare policymakers, clinicians, medical institutions, and communities must work to ensure that medical decision-making for this population proceeds ethically and equitably and that all available evidence, including cultural and ethnic factors, is available during deliberations about treatment decisions.[80]

Futile Care

This final section will explore whether futile care can be considered beneficence. Medical futility refers to actions that are unlikely to make the patient well. This definition seems simplistic, but it is often controversial in practice. Physicians should be the guarantors of whether a treatment has a therapeutic advantage. If a treatment does not have a benefit, it should not be offered.[81] However, as stated earlier in this chapter, the beneficent act is relational and always involves at least two people: healthcare providers and patients.[82] Therefore, this problem should be discussed from two approaches: the patient/family or the clinicians advocating for the inappropriate care, although in both incidences, the clinicians are ultimately responsible. The first approach discussed will be when the patient or their family requests medically ineffective treatment.

Many ethicists now frown on the term *futile* and prefer the phrases *potentially inappropriate* or *medically inappropriate* care. The feeling is that the term *futile* is too restrictive and may label an action too harshly. A 2015 article, "An Official ATS/AACN/ACCP/ ESICM/SCCM Policy Statement: Responding to Requests for Potentially Inappropriate Treatments Intensive Care Units,"[83] states:

> *inappropriate conveys more clearly than the word "futile" or "ineffective" that the assertion being made by clinicians depends both on technical, medical expertise and a value-laden claim, rather than strictly a technical judgment. Second, the word "potentially" signals that the judgments are preliminary rather than final.*

Although I understand their concern, this labeling discussion does little to help clinicians decide whether to do a treatment or not! In the same article, the authors try to describe a genuinely futile treatment. They give the example of not doing CPR on a person who has died several hours ago. I must admit that this is the strictest definition I have ever heard, and I am not sure it fully answers the question. Yes, we should not do any medical interventions on a corpse! However, how do they determine if a patient died several hours ago in real time? What about cold water drownings or patients that have suffered a neurological death (i.e., are brain dead)? Even their definition of futile is not clear.

Healthcare providers often provide ineffective or probably futile treatments. Much of the literature documents the frequency and cost of this treatment from the Intensive Care Unit (ICU). The ICU has likely been explicitly studied because of the high cost of providing aggressive and acute care.[84] Nevertheless, other types of treatment can be placed in this category, including cancer treatment.[85] Recently, laws have been passed that permit terminally ill people the right to try and grant terminally ill patients greater access to experimental or not yet fully approved treatments and medications. The Right to Try Act raises concerns that drugs that would become more widely available to terminally ill patients have no proven effectiveness.[86] Questions remain about why physicians allow this and whether this follows beneficence.

Some physicians feel that they are just following the principle of autonomy as long as the discussion between physician and patient is rational, where all relevant facts, preferences, and reasons are discussed. Of note, 28.6% of clinicians in one study would provide a treatment not medically indicated at the patient's request.[87] Other reasons given were a family request for the treatment, fear of litigation and legal consequences, and reluctance to have an end-of-life conversation with the patient.[88] Unfortunately, this reluctance often makes patients poorly informed about their situation and tend to see their prognosis in overly optimistic terms. Another reason for this misunderstanding is that physicians can also overestimate survival and fail to explicitly explain the treatment's prognosis or palliative goal. Therefore, the physician should explain the situation and provide prognostic information and psychological support to enable the patient to understand their situation better.[89] This conversation would allow the patient to make a truly autonomous decision. Regrettably, some physicians admit that doing what the patient wishes is easier than having these discussions.[90]

The situation becomes even more challenging when the patient is not competent, and the decisions have to be made by surrogates. Patients' families often have unrealistic expectations, and treatment decisions often come down to how aggressive the family is and the physician's willingness to deal with that.[91] Family members are often ill-equipped to make end-of-life decisions. Often, they have not had these discussions with their loved ones for fear of upsetting them. These conversations are difficult and too often avoided until it is too late. Families then have the difficult task of dealing with a loved one's severe illness and making difficult choices.[92] Frequently, relatives are emotionally unprepared to make these decisions and choose aggressive care to buy time. Unfortunately, that may lead to another difficult decision to remove life support. Additionally, physicians often prolong aggressive care to avoid conflict, wasting time, effort, and resources.[93] There is also a tendency to avoid these conversations because physicians are concerned about removing hope.[94]

Whether the patient or the family requests treatments deemed medically ineffective, one thing is clear: the need for better communication. Although autonomy, the ability of a competent patient to make decisions regarding their care, is essential, it is also necessary that the decision-makers are fully informed. Therefore, clinicians must address their avoidance of these conversations and seek to improve their communication competencies.[95]

However, families may still request inappropriate treatments even when appropriate discussions occur, especially when children are involved. For example, the Charlie Gard case gained international attention. Charlie was an infant born with a terminal illness and on life support in a British hospital. His family wanted him transported to the United States for a highly experimental treatment (the treatment had never been tested on humans for this condition.).[96] The Charlie Gard case underscored the legal concerns that occur when parents consider subjecting a child without capacity to treatment that the medical community considered futile.[97] Unfortunately, situations will become more common in America with the Right to Try Act passed. Under this new law, clinicians will be asked to give drugs and treatments to terminally ill patients at their request, for which there is no guarantee of regulation or safety. This action will challenge the concept of beneficence.

The above discussion dealt with physicians dealing with patients' and families' requests for treatments deemed medically ineffective and perhaps dangerous. These arguments illustrate the conflict between autonomy and beneficence. However, it is easy to sympathize with patients and families desperately clinging to life. Therefore, clinicians are put in the unenviable position of going against the wishes of these desperate people and feel pressured to go along with treatments that they would not recommend under ordinary circumstances. What is less understood is why physicians still impose futile therapies even when there is no outside pressure to do so.

It is challenging for clinicians to remove life support on a terminally ill patient when the family demands to continue these therapies, even though they are medically ineffective. For example, a child was born in Texas with a fatal congenital condition in 2005. His condition required placing him on life support while the medical team decided his disposition. The clinicians determined that continued ventilator support was futile, although his mother wanted the ventilator support to be continued. However, since no medical facility was willing to accept the transfer of the child, life support was removed, and the child very quickly died.[98] However, there are other cases where there is no patient or familial request to continue futile life support, yet the clinicians are still reluctant to remove it.

Some Asian countries find this reluctance of clinicians to remove life support extremely problematic. In one study, 56.1% of respondents were uncomfortable discussing stopping life-sustaining treatments, and 22.1% did not consider families' or surrogates' requests important. The study also found that 35.6% felt these family requests to remove life support were almost always inappropriate. Unlike the United States, many Asian countries have no established medicolegal system to guide end-of-life care, which likely increases the insecurity of removal of life support.[99] Taiwan should be noted as one of the first Asian countries to create a law that allows for stopping life-sustaining treatment (LST). The Hospice and Palliative Care Act was enacted in 2000 and legalized LST withholding from terminally ill patients per their family's consent.[100]

By contrast, in the United States, medical futility has been emphasized earlier and in more detail than in most other countries. It is agreed that medically ineffective treatments do not need to be administered. Clinicians are not morally, deontologically, or legally obliged to initiate or continue LST. Instead, these treatments should be removed, and palliative care should be undertaken to prevent unnecessary suffering and allow patients dignity at the end of life.[101] Beneficence is the obligation to further the welfare or well-being of others. This principle also includes the responsibility to prevent and remove harm and weigh and balance the action's risks and benefits. Beneficence promotes positive outcomes and avoids unnecessary suffering and other forms of harm.[102] Therefore, there is little justification for a clinician to unilaterally continue futile LST morally, deontologically, or legally, particularly in the United States. This argument also includes non-LST as well.

Medication de-escalation is considered beneficial in dying patients, for example, medications for chronic diseases such as hypertension or diabetes. There should be a reasonable expectation of benefit before starting or continuing a medical intervention in this group. Still, the evidence need not be overwhelming because the iatrogenic burden is usually low, and the intervention can generally be stopped easily.[103] One study looked at statin use (medications that lower cholesterol) among patients with brain metastases receiving whole-brain radiotherapy; 26% of patients were taking a statin at their initial radiation oncology consultation. Most patients (77%) had an expected survival time of four months. Despite their short life expectancy and care from oncologists who presumably knew their prognosis, 19% of patients were still on a statin at their last follow-up visit.[104]

Furthermore, the continuation of fluids, electrolytes, and nutrition should also be considered futile in a dying patient. This topic is controversial and heavily weighted with historical symbolism and decisive religious, societal, and cultural conflicts. The patient's legal right to forgo hydration is of prime importance. Forced hydration is against the autonomy, liberty, and dignity of a competent patient who is unmistakably refusing, and as in other futile treatments, it is against beneficence. Clinicians have a duty to respect and protect this decision and provide adequate care and comfort during the dying process.[105]

In closing, doctors attributed the provision of futile treatment to a wide range of interrelated factors. First, the impact of the patient and family wishes includes demands for further treatment, prognostic uncertainty, and lack of information about patient wishes. Clinicians who have named family or patient requests and are locked into a curative role are the main reasons for futile care. Second was the characteristics of treating doctors, including their orientation towards curative treatment, discomfort or inexperience with death and dying, concerns about legal risk, and poor communication skills leading to avoiding having conversations about removing LST, but even common medications, fluids, and nutrition. For this to change, more education is needed for clinicians regarding beneficence and futile care, especially for dying patients.[106] The disease-centered model so often taught to students fails to address what matters most to patients who vary in their health priorities.[107] For example, giving a statin to prevent cardiovascular events in the future may have little value to someone dying of a brain tumor. However, a patient-centered focus looks to help clinicians be sympathetic to the needs of the people they care for to genuinely provide care consistent with beneficence.[108]

CONCLUSION

Beneficence is doing good for the patient. As Carl Jung put it, "Medicines cure diseases, but only doctors can cure patients."[109] Although this often means treating and curing diseases that may occur in the patient, clinicians must emphasize the patient, not the diseases. This task is much more challenging than just treating the disease, which in itself is already demanding. However, as we have tried to illustrate, this gets to the heart of the meaning. In the first section, beneficence was discussed in the context of Casuistry, Deontology, and Consequentialism. It was found that just past cases, rules, or results cannot adequately define beneficence. Although helpful, these disciplines fail to see the person in the now. Therefore, the concept of well-being was also discussed to offset these ideas.

The second section looked at some common pitfalls clinicians face when trying to act beneficently. For example, with paternalism, the physician means well, just as a father looking after his children. However, this approach fails to allow the patient to help decide what is genuinely right for them. This section also discussed potentially inappropriate treatment care from the patient- or physician-driven perspective. With both these perspectives, clinicians are encouraged to make decisions that are indeed in the patient's best interest. Both clinicians and healthcare systems strive to do what is best for patients, and the goal of this chapter was to widen the understanding of the principle of beneficence.

TAKE-HOME POINTS

- Beneficence states that what is done to the patient by the provider should benefit the patient.
- Defining what is beneficial to patients who are chronically ill can be complex, with no clear answers.
- The ethical theory of casuistry interprets and resolves moral problems by comparing a current case with a paradigmatic one rather than applying ethical theories and principles. It describes what is good for a person based on what has been good for others.

- The deontological approach, also called Kantian (after Immanuel Kant), is based on strict adherence to rules about what is right or wrong.
- A final theory, consequentialism, states that the correct act in any situation is the one that generates the best overall result, as determined from an impersonal perspective that gives equal weight to the interests of each affected party (or parties). The concept of well-being takes in the duality of beneficence. It involves doing what is physically best for the patient and also considering their goals, values, and beliefs.
- Paternalism involves interference with or refusal to conform to another person's preferences regarding their welfare. In theory, it is done to benefit the patient, much like a father would make decisions for his child.
- Patients who lack capacity and have no family or advance directives often depend on the healthcare system to make decisions for them.
- The term potentially inappropriate treatment is preferable to futile care because it shows that the decision is based on technical, medical expertise and a value-laden claim rather than strictly a technical judgment.
- Although most clinicians attest that potentially inappropriate treatments should be avoided, many reasons can be given as to why it occurs.

NOTES

1 Tom L. Beauchamp and James F. Childress, *Principles of Biomedical Ethics*, seventh edition (Oxford: Oxford University Press, 2013), page 217.
2 Merriam-Webster, *Merriam-Webster's Intermediate Dictionary* (Springfield, MA: Merriam-Webster, 2020).
3 Johan Christiaan Bester, "Beneficence, Interests, and Wellbeing in Medicine: What It Means to Provide Benefit to Patients," *The American Journal of Bioethics : AJOB* 20, no. 3 (March 2020): 53–62, https://doi.org/10.1080/15265161.2020.1714793, page 53.
4 Daniel S. Eiferman and Christian Jones, "Of Course, Futile Care Is Wasteful-Are We Ready to Act on This Knowledge?," *Critical Care Medicine* 43, no. 2 (February 2015): e58–e59.
5 Dorothy Rasinski Gregory and Miriam Piven Cotler, "The Problem of Futility: III. The Importance of Physician-Patient Communication and a Suggested Guide through the Minefield," *Cambridge Quarterly of Healthcare Ethics* 3, no. 2 (1994): 257–269, page 257.
6 Albert R. Jonsen, "Casuistry: An Alternative or Complement to Principles?," *Kennedy Institute of Ethics Journal* 5, no. 3 (1995): 237–251, https://doi.org/10.1353/ken.0.0016, page 127.
7 Bernard Lo, *Resolving Ethical Dilemmas: A Guide for Clinicians*, sixth edition (Philadelphia: Wolters Kluwer, 2020), page 15.
8 Bernard Lo, *Resolving Ethical Dilemmas: A Guide for Clinicians*, sixth edition (Philadelphia: Wolters Kluwer, 2020), page 17.
9 Albert R. Jonsen, "Casuistry: An Alternative or Complement to Principles?," *Kennedy Institute of Ethics Journal* 5, no. 3 (1995): 237–251, https://doi.org/10.1353/ken.0.0016, page 245.
10 Bernhard Bleyer, "Casuistry: On a Method of Ethical Judgement in Patient Care," *HEC Forum* 32, no. 3 (September 2020): 211–226, https://doi.org/10.1007/s10730-020-09396-7, page 222.

11 Stephen J. Freeman and Perry C. Francis, "Casuistry: A Complement to Principle Ethics and a Foundation for Ethical Decisions," *Counseling and Values* 50, no. 2 (January 2006): 142–153, page 149.

12 Merriam-Webster, *Merriam-Webster's Intermediate Dictionary* (Springfield, MA: Merriam-Webster, 2020).

13 Horace Gerald Danner, *A Thesaurus of English Word Roots* (Lanham, MD: Rowman & Littlefield Publishers, 2014).

14 David F. Kelly, Gerard Magill, and H. ten Have, *Contemporary Catholic Health Care Ethics*, second edition (Washington, DC: Georgetown University Press, 2013), page 66.

15 David F. Kelly, Gerard Magill, and H. ten Have, *Contemporary Catholic Health Care Ethics*, second edition (Washington, DC: Georgetown University Press, 2013), page 16.

16 Emilian Mihailov, "Measuring Impartial Beneficence: A Kantian Perspective on the Oxford Utilitarianism Scale," *Review of Philosophy and Psychology*, January 7, 2022, 1–16, https://doi.org/10.1007/s13164-021-00600-2, page 13.

17 Tom L. Beauchamp and James F. Childress, *Principles of Biomedical Ethics*, seventh edition (Oxford: Oxford University Press, 2013), page 395.

18 Emilian Mihailov, "Measuring Impartial Beneficence: A Kantian Perspective on the Oxford Utilitarianism Scale," *Review of Philosophy and Psychology*, January 7, 2022, 1–16, https://doi.org/10.1007/s13164-021-00600-2, page 8.

19 Immananuel Kant, *Practical Philosophy*, vol. 6 (Cambridge: Cambridge University Press, 1999), page 451.

20 David F. Kelly, Gerard Magill, and H. ten Have, *Contemporary Catholic Health Care Ethics*, second edition (Washington, DC: Georgetown University Press, 2013), page 62.

21 James F. Childress, *Practical Reasoning in Bioethics*, Medical Ethics Series (Bloomington: Indiana University Press, 1997), page 26.

22 Tom L. Beauchamp and James F. Childress, *Principles of Biomedical Ethics*, seventh edition (Oxford: Oxford University Press, 2013), pages 398–399.

23 Merriam-Webster, *Merriam-Webster's Intermediate Dictionary* (Springfield, MA: Merriam-Webster, 2020).

24 Tom L. Beauchamp and James F. Childress, *Principles of Biomedical Ethics*, seventh edition (Oxford: Oxford University Press, 2013), page 388.

25 David F. Kelly, Gerard Magill, and H. ten Have, *Contemporary Catholic Health Care Ethics*, second edition (Washington, DC: Georgetown University Press, 2013), page 68.

26 David F. Kelly, Gerard Magill, and H. ten Have, *Contemporary Catholic Health Care Ethics*, second edition (Washington, DC: Georgetown University Press, 2013), page 62.

27 Hugh Upton, "Moral Theory and Theorizing in Health Care Ethics," *Ethical Theory and Moral Practice* 14, no. 4 (August 2011): 431–443, https://doi.org/10.1007/s10677-011-9295-6, page 433.

28 Tom L. Beauchamp and James F. Childress, *Principles of Biomedical Ethics*, seventh edition (Oxford: Oxford University Press, 2013), page 389.

29 William Jackson Epperson, Susan Fink Childs, and Gordon Wilhoit, "Provider Burnout and Patient Engagement: the Quadruple and Quintuple Aims," 2016, www.physicianleaders.org/articles/provider-burnout-and-patient-engagement-quadruple-and-quintuple-aims,

30 Tom L. Beauchamp and James F. Childress, *Principles of Biomedical Ethics*, seventh edition (Oxford: Oxford University Press, 2013), page 393.

31 David F. Kelly, Gerard Magill, and H. ten Have, *Contemporary Catholic Health Care Ethics*, second edition (Washington, DC: Georgetown University Press, 2013), page 68.

32 David F. Kelly, Gerard Magill, and H. ten Have, *Contemporary Catholic Health Care Ethics*, second edition (Washington, DC: Georgetown University Press, 2013), page 88.

33 Morgan J. Katz et al., "Implementation of an Antibiotic Stewardship Program in Long-Term Care Facilities Across the US," *JAMA Network Open* 5, no. 2 (February 28, 2022): e220181–e220181, https://doi.org/10.1001/jamanetworkopen.2022.0181, page 1.

34 Morgan J. Katz et al., "Implementation of an Antibiotic Stewardship Program in Long-Term Care Facilities Across the US," *JAMA Network Open* 5, no. 2 (February 28, 2022): e220181–e220181, https://doi.org/10.1001/jamanetworkopen.2022.0181, page 2.

35 Katrien Latour et al., "Nursing Home Residents with Suspected Urinary Tract Infections: A Diagnostic Accuracy Study," *BMC Geriatrics* 22, no. 1 (March 7, 2022), https://doi.org/10.1186/s12877-022-02866-2, page 1.

36 Myriam Gharbi et al., "Antibiotic Management of Urinary Tract Infection in Elderly Patients in Primary Care and Its Association with Bloodstream Infections and All Cause Mortality: Population Based Cohort Study," *BMJ*, February 27, 2019, l525, https://doi.org/10.1136/bmj.l525, page 11.

37 Christine Cassel and Terry Fulmer, "Achieving Diagnostic Excellence for Older Patients," *JAMA* 327, no. 10 (March 8, 2022): 919, https://doi.org/10.1001/jama.2022.1813, page 920.

38 Maya Warrier, "Āyurveda and Mind-Body Healing: Legitimizing Strategies in the Autobiographical Writing of Deepak Chopra," *International Journal of Hindu Studies* 23, no. 2 (August 2019): 123–145, page 135.

39 Tom L. Beauchamp and James F. Childress, *Principles of Biomedical Ethics*, seventh edition (Oxford: Oxford University Press, 2013), page 219.

40 Joshua J. Fenton, "The Cost of Satisfaction: A National Study of Patient Satisfaction, Health Care Utilization, Expenditures, and Mortality," *Archives of Internal Medicine* 172, no. 5 (March 12, 2012): 405, https://doi.org/10.1001/archinternmed.2011.1662, pages 407–408.

41 Dorothy Rasinski Gregory and Miriam Piven Cotler, "The Problem of Futility: III. The Importance of Physician-Patient Communication and a Suggested Guide through the Minefield," *Cambridge Quarterly of Healthcare Ethics* 3, no. 2 (1994): 257–269.

42 Johan Christiaan Bester, "The Two Components of Beneficence and Wellbeing in Medicine: A Restatement and Defense of the Argument," *American Journal of Bioethics* 20, no. 5 (June 2020): W4–W11, https://doi.org/10.1080/15265161.2020.1745947.

43 Johan Christiaan Bester, "The Two Components of Beneficence and Wellbeing in Medicine: A Restatement and Defense of the Argument," *American Journal of Bioethics* 20, no. 5 (June 2020): W4–W11, https://doi.org/10.1080/15265161.2020.1745947.

44 Johan Christiaan Bester, "The Two Components of Beneficence and Wellbeing in Medicine: A Restatement and Defense of the Argument," *American Journal of Bioethics* 20, no. 5 (June 2020): W4–W11, https://doi.org/10.1080/15265161.2020.1745947.

45 Johan Christiaan Bester, "Beneficence, Interests, and Wellbeing in Medicine: What It Means to Provide Benefit to Patients," *The American Journal of Bioethics : AJOB* 20, no. 3 (March 2020): 53–62, https://doi.org/10.1080/15265161.2020.1714793.

46 Johan Christiaan Bester, "Beneficence, Interests, and Wellbeing in Medicine: What It Means to Provide Benefit to Patients," *The American Journal of Bioethics : AJOB* 20, no. 3 (March 2020): 53–62, https://doi.org/10.1080/15265161.2020.1714793, page 54.

47 Laurence B. McCullough, "Beneficence and Wellbeing: A Critical Appraisal," *The American Journal of Bioethics : AJOB* 20, no. 3 (March 2020): 65–68, https://doi.org/10.1080/15265161.2020.1714817, page 66.

48 Tom L. Beauchamp and James F. Childress, *Principles of Biomedical Ethics*, seventh edition (Oxford: Oxford University Press, 2013), page 220.

49 Laurence B. McCullough, "Beneficence and Wellbeing: A Critical Appraisal," *The American Journal of Bioethics : AJOB* 20, no. 3 (March 2020): 65–68, https://doi.org/10.1080/15265161.2020.1714817, pages 65–67.

50 Nora Jacobson and Diego S. Silva, "Dignity Promotion and Beneficence," *Journal of Bioethical Inquiry* 7, no. 4 (December 2010): 365–372, https://doi.org/10.1007/s11673-010-9258-y, page 370.

51 Nora Jacobson and Diego S. Silva, "Dignity Promotion and Beneficence," *Journal of Bioethical Inquiry* 7, no. 4 (December 2010): 365–372, https://doi.org/10.1007/s11673-010-9258-y, pages 365–373.

52 M. Jawad Hashim, "Patient-Centered Communication: Basic Skills," *American Family Physician* 95, no. 1 (January 1, 2017): 29–34, page 29.
53 Eric J. Cassell, *The Nature of Suffering: And the Goals of Medicine* (Oxford: Oxford University Press, 1991), page 132.
54 Pernilla Liedgren, "Minorities with Different Values at School—the Case of Jehovah's Witnesses," *British Journal of Religious Education* 40, no. 1 (January 2, 2018): 31–43, https://doi.org/10.1080/01416200.2016.1150253.
55 Douglas R. Migden and G. Richard Braen, "The Jehovah's Witness Blood Refusal Card: Ethical and Medicolegal Considerations for Emergency Physicians," *Academic Emergency Medicine* 5, no. 8 (August 1998): 815–824, https://doi.org/10.1111/j.1553-2712.1998.tb02510.x.
56 Jan Domaradzki, Katarzyna Głodowska, and Piotr Jabkowski, "Between Autonomy and Paternalism: Attitudes of Nursing Personnel Towards Jehovah's Witnesses' Refusal of Blood Transfusion," *International Journal of Public Health* 68 (August 3, 2023): 1606291, https://doi.org/10.3389/ijph.2023.1606291.
57 James M. West, "Ethical Issues in the Care of Jehovah's Witnesses," *Current Opinion in Anaesthesiology* 27, no. 2 (April 2014): 170–176, https://doi.org/10.1097/ACO.0000000000000053.
58 Caroline Bridge, "Religious Beliefs and Teenage Refusal of Medical Treatment," *The Modern Law Review* 62, no. 4 (July 1, 1999): 585–594, https://search.ebscohost.com/login.aspx?direct=true&AuthType=sso&db=edsjsr&AN=edsjsr.1097111&site=eds-live&scope=site&custid=s9004660.
59 James M. West, "Ethical Issues in the Care of Jehovah's Witnesses," *Current Opinion in Anaesthesiology* 27, no. 2 (April 2014): 170–176, https://doi.org/10.1097/ACO.0000000000000053.
60 J. M. T. Finney, "The standardization of the Surgeon," *JAMA* 63, no. 17 (1914).
61 Lucia D. Wocial et al., "Factors Associated with Physician Moral Distress Caring for Hospitalized Elderly Patients Needing a Surrogate Decision-Maker: A Prospective Study," *Journal of General Internal Medicine* 35, no. 5 (May 2020): 1405–1412, https://doi.org/10.1007/s11606-020-05652-1, page 1405.
62 Diane Lynn Redleaf, Suzanne Baillie Schmitt, and William Charles Thompson, "The California Natural Death Act: An Empirical Study of Physicians' Practices," *Stanford Law Review* 31, no. 5 (May 1979): 913–945, page 918.
63 E. H. Bradley and J. A. Rizzo, "Public Information and Private Search: Evaluating the Patient Self-Determination Act," *Journal of Health Politics, Policy and Law* 24, no. 2 (April 1999): 239–273, https://doi.org/10.1215/03616878-24-2-239, page 242.
64 Tom L. Beauchamp and James F. Childress, *Principles of Biomedical Ethics*, seventh edition (Oxford: Oxford University Press, 2013), page 228.
65 Shlomo Cohen, "The Logic of the Interaction between Beneficence and Respect for Autonomy," *Medicine, Health Care, and Philosophy* 22, no. 2 (June 2019): 297–304, https://doi.org/10.1007/s11019-018-9876-4, page 299.
66 Niels Lynøe, Ingemar Engström, and Niklas Juth, "How to Reveal Disguised Paternalism: Version 2.0," *BMC Medical Ethics* 22, no. 1 (December 1, 2021), https://doi.org/10.1186/s12910-021-00739-8, page 2.
67 Niels Lynøe, Ingemar Engström, and Niklas Juth, "How to Reveal Disguised Paternalism: Version 2.0," *BMC Medical Ethics* 22, no. 1 (December 1, 2021), https://doi.org/10.1186/s12910-021-00739-8, page 1.
68 Søren Holm, "Authenticity, Best Interest, and Clinical Nudging," *Hastings Center Report* 47, no. 2 (April 3, 2017): 38–40, page 39.
69 Søren Holm, "Authenticity, Best Interest, and Clinical Nudging," *Hastings Center Report* 47, no. 2 (April 3, 2017): 38–40, page 38.
70 Niels Lynøe, Ingemar Engström, and Niklas Juth, "How to Reveal Disguised Paternalism: Version 2.0," *BMC Medical Ethics* 22, no. 1 (December 1, 2021), https://doi.org/10.1186/s12910-021-00739-8, page 2.

71 Brian C. Drolet and Candace L White, "Selective Paternalism," *The Virtual Mentor* 14, no. 7 (July 1, 2012): 582–588, https://doi.org/10.1001/virtualmentor.2012.14.7.oped2–1207, page 583.
72 Brian C. Drolet and Candace L White, "Selective Paternalism," *The Virtual Mentor* 14, no. 7 (July 1, 2012): 582–588, https://doi.org/10.1001/virtualmentor.2012.14.7.oped2–1207, page 586.
73 Søren Holm, "Authenticity, Best Interest, and Clinical Nudging," *Hastings Center Report* 47, no. 2 (April 3, 2017): 38–40, page 39.
74 Jessica Bryant et al., "The Accuracy of Surrogate Decision Makers: Informed Consent in Hypothetical Acute Stroke Scenarios," *BMC Emergency Medicine* 13 (November 13, 2013): 18, https://doi.org/10.1186/1471-227X-13–18, page 1.
75 M. Hoffmann et al., "Psychological Symptoms in Relatives of Critically Ill Patients (ICU Families): A Prospective Multicenter Study," *Intensive Care Medicine* 46, no. 5 (May 2020): 1060–1062, https://doi.org/10.1007/s00134-020-05997-5, page 1060.
76 Brian C. Drolet and Candace L White, "Selective Paternalism," *The Virtual Mentor* 14, no. 7 (July 1, 2012): 582–588, https://doi.org/10.1001/virtualmentor.2012.14.7.oped2–1207, page 584.
77 Cynthia Griggins et al., "Making Medical Decisions for Incapacitated Patients Without Proxies: Part I," *HEC Forum: HealthCare Ethics Committee Forum: An Interprofessional Journal on Healthcare Institutions' Ethical and Legal Issues* 32, no. 1 (March 1, 2020): 33–45, https://doi.org/10.1007/s10730-019-09387-3, page 34.
78 Erin S. DeMartino, Cavan K. Doyle, David M. Dudzinski, Beau P. Sperry, Mark Siegler, Daniel B. Kramer, Paul S. Mueller, Daniel P. Sulmasy, "Legal Aspects of the Physician's Role in Caring for Incapacitated Patients: A Review of US State Statutes," *American Journal of Critical Care Medicine* 195 (2017).
79 Timothy M. Dempsey and Erin Sullivan DeMartino, "How Should Clinicians Navigate Decision Making for Unrepresented Patients?," *AMA Journal of Ethics* 21, no. 7 (July 2019): 559–565.
80 Timothy W. Farrell et al., "AGS Position Statement: Making Medical Treatment Decisions for Unbefriended Older Adults," *Journal of the American Geriatrics Society* 65, no. 1 (2017), page 15.
81 David F. Kelly, Gerard Magill, and H. ten Have, *Contemporary Catholic Health Care Ethics*, second edition (Washington, DC: Georgetown University Press, 2013).
82 Nora Jacobson and Diego S. Silva, "Dignity Promotion and Beneficence," *Journal of Bioethical Inquiry* 7, no. 4 (December 2010): 365–372, https://doi.org/10.1007/s11673-010-9258-y, pages 365–373.
83 Gabriel T. Bosslet et al., "An Official ATS/AACN/ACCP/ESICM/SCCM Policy Statement: Responding to Requests for Potentially Inappropriate Treatments in Intensive Care Units," *American Journal of Respiratory and Critical Care Medicine* 191, no. 11 (June 1, 2015): 1318–1330, https://doi.org/10.1164/rccm.201505-0924ST.
84 Joshua T. Landry, "Is Shared Decision-making to Blame for the Provision of Ethically Inappropriate Treatment? Results of a Multi-site Study Exploring Physician Understanding of the 'Shared' Model of Decision Making," *Journal of Evaluation in Clinical Practice* 27, no. 4 (August 2021): 826–835, page 827.
85 Zoe Keon-Cohen, Paul Farquhar-Smith, and Timothy Wigmore, "Ethical Challenges in Caring for Cancer Patients in the Intensive Care Unit: Advanced Care Pathways and Avoidance of Futility," *Current Anesthesiology Reports* 5, no. 3 (September 2015): 354–360, https://doi.org/10.1007/s40140-015-0116–7, page 354.
86 K. Hansen, "Futile Care, Experimental Treatments, and the Right to Try Movement: Could the Charlie Gard Case Happen in America?," *Suffolk University Law Review* 52, no. 1 (2019): 87–108, page 98.
87 Joshua T. Landry, "Is Shared Decision-making to Blame for the Provision of Ethically Inappropriate Treatment? Results of a Multi-site Study Exploring Physician Understanding of

the 'Shared' Model of Decision Making," *Journal of Evaluation in Clinical Practice* 27, no. 4 (August 2021): 826–835, page 834.

88 Lindy Willmott et al., "Reasons Doctors Provide Futile Treatment at the End of Life: A Qualitative Study," *Journal of Medical Ethics* 42, no. 8 (August 1, 2016): 496, https://doi.org/10.1136/medethics-2016–103370, page 498.

89 Eva C. Winkler, Wolfgang Hiddemann, and Georg Marckmann, "Evaluating a Patient's Request for Life-Prolonging Treatment: An Ethical Framework," *Journal of Medical Ethics* 38, no. 11 (November 2012): 647–651, https://doi.org/10.1136/medethics-2011–100333, page 649.

90 Amalie M. Hauge, "One Last Round of Chemo? Insights from Conversations between Oncologists and Lung Cancer Patients about Prognosis and Treatment Decisions," *Social Science & Medicine* 266 (December 1, 2020).

91 Lindy Willmott et al., "Reasons Doctors Provide Futile Treatment at the End of Life: A Qualitative Study," *Journal of Medical Ethics* 42, no. 8 (August 1, 2016): 496, https://doi.org/10.1136/medethics-2016–103370, page 498.

92 Dragana Bolcic-Jankovic et al., "Exploring Determinants of Surrogate Decision-Maker Confidence : An Example From the ICU," *Journal of Empirical Research on Human Research Ethics: An International Journal* 9, no. 4 (2014): 76.

93 Erwin J. O. Kompanje, Ruth D. Piers, and Dominique D. Benoit, "Causes and Consequences of Disproportionate Care in Intensive Care Medicine," *Current Opinion in Critical Care* 19, no. 6 (December 2013): 630–635, https://doi.org/10.1097/MCC.0000000000000026.

94 Carmen P. Escalante et al., "Medical Futility and Appropriate Medical Care in Patients Whose Death Is Thought to Be Imminent," *Support Care Cancer* 5 (1997): 274–280, page 276.

95 Lindy Willmott et al., "Reasons Doctors Provide Futile Treatment at the End of Life: A Qualitative Study," *Journal of Medical Ethics* 42, no. 8 (August 1, 2016): 496, https://doi.org/10.1136/medethics-2016–103370.

96 Kaitlyn Hansen, "Futile Care, Experimental Treatments, and the Right to Try Movement: Could the Charlie Gard Case Happen in America?," *Suffolk University Law Review* 52, no. 1 (January 1, 2019), page 88

97 Kaitlyn Hansen, "Futile Care, Experimental Treatments, and the Right to Try Movement: Could the Charlie Gard Case Happen in America?," *Suffolk University Law Review* 52, no. 1 (January 1, 2019), page 99.

98 Matthew H. Armstrong, Joseph K. Poku, and Christopher M. Burkle, "Medical Futility and Nonbeneficial Interventions: An Algorithm to Aid Clinicians," *Mayo Clinic Proceedings* 89, no. 12 (December 1, 2014): 1599, https://doi.org/10.1016/j.mayocp.2014.08.017, page 1602.

99 Jason Phua et al., "Withholding and Withdrawal of Life-Sustaining Treatments in Intensive Care Units in Asia," *JAMA Internal Medicine* 175, no. 3 (March 1, 2015): 363, https://doi.org/10.1001/jamainternmed.2014.7386, page 369.

100 Miho Tanaka et al., "Forgoing Life-Sustaining Treatment—a Comparative Analysis of Regulations in Japan, Korea, Taiwan, and England," *BMC Medical Ethics* 21, no. 1 (December 2020): 99, https://doi.org/10.1186/s12910-020-00535-w.

101 Patrizia Borsellino, "Limitation of the Therapeutic Effort: Ethical and Legal Justification for Withholding and/or Withdrawing Life Sustaining Treatments," *Multidisciplinary Respiratory Medicine* 10, no. 1 (December 2015): 5, https://doi.org/10.1186/s40248-015-0001–8, page 4.

102 C. P. Escalante et al., "Medical Futility and Appropriate Medical Care in Patients Whose Death Is Thought to Be Imminent," *Supportive Care in Cancer* 5, no. 4 (July 1997): 274–280, page 275.

103 Jill A. Rhymes, "Withdrawing Very Low-Burden Interventions in Chronically Ill Patients," *JAMA* 283, no. 8 (February 23, 2000): 1061, https://doi.org/10.1001/jama.283.8.1061, page 1062.

104 Jacqueline A. Mullvain et al., "Statin Use in Cancer Patients with Brain Metastases: A Missed Communication Opportunity at the End of Life," *Supportive Care in Cancer* 23, no. 9 (September 2015): 2643–2648, https://doi.org/10.1007/s00520-015-2624-x, page 2644.

105 Joan L. Huffman and Geoffrey P. Dunn, "The Paradox of Hydration in Advanced Terminal Illness," *Journal of the American College of Surgeons* 194, no. 6 (June 2002): 835–839, https://doi.org/10.1016/S1072-7515(02)01152-3, page 838.

106 Lindy Willmott et al., "Reasons Doctors Provide Futile Treatment at the End of Life: A Qualitative Study," *Journal of Medical Ethics* 42, no. 8 (August 1, 2016): 496, https://doi.org/10.1136/medethics-2016-103370, pages 496–503.

107 Mary E. Tinetti, Aanand D. Naik, and John A. Dodson, "Moving From Disease-Centered to Patient Goals: Directed Care for Patients With Multiple Chronic Conditions: Patient Value-Based Care," *JAMA Cardiology* 1, no. 1 (April 1, 2016): 9, https://doi.org/10.1001/jamacardio.2015.0248.

108 Jasmine Hearn et al., "Patient-Centered Medical Education: A Proposed Definition," *Medical Teacher* 41, no. 8 (August 2019): 934–938.

109 Paul Bishop, *Carl Jung*, Critical Lives (Reaktion Books, 2014).

BIBLIOGRAPHY

Armstrong, Matthew H., Joseph K. Poku, and Christopher M. Burkle. "Medical Futility and Non-beneficial Interventions: An Algorithm to Aid Clinicians." *Mayo Clinic Proceedings* 89, no. 12 (December 1, 2014): 1599. https://doi.org/10.1016/j.mayocp.2014.08.017.

Beauchamp, Tom L., and James F. Childress. *Principles of Biomedical Ethics.* Seventh edition. Oxford: Oxford University Press, 2013.

Bester, Johan Christiaan. "Beneficence, Interests, and Wellbeing in Medicine: What It Means to Provide Benefit to Patients." *The American Journal of Bioethics : AJOB* 20, no. 3 (March 2020): 53–62. https://doi.org/10.1080/15265161.2020.1714793.

Bester, Johan Christiaan. "The Two Components of Beneficence and Wellbeing in Medicine: A Restatement and Defense of the Argument." *American Journal of Bioethics* 20, no. 5 (June 2020): W4–W11. https://doi.org/10.1080/15265161.2020.1745947.

Bishop, Paul. *Carl Jung.* Reaktion Books, 2014.

Bleyer, Bernhard. "Casuistry: On a Method of Ethical Judgement in Patient Care." *HEC Forum* 32, no. 3 (September 2020): 211–226. https://doi.org/10.1007/s10730-020-09396-7.

Bolcic-Jankovic Dragana, Brian R. Clarridge, Jessica L. LeBlanc, Rumel S. Mahmood, Anthony M. Roman, and Bradley D. Freeman. "Exploring Determinants of Surrogate Decision Maker Confidence : An Example From the ICU." *Journal of Empirical Research on Human Research Ethics: An International Journal* 9, no. 4 (2014): 76.

Borsellino, Patrizia. "Limitation of the Therapeutic Effort: Ethical and Legal Justification for Withholding and/or Withdrawing Life Sustaining Treatments." *Multidisciplinary Respiratory Medicine* 10, no. 1 (December 2015): 5. https://doi.org/10.1186/s40248-015-0001-8.

Bosslet, Gabriel T., Thaddeus M. Pope, Gordon D. Rubenfeld, Bernard Lo, Robert D. Truog, Cynda H. Rushton, J. Randall Curtis, et al. "An Official ATS/AACN/ACCP/ESICM/SCCM Policy Statement: Responding to Requests for Potentially Inappropriate Treatments in Intensive Care Units." *American Journal of Respiratory and Critical Care Medicine* 191, no. 11 (June 1, 2015): 1318–1330. https://doi.org/10.1164/rccm.201505-0924ST.

Bradley, E H, and J A Rizzo. "Public Information and Private Search: Evaluating the Patient Self-Determination Act." *Journal of Health Politics, Policy and Law* 24, no. 2 (April 1999): 239–273. https://doi.org/10.1215/03616878-24-2-239.

Bridge, Caroline. "Religious Beliefs and Teenage Refusal of Medical Treatment." *The Modern Law Review* 62, no. 4 (July 1, 1999): 585–594.

Bryant, Jessica, Lesli E Skolarus, Barbara Smith, Eric E Adelman, and William J Meurer. "The Accuracy of Surrogate Decision Makers: Informed Consent in Hypothetical Acute Stroke Scenarios." *BMC Emergency Medicine* 13 (November 13, 2013): 18. https://doi.org/10.1186/1471-227X-13-18.

Cassel, Christine, and Terry Fulmer. "Achieving Diagnostic Excellence for Older Patients." *JAMA* 327, no. 10 (March 8, 2022): 919. https://doi.org/10.1001/jama.2022.1813.

Cassell, Eric J. *The Nature of Suffering: And the Goals of Medicine.* Oxford: Oxford University Press, 1991.

Childress, James F. *Practical Reasoning in Bioethics*. Medical Ethics Series. Bloomington: Indiana University Press, 1997.

Cohen, Shlomo. "The Logic of the Interaction between Beneficence and Respect for Autonomy." *Medicine, Health Care, and Philosophy* 22, no. 2 (June 2019): 297–304. https://doi.org/10.1007/s11019-018-9876-4.

Danner, Horace Gerald. *A Thesaurus of English Word Roots*. Lanham, MD: Rowman & Littlefield Publishers, 2014.

DeMartino, Erin S., Cavan K. Doyle, David M. Dudzinski, Beau P. Sperry, Mark Siegler, Daniel B. Kramer, Paul S. Mueller, Daniel P. Sulmasy. "Legal Aspects of the Physician's Role in Caring for Incapacitated Patients: A Review of US State Statutes." *American Journal of Critical Care Medicine* 195 (2017).

Dempsey, Timothy M., and Erin Sullivan DeMartino. "How Should Clinicians Navigate Decision Making for Unrepresented Patients?" *AMA Journal of Ethics* 21, no. 7 (July 2019): 559–565.

Domaradzki, Jan, Katarzyna Głodowska, and Piotr Jabkowski. "Between Autonomy and Paternalism: Attitudes of Nursing Personnel Towards Jehovah's Witnesses' Refusal of Blood Transfusion." *International Journal of Public Health* 68 (August 3, 2023): 1606291. https://doi.org/10.3389/ijph.2023.1606291.

Drolet, Brian C, and Candace L White. "Selective Paternalism." *The Virtual Mentor : VM* 14, no. 7 (July 1, 2012): 582–588. https://doi.org/10.1001/virtualmentor.2012.14.7.oped2-1207.

Eiferman, Daniel S., and Christian Jones. "Of Course, Futile Care Is Wasteful-Are We Ready to Act on This Knowledge?" *Critical Care Medicine* 43, no. 2 (February 2015): e58–e59.

Escalante, C. P., Charles G. Martin, Linda S. Elting, Edward B. Rubenstein, C G Martin, L S Elting, and E B Rubenstein. "Medical Futility and Appropriate Medical Care in Patients Whose Death Is Thought to Be Imminent." *Supportive Care in Cancer* 5, no. 4 (July 1997): 274–280.

Farrell, Timothy W., et al. "AGS Position Statement: Making Medical Treatment Decisions for Unbefriended Older Adults." *Journal of the American Geriatrics Society* 65, no. 1 (2017).

Fenton, Joshua J. "The Cost of Satisfaction: A National Study of Patient Satisfaction, Health Care Utilization, Expenditures, and Mortality." *Archives of Internal Medicine* 172, no. 5 (March 12, 2012): 405. https://doi.org/10.1001/archinternmed.2011.1662.

Freeman, Stephen J; Francis, Perry C. "Casuistry: A Complement to Principle Ethics and a Foundation for Ethical Decisions." *Counseling and Values* 50, no. 2 (January 2006): 142–153.

Gharbi, Myriam, Joseph H Drysdale, Hannah Lishman, Rosalind Goudie, Mariam Molokhia, Alan P Johnson, Alison H Holmes, and Paul Aylin. "Antibiotic Management of Urinary Tract Infection in Elderly Patients in Primary Care and Its Association with Bloodstream Infections and All Cause Mortality: Population Based Cohort Study." *BMJ*, February 27, 2019, 1525. https://doi.org/10.1136/bmj.l525.

Gregory, Dorothy Rasinski, and Miriam Piven Cotler. "The Problem of Futility: III. The Importance of Physician-Patient Communication and a Suggested Guide through the Minefield." *Cambridge Quarterly of Healthcare Ethics* 3, no. 2 (1994): 257–269.

Griggins, Cynthia, Eric Blackstone, Lauren McAliley, and Barbara Daly. "Making Medical Decisions for Incapacitated Patients Without Proxies: Part I." *HEC Forum: HealthCare Ethics Committee Forum: An Interprofessional Journal on Healthcare Institutions' Ethical and Legal Issues* 32, no. 1 (March 1, 2020): 33–45. https://doi.org/10.1007/s10730-019-09387-3.

Hansen, K. ""Futile Care, Experimental Treatments, and the Right to Try Movement: Could the Charlie Gard Case Happen in America?" *Suffolk University Law Review* 52, no. 1 (2019): 87–108.

Hansen, Kaitlyn. "Futile Care, Experimental Treatments, and the Right to Try Movement: Could the Charlie Gard Case Happen in America?" *Suffolk University Law Review* 52, no. 1 (January 1, 2019): 87.

Hashim, M. Jawad. "Patient-Centered Communication: Basic Skills." *American Family Physician* 95, no. 1 (January 1, 2017): 29–34.

Hauge, Amalie M. "One Last Round of Chemo? Insights from Conversations between Oncologists and Lung Cancer Patients about Prognosis and Treatment Decisions." *Social Science & Medicine* 266 (December 1, 2020).

Hearn, Jasmine, Mohamed Dewji, Claire Stocker, and Greg Simons. "Patient-Centered Medical Education: A Proposed Definition." *Medical Teacher* 41, no. 8 (August 2019): 934–938.

Hoffmann, M., M.-M. Jeitziner, R. Riedl, P. Eller, K. Amrein, ICU-Families Study Group, J. C. Schefold, et al. "Psychological Symptoms in Relatives of Critically Ill Patients (ICU Families): A Prospective Multicenter Study." *Intensive Care Medicine* 46, no. 5 (May 2020): 1060–1062. https://doi.org/10.1007/s00134-020-05997-5.

Holm, Søren. "Authenticity, Best Interest, and Clinical Nudging." *Hastings Center Report* 47, no. 2 (April 3, 2017): 38–40.

Huffman, Joan L., and Geoffrey P. Dunn. "The Paradox of Hydration in Advanced Terminal Illness." *Journal of the American College of Surgeons* 194, no. 6 (June 2002): 835–839. https://doi.org/10.1016/S1072-7515(02)01152-3.

Jacobson, Nora, and Diego S. Silva. "Dignity Promotion and Beneficence." *Journal of Bioethical Inquiry* 7, no. 4 (December 2010): 365–372. https://doi.org/10.1007/s11673-010-9258-y.

Jonsen, Albert R. "Casuistry: An Alternative or Complement to Principles?" *Kennedy Institute of Ethics Journal* 5, no. 3 (1995): 237–251. https://doi.org/10.1353/ken.0.0016.

Kant, Immanuel. *Practical Philosophy*. Vol. 6. Cambridge: Cambridge University Press, 1999.

Katz, Morgan J., Pranita D. Tamma, Sara E. Cosgrove, Melissa A. Miller, Prashila Dullabh, Therese A. Rowe, Roy Ahn, et al. "Implementation of an Antibiotic Stewardship Program in Long-Term Care Facilities Across the US." *JAMA Network Open* 5, no. 2 (February 28, 2022): e220181–e220181. https://doi.org/10.1001/jamanetworkopen.2022.0181.

Kelly, David F., Gerard Magill, and H. ten Have. *Contemporary Catholic Health Care Ethics.* Second edition. Georgetown University Press, 2013.

Keon-Cohen, Zoe, Paul Farquhar-Smith, and Timothy Wigmore. "Ethical Challenges in Caring for Cancer Patients in the Intensive Care Unit: Advanced Care Pathways and Avoidance of Futility." *Current Anesthesiology Reports* 5, no. 3 (September 2015): 354–360. https://doi.org/10.1007/s40140-015-0116-7.

Kompanje, Erwin J O, Ruth D Piers, and Dominique D Benoit. "Causes and Consequences of Disproportionate Care in Intensive Care Medicine." *Current Opinion in Critical Care* 19, no. 6 (December 2013): 630–635. https://doi.org/10.1097/MCC.0000000000000026.

Landry, Joshua T. "Is Shared Decision-making to Blame for the Provision of Ethically Inappropriate Treatment? Results of a Multi-site Study Exploring Physician Understanding of the 'Shared' Model of Decision Making." *Journal of Evaluation in Clinical Practice* 27, no. 4 (August 2021): 826–835.

Latour, Katrien, Jan De Lepeleire, Boudewijn Catry, and Frank Buntinx. "Nursing Home Residents with Suspected Urinary Tract Infections: A Diagnostic Accuracy Study." *BMC Geriatrics* 22, no. 1 (March 7, 2022). https://doi.org/10.1186/s12877-022-02866-2.

Liedgren, Pernilla. "Minorities with Different Values at School—the Case of Jehovah's Witnesses." *British Journal of Religious Education* 40, no. 1 (January 2, 2018): 31–43. https://doi.org/10.1080/01416200.2016.1150253.

Lo, Bernard. *Resolving Ethical Dilemmas: A Guide for Clinicians*. Sixth edition. Philadelphia: Wolters Kluwer, 2020.

Lynøe, Niels, Ingemar Engström, and Niklas Juth. "How to Reveal Disguised Paternalism: Version 2.0." *BMC Medical Ethics* 22, no. 1 (December 1, 2021). https://doi.org/10.1186/s12910-021-00739-8.

McCullough, Laurence B. "Beneficence and Wellbeing: A Critical Appraisal." *The American Journal of Bioethics : AJOB* 20, no. 3 (March 2020): 65–68. https://doi.org/10.1080/15265161.2020.1714817.

Merriam-Webster. *Merriam-Webster's Intermediate Dictionary*. Springfield, MA: Merriam-Webster, Incorporated, 2020.

Migden, Douglas R., and G. Richard Braen. "The Jehovah's Witness Blood Refusal Card: Ethical and Medicolegal Considerations for Emergency Physicians." *Academic Emergency Medicine* 5, no. 8 (August 1998): 815–824. https://doi.org/10.1111/j.1553-2712.1998.tb02510.x.

Mihailov, Emilian. "Measuring Impartial Beneficence: A Kantian Perspective on the Oxford Utilitarianism Scale." *Review of Philosophy and Psychology*, January 7, 2022, 1–16. https://doi.org/10.1007/s13164-021-00600-2.

Mullvain, Jacqueline A., Kevin R. Kozak, John S. Moody, and Toby C. Campbell. "Statin Use in Cancer Patients with Brain Metastases: A Missed Communication Opportunity at the End of Life." *Supportive Care in Cancer* 23, no. 9 (September 2015): 2643–2648. https://doi.org/10.1007/s00520-015-2624-x.

Phua, Jason, Gavin M. Joynt, Masaji Nishimura, Yiyun Deng, Sheila Nainan Myatra, Yiong Huak Chan, Nguyen Gia Binh, et al. "Withholding and Withdrawal of Life-Sustaining Treatments in Intensive Care Units in Asia." *JAMA Internal Medicine* 175, no. 3 (March 1, 2015): 363. https://doi.org/10.1001/jamainternmed.2014.7386.

Redleaf, Diane Lynn, Suzanne Baillie Schmitt and William Charles Thompson. "The California Natural Death Act: An Empirical Study of Physicians' Practices." *Stanford Law Review* 31, no. 5 (May 1979): 913–945.

Rhymes, Jill A. "Withdrawing Very Low-Burden Interventions in Chronically Ill Patients." *JAMA* 283, no. 8 (February 23, 2000): 1061. https://doi.org/10.1001/jama.283.8.1061.

Rusinko, Susan. "Plautus." In *Salem Press Biographical Encyclopedia*. Salem Press, 2021. Research Starters.

Tanaka, Miho, Satoshi Kodama, Ilhak Lee, Richard Huxtable, and Yicheng Chung. "Forgoing Life-Sustaining Treatment—a Comparative Analysis of Regulations in Japan, Korea, Taiwan, and England." *BMC Medical Ethics* 21, no. 1 (December 2020): 99. https://doi.org/10.1186/s12910-020-00535-w.

Tinetti, Mary E., Aanand D. Naik, and John A. Dodson. "Moving From Disease-Centered to Patient Goals–Directed Care for Patients With Multiple Chronic Conditions: Patient Value-Based Care." *JAMA Cardiology* 1, no. 1 (April 1, 2016): 9. https://doi.org/10.1001/jamacardio.2015.0248.

Upton, Hugh. "Moral Theory and Theorizing in Health Care Ethics." *Ethical Theory and Moral Practice* 14, no. 4 (August 2011): 431–443. https://doi.org/10.1007/s10677-011-9295-6.

Warrier, Maya. "Āyurveda and Mind-Body Healing: Legitimizing Strategies in the Autobiographical Writing of Deepak Chopra." *International Journal of Hindu Studies* 23, no. 2 (August 2019): 123–145.

West, James M. "Ethical Issues in the Care of Jehovah's Witnesses." *Current Opinion in Anaesthesiology* 27, no. 2 (April 2014): 170–176. https://doi.org/10.1097/ACO.0000000000000053.

Willmott, Lindy, Benjamin White, Cindy Gallois, Malcolm Parker, Nicholas Graves, Sarah Winch, Leonie Kaye Callaway, Nicole Shepherd, and Eliana Close. "Reasons Doctors Provide Futile Treatment at the End of Life: A Qualitative Study." *Journal of Medical Ethics* 42, no. 8 (August 1, 2016): 496. https://doi.org/10.1136/medethics-2016-103370.

Winkler, Eva C, Wolfgang Hiddemann, and Georg Marckmann. "Evaluating a Patient's Request for Life-Prolonging Treatment: An Ethical Framework." *Journal of Medical Ethics* 38, no. 11 (November 2012): 647–651. https://doi.org/10.1136/medethics-2011-100333.

Wocial, Lucia D., James E. Slaven, Kianna Montz, Patrick O. Monahan, Susan E. Hickman, Christopher M. Callahan, Paul R. Helft, et al. "Factors Associated with Physician Moral Distress Caring for Hospitalized Elderly Patients Needing a Surrogate Decision-Maker: A Prospective Study." *Journal of General Internal Medicine* 35, no. 5 (May 2020): 1405–1412. https://doi.org/10.1007/s11606-020-05652-1.

Chapter 3

The Ethical Principle of Nonmaleficence

INTRODUCTION

This chapter will discuss the ethical principle of nonmaleficence. As with autonomy and beneficence, this important bioethical principle will be presented in a way that is useful for the varied professionals who often deal with healthcare bioethics. The chapter on beneficence deals with providing healthcare to a patient that provides a good or benefit. However, this principle was not considered adequate, and another guide, nonmaleficence, was added to emphasize the importance of not delivering harm.

NONMALEFICENCE

For clinicians, nonmaleficence means not doing bad things to your patients. From the Latin word *maleficentia*, a mix formed from *malum* (evil) and *facere* (to do), nonmaleficence is the moral imperative of not committing harm or evil in one's actions.[1] The *Merriam-Webster Dictionary* defines maleficence "as the act of committing harm or evil," [2] so nonmaleficence would simply dictate not to do that. In their book *Principles of Biomedical Ethics*, Drs. Beauchamp and Childress further define it "as an obligation not to inflict harm on others" and note that it is often linked to the maxim *primum non nocere*, which will be discussed in the next section.[3]

Primum Non Nocere

Healthcare professionals frequently use this phrase to warn students, but its origin is unclear. Its translation simply is, "The first thing is to do no harm." Many are surprised to learn that it does not appear in the Hippocratic oath, much like Darth Vader never said, "Luke, I am your father." The closest line from Hippocrates

DOI: 10.4324/9781003654124-4

states, "At least, do no harm," which does not carry the same impact. However, the Hippocratic oath does designate a duty of nonmaleficence when it says, "I will use treatment to help the sick according to my ability and judgment, but I will never use it to injure or wrong them."[4] Another possible origin is in Hippocrates' book *Epidemics*, which states that when treating diseases, it is vital to "help or not to harm." Later, when Galen translated *Epidemics*, he attached the "above all" to the helping part rather than the avoiding harm part. Therefore, the idea that preventing harm must take precedence in medical practice does not have a clear background with either Hippocrates or Galen, although it still remains appropriate. [5]

For example, the phrase is still prevalent in contemporary medical articles. "Primum Non Nocere (First Do No Harm) with Oxygen Therapy" was published in 2022.[6] Two articles about the pandemic, "Primum Non Nocere—First Do No Harm—in the Time of SARS-CoV-2/COVID-19 Pandemic,"[7] and "Hydroxychloroquine/ Chloroquine as a Treatment Choice or Prophylaxis for Covid-19 at the Primary Care Level in Developing Countries: A Primum Non Nocere Dilemma,"[8] were also seen in academic journals in recent years. The phrase was also seen in several articles regarding the treatment of elderly patients, "TAVR—Primum Non Nocere: The Issue of Nonmaleficence in an Era of Modern Medical Advances," "Elderly Patients with Comorbidities and Acute Coronary Syndrome: Primum Non Nocere,"[9] and "Multidisciplinary Management of Breast Cancer in a 103 Years Old Patient: The Ultimate 'Primum Non Nocere' Challenge."[10] Finally, several articles about medical therapies invoked the same principle, "Asymptomatic Hypertension in the Hospital Setting: Primum Non Nocere," "Steroids for Tinea Incognito: Primum Non Nocere," "Primum Non Nocere: Is It Really True with Corticosteroid Hip Injections?"[11] and the editorial, "Opioids in Inflammatory Bowel Disease—Primum Non Nocere."[12] However, what does this imply for medical professionals?

The problem for clinicians is that every medical intervention has the potential to evoke harm. Therefore, if the phrase "first do no harm" were really to govern medicine, doctors would have to avoid intervening whenever there was a risk of hurting their patients (or others)-which would be almost always. This practice would lead to therapeutic nihilism or minimalism (do very little or nothing) regardless of the potential benefits of taking a risk. Nonmaleficence's most significant importance is as a balance to a clinician's primary obligation to do good for their patients. Even St. Thomas Aquinas is reputed to have said, "If the highest aim of a captain were to preserve his ship, he would keep it in port forever." Such benefit must be considered in the context of the possible harm that medical treatments often involve. Moreover, that benefit should be assessed with respect to autonomy and the potential harm that may occur.[13] This action requires a conversation between the clinicians and the patient regarding how much harm the patient is willing to endure to achieve a specific goal.

An excellent example of this is seen in the surgical treatment of head and neck cancers. Indeed, there is a need to balance burdens and benefits in formulating a treatment plan. The chances of treatment failure are balanced against the risks of morbidity and mortality from proposed surgical interventions. The term "unresectable" is sometimes used to state that a surgical procedure involves a degree of harm deemed unacceptable relative to the perceived benefit of the procedure.[14] The amount of acceptable harm should be discussed with the patient and the surgeon. Patients considering surgery for head and neck cancer are often concerned about changes in their appearance and functional impairments. There is a worry about body image difficulties, higher levels of anxiety, and perceived lower quality of life. Changes in appearance and functional impairments could become a barrier to social interactions and gaining back one's identity.[15] Indeed, for some, a post-surgical appearance that would frighten the grandchildren may take precedence over any increased life expectancy advantage. For others, the prospect of surviving longer and seeing their grandchildren grow up would be valued despite the cost. Clinicians, therefore, must work with these patients to set appropriate goals of care based on the patient's values. The following section will discuss this balance between nonmaleficence and the other principles.

Nonmaleficence and the Other Ethical Principles

It is tempting to think that if the primary goal is to do no harm, then why do anything at all? Doing nothing would remove all chances of causing harm and, therefore, comply with the maxim. This section will explore this critical question about nonmaleficence versus the other principles. Thus, nonmaleficence is formulated on the assumption that it is possible to distinguish not inflicting harm from beneficence, doing good. However, if the two should come into conflict, then nonmaleficence considerations will generally have priority over considerations of beneficence.[16]

Several articles about vaccines were considered to explore the interaction between nonmaleficence and beneficence further. One study looked at pre-pandemic vaccination concerns. Before the COVID-19 pandemic, most people had no experience with infectious disease outbreaks, and vaccine hesitancy was not uncommon. There were also concerns about vaccine side effects such as autism and the belief that pharmaceutical companies were profit-driven and untrustworthy.[17] These concerns were exacerbated during the pandemic when many people, especially healthcare workers, were urged to vaccinate. For instance, the lowest rates of COVID-19 vaccinations in the general population were reported for Kuwait, Jordan, Italy, Russia, Poland, the United States, and France.[18] The study also found that 22.51% of 76,417 healthcare workers worldwide hesitated about the available vaccines. The main concerns cited (safety, efficacy, and side effects) were very similar to those identified by the general public. Given the high rate of COVID-19 vaccination hesitancy in the general population already, this reluctance by healthcare workers makes this dilemma worse.[19] Because of this, some would argue for mandatory vaccinations for healthcare workers. In France, a 2021 law mandating vaccination for healthcare workers led to a massive increase in vaccination rates, from 60% in July (when the new requirement was announced) to over 99% in October. It was also noted that no more than 0.1% of healthcare staff refusing to be vaccinated left their jobs.[20] Closer to home, when Houston Methodist Hospital required its workers to be vaccinated, 99.5% received the vaccine, with few resigning rather than getting vaccinated.[21]

Mandating COVID-19 vaccination for healthcare workers would hypothetically decrease viral transmission from healthcare workers to vulnerable patients. It would also set a good example that could encourage vaccination in the general population. [22] Nevertheless, despite these claims, there is a downside to mandatory vaccinations. While educational campaigns emphasizing the benefits of mandates for public health, herd immunity, and the economy may decrease negativity, any mandatory regulation affecting health professionals could trigger harmful behaviors that put public health at risk. One study showed that a mandate's response could elicit activism and tendencies to avoid new vaccines and skip voluntary flu shots. The paper demonstrated the complex relationship between risk, policies, and behavior as defensive behaviors against COVID-19 and flu vaccinations are still crucial even when COVID-19 vaccines are available.[23] The ethical question, therefore, is whether mandating vaccinations is justified by the principle of nonmaleficence.

The study also found that these articles also discussed the principle of autonomy concerning nonmaleficence. To further explore nonmaleficence versus autonomy, a discussion regarding physician-assisted suicide (PAS), sometimes called physician-assisted death, will be introduced later in this chapter. Ethical principles are needed to guide terminally ill patients in exploring end-of-life options that could include PAS when it is legally viable. Furthermore, additional recommendations are required for increasing intellectual and emotional concerns regarding euthanasia.[24] However, the question is whether doing something harmful even when an autonomous patient requests it is ethical.

Justice is another ethical principle that will be discussed fully in another chapter. Nevertheless, it should be mentioned in context with nonmaleficence. Justice means treating people fairly, which is significant when talking about nonmaleficence.[25] One author describes the principle of justice as nonmaleficence: "The primary goal of just institutions in the distribution of goods and resources, opportunities and rights, is to fulfill a natural duty of justice not to cause (or to reduce) harm."[26] The problem occurs when decisions need to be made by institutions because of financial constraints. The example cited discusses a hypothetical medication that could reduce harm in both children and elderly patients born with a rare genetic disease, but because of "resource scarcity," a decision needs to be made. The choice could be to treat one group, the children or elderly patients, or to find a strategy that reduces harm in both groups but does not treat either group ideally.[27] Therefore, the consequence is that a choice to help the children could negatively impact the elderly patients and vice versa. This scenario also became evident early in the pandemic, when health systems had to decide on ventilators and intensive care units (ICUs) when these resources were finite.[28]

Nonmaleficence and Patient Safety

Clinicians, especially hospital-based ones, know how much this has been emphasized in the last twenty years. In 2000, the Institute of Medicine (IOM) published a book about the importance of patient safety, *To Err Is Human: Building a Safer Health System*. Building a safer system in healthcare means designing care processes to ensure that patients are safe from accidental injury. For example, when an agreement has been reached to pursue medical treatment, patients should be assured that it will proceed correctly and safely so they have the best chance of achieving the desired outcome.[29]

Since then, state legislatures have enacted requirements for physician training in patient safety. Act 13, passed by the Pennsylvania General Assembly in 2002, mandated CME requirements for physician licensure renewal to include credit hours in patient safety or risk management. The complete requirements took effect for physicians licensed through the State Board of Medicine beginning January 1, 2005. For physicians licensed through the State Board of Osteopathic Medicine, requirements for CME in patient safety or risk management were implemented during the licensure cycle beginning November 1, 2004.[30] There are reasons why professional organizations emphasize patient safety.

According to the Institute of Medicine, 44,000 to 98,000 Americans die annually from preventable medical errors. Even if the lower estimates are used, medical mistakes become the eighth leading cause of American death. The annual cost of adverse and preventable adverse events is between $54.6 and $79 billion, accounting for 6% of national healthcare expenditures.[31] The continuing safety problems were highlighted by investigative news reports about chronic safety problems leading to patient deaths and injuries at prestigious hospitals such as Baylor St. Luke's Medical Center, Johns Hopkins All Children's Hospital, UNC Health Care System, and University of Texas MD Anderson Cancer Center. In some cases, system leaders knew of the problems while they were occurring but did little until details were published in the news reports.[32]

A tragic case at Vanderbilt University Medical Center in Nashville, Tennessee, resulted in a patient's death, which should never have happened. According to a federal investigative report, in December 2017 a nurse, RaDonda Vaught, was caring for a 75-year-old patient, Charlene Murphey, who needed a magnetic resonance imaging (MRI) study.[33] Like many patients, Ms. Murphey was hesitant about going into the tubelike machine, and Versed, a medication similar to Valium, was prescribed to ease her anxiety. Vaught typed VE, for Versed, into the automated dispensing cabinet (ADC), a computerized device that gives out medicine in a hospital. However, Vecuronium came up first on the list. Not realizing the error, her nurse manually overrides the ADC's warnings and obtains the medication to give her patient.[34]

Vecuronium is a powerful muscle-paralyzing agent used for general anesthesia in surgical patients. It is also sometimes used in mechanically ventilated intensive care unit (ICU) patients. Unfortunately, Ms. Murphey died of respiratory failure because the medication paralyzed her breathing muscles. She, regrettably, was most likely fully awake. Vaught reported the incident immediately; she was fired a few days later and eventually lost her nursing license.[35] However, that was not the end.

In February, RaDonda Vaught was indicted on charges of reckless homicide and impaired adult abuse concerning her fatal error. On March 25, 2022, a Tennessee jury convicted Vaught of reckless homicide and abuse of an impaired adult. Although she could have been sentenced to up to 12 years in prison for the medication error, the judge sentenced her to supervised probation for three years on May 13, 2022.[36] After the trial results were disclosed, nurses and nursing organizations condemned the verdict through thousands of social media posts, shares, comments, and videos. They warn that the fallout will ripple through their profession, demoralizing and depleting the ranks of nurses already stretched thin by the pandemic.[37] Ultimately, they say, it will worsen healthcare for all. Linda Aiken, a nursing and sociology professor at the University of Pennsylvania, states it will make nurses less forthcoming about mistakes.[38]

From a nonmaleficence view, many questions remain unanswered. This fatal accident was blamed almost exclusively on the mistakes made by Vaught. However, the system at Vanderbilt should also be examined. The most obvious error was the nurse's ability to override the safety measures programmed into the ADC singlehandedly. Medical practices requiring a second person, such as a pharmacist, to supersede the computer's warnings would most likely have prevented this tragedy. Allowing one person's mistake without support from anyone else discloses a fatal flaw in the technology used by Vanderbilt. Making Nurse Vaught or any nurse the lone scapegoat may also have the additional effect of hiding medication errors.[39] Aikens is further quoted as saying, "The only way you can really learn about errors in these complicated systems is to have people say, 'Oh, I almost gave the wrong drug because …' Well, nobody is going to say that now."[40]

In an oddly related issue, the Supreme Court, on June 27, 2022, made it less likely for physicians to be convicted for overprescribing opioids. The Court unanimously set aside the convictions of two physicians accused of operating opioid "pill mills." Instead, the Justices decided that the government must prove beyond a reasonable doubt that the doctor knew or intended to prescribe the drugs in an unauthorized manner.[41] So, on the one hand, the criminal justice system prosecuted a nurse who made a terrible mistake but then made it difficult to prosecute physicians unless it is proven beyond a reasonable doubt that a doctor knew what they were doing was illegal when the prescription was issued. It is sensible, therefore, to conclude that the criminal justice system is unlikely to solve the patient safety issue.[42]

Solutions for the patient safety problem are not simple. The ethical principle of nonmaleficence emphasizes the obligation of those involved in healthcare to adopt technologies that promote benefits and avoid harm to patients.[43] Over twenty years ago, the IOM report set patient safety standards, but hospitals still fall short of these goals.[44] Although much has been achieved, little has changed. A growing realization has emerged that system-level change and cultural transformation are required to affect patient safety significantly.[45] For healthcare systems, creating a culture of safety is challenging. Safety culture is not fully understood, and people have not rallied around a single definition or set of concepts. However, it also reflects several vital facets of safety culture, as seen in the various examples of absent or inadequate safety culture. The tendency to blame people for errors with severe outcomes is often unwarranted and certainly not in the long-term interests of patient safety.[46]

To Err Is Human listed five types of medical errors: operative, drug-related, diagnostic, therapeutic, procedure-related, and other.[47] Defensive medicine, overprescribing tests, medications, procedures, and operations "just to be sure" will not solve the patient safety dilemma. Overutilizing medical resources will impose financial burdens on our healthcare system and increase patient risks due to increased exposure to unwarranted invasive testing. Clinicians, therefore, need to be prudent when ordering tests, medications, and procedures and openly discuss these elements' risks and benefits with their patients. Clinicians who recognize that their patients will have different health literacy abilities and aim to accommodate them through better informative communication strategies are best placed to support their patients in choosing wisely.[48] In 2012, the widely publicized American Board of Internal Medicine (ABIM) Foundation's "Choosing Wisely" campaign was initiated to provide direction for physicians to address pervasive overuse in healthcare. These initiatives are profoundly needed, as practicing physicians and trainees have poor knowledge of medical costs and the consequences of excessive ordering.[49]

Various proposals to improve patient safety have been explored to conclude this section. Although it was published over twenty years ago, the IOM report on patient safety has recommendations that are still relevant.[50] Medication errors remain problematic, and identifying barriers to reporting medication administration errors would be helpful.[51] In addition, something as straightforward as knowing a patient's weight would cause fewer medication errors.[52] Nevertheless, other solutions will prove to be more challenging. Building a culture that educates, perceives, and practices the fundamental ethical values must be fostered with mutual efforts by the government, people, healthcare institutions, and healthcare professionals to lift healthcare providers' ethical awareness and perception of patient safety culture.[53] This practice would involve removing the negative aspects of reporting errors and proactively taking steps to reduce the mistakes.[54] As previously stated in the Vaught case, criminalizing errors will not make patients safer.[55] Solutions to help prevent medical mistakes would also involve input from those not involved with patient care, such as policymakers, leadership, and managers.[56] Other solutions to be explored are safety procedures outside the hospital setting, where medication errors also occur alarmingly.[57] These studies are ongoing and will continue to look to make patients safer by decreasing medical errors, a result that is consistent with the ethical principle of nonmaleficence.

THE PRINCIPLE OF DOUBLE EFFECT

Another respected attempt to explain the principle of nonmaleficence appears in the principle of double effect (PDE). This rule incorporates a critical distinction between intended and merely foreseen effects, where effects are consequences of actions. This discussion should help clinicians with complex decision-making in medicine, especially concerning the beginning and end of life. However, let us first look at a debate about St. Thomas Aquinas and how this principle he developed to justify wars is used in medicine.

Saint Thomas Aquinas

St. Thomas was born in 1225 in the little town of Aquino, equidistant between Rome and Naples.[58] His most famous writing is *Summa Theologica* (Summary of Theology), which he wrote towards the end of his life in 1274. In this work, he introduces the PDE idea about whether one can kill another in self-defense. First, Aquinas refers to the position of St. Augustine (354–430 AD), which states that homicide is forbidden even in self-defense since the purpose of such self-defense is to save his own life, and therefore, the motives of this action are selfish.[59] He then proposes that killing someone in self-defense could be morally justified under certain circumstances. Thus, Aquinas developed PDE in its earliest form to explain the conditions in which it is ethically legitimate to cause or permit evil in pursuing good. One of his key points is between intentionally causing something bad, for example, bringing about another person's death, versus merely seeing it as a possible consequence.[60] He adds, "A particular action coming from a good intention can be unlawful if it should not be proportionate to the end. Thus, if one uses greater violence than is necessary for defending one's life, it will be unlawful." But he further writes that it is not "necessary for salvation that a man omit an action of moderate self-defense to avoid killing another because a man is more obliged to provide for his own life than the life of another."[61] He then delineates the requirements needed to justify such an act. The elements of PDE are listed as follows:

a. The object of the action must be correct or indifferent in itself; it cannot be intrinsically wrong.
b. The wrong effect, though foreseen, cannot be intended.
c. The wrong effect cannot be the means to the good effect.
d. There must be a proportionate reason for allowing the wrong effect to occur.[62]

For example, in self-defense, the object is to save one's life, and although there is a possibility that the attacker may die in the ensuing struggle, the goal is to use just enough force to preserve one's own life. So, how did a self-defense argument go on to be used as a justification for medical practices?

The crucial debate is what is morally acceptable to preserve life in a medical context. Aquinas uses the justification of self-defense to analyze many moral procedures, including amputations and sterilization, if their purpose was saving a life. Ultimately, even if death is the outcome, these ordinarily forbidden evils might be justified under particular circumstances.[63]

The problem occurs in defining what is intentional versus what is merely foreseen. PDE analyzes and evaluates actions with many consequences, some of which qualify as correct from a moral point of view, while others qualify as wrong. The distinction between intended and only anticipated effects is the basis of the present-day formulations of the discussed principle. Contemporary medical descriptions of the described principle state that actions in which good results are intended and bad ones anticipated but not intended are justified (with certain conditions) from a moral point of view. PDE recognizes activities in which the individual only predicts, even with a high degree of probability or even certainty, that the unjust effects of his actions are more justified than those whose bad effects are the direct intention of the clinician.[64]

Indeed, not all medical acts are justifiable under PDE. Beauchamp and Childress use the example of an abortion to save a mother's life with severe heart disease. Suppose the procedure is to crush the fetus's skull to enable passing through the birth canal.[65] One could argue that the unborn child's death was foreseen but not intended; the intent was to save the mother's life. However, the essential lesson for medical ethics that emerges from PDE is that actions cannot be morally judged solely in terms of their consequences. The circumstances under which they are performed, including the intention and the reason they are carried out, is a vital aspect of their moral assessment.[66]

However, scholars disagree about how to interpret these conditions. In medicine, it is difficult to explain a causal connection, where there is one, between effects a proposed treatment might produce. Therefore, is it justifiable for a clinician to exclude a harmful effect, even if temporary, before the good effect? Likewise, how does a clinician decide the proportionality of a harmful versus a good effect? Finally, even if there is an agreement about intentionality and proportionality, the final decision may still be problematic. These are issues that even the experts find debatable.[67]

At this point, healthcare professionals might ask, if the experts cannot agree on these issues, what am I supposed to do when there is a responsibility to decide what is good for my patient? Going back to St. Thomas Aquinas, he believed that every person has the ability to "perceive duty accurately if they truly want to. The private person genuinely concerned with the common good would then see that his duty is to act."[68] Several centuries later, a Medieval ethicist and physician, Gabriele de Zerbi, wrote a book, *De Cautelis Medicorum* (Advice to Physicians).

Zerbi's theme is this: "The doctor is the faithful companion of his patient's body, suffers with him, and rejoices in his health. However, the physician's obligation extends beyond the patient; the physician must be faithful to the intellectual tradition of medicine, other learned and moral colleagues, and the teaching of the Holy Church, for the rules of morality and medical ethics rests ultimately on the law of the Gospel." Zerbi's ethics, says a modern historian, "seem to be one of the earliest expressions of a group's self-regulatory rules of the Renaissance period ... a self-conscious discussion of how medical men should behave."[69]

The argument is that clinicians need to be familiar with ethical challenges, including PDE, from a clinical point of view. The following two sections further illustrate this idea and will look at PDE from two very different situations: the beginning and end of life. Both scenarios rely heavily on PDE to define the Principle of Nonmaleficence. For healthcare providers, shifting this discussion from purely academic to clinical may clarify some of the questions associated with these critical principles.

The Principle of Double Effect and Beginning-of-Life Issues

This section will look at how PDE is utilized for beginning-of-life (reproductive health) issues, and this discussion has never been more timely. In a historic decision, the US Supreme Court officially reversed *Roe v Wade* on June 24, 2022, declaring that the constitutional right to abortion no longer exists.[70] The judgment will be under what conditions, if any, will Federal and State laws justify abortion.[71] Many Americans are concerned about what is now legal regarding abortion when they go to the hospital, and the results will now vary from state to state. However, there is still a federal law that should offer some protection if a woman's life is in danger because of her pregnancy. Congress passed the Emergency Medical Treatment & Labor Act (EMTALA) in 1986. This act ensures public access to emergency healthcare services regardless of the ability to pay.[72] The United States Department of Justice maintains that bans on abortion that do not include exceptions for saving the life or the health of the pregnant individual are preempted by federal law, according to the Supremacy Clause of the US Constitution.[73] Because of this law, Catholic hospitals will also be scrutinized when faced with a woman with a complicated pregnancy and what procedures are permissible to save the woman's life if it should come to that. As previously discussed, PDE allows for taking one life to protect another under some very rigorous conditions.[74] With beginning-of-life issues, this often comes down to whether there is a need to sacrifice the unborn child's life to save the mother. These decisions can get complicated, and as the author C. S. Lewis quipped, "History isn't just the story of bad people doing bad things. It's quite as much a story of people trying to do good things. But somehow, something goes wrong."[75]

This section will only briefly discuss the Catholic Church's position on abortion; however, the idea of a justifiable abortion will be explored. This position has relevance even outside Catholic hospitals, as it is now up to the individual states to decide what constitutes a defensible abortion to save a woman's life. In states like Michigan, a 1931 law allows abortion only to preserve the mother's life and makes no exceptions for families that learn their infants have serious illnesses or anomalies, even ones incompatible with life.[76] Unless amended, this law is in effect in all Michigan hospitals, not just Catholic ones.

It is sensible to begin with the Catholic Church's position on beginning-of-life issues. These teachings can be found in the documents endorsed by the National Conference of Catholic Bishops known as the *Ethical and Religious Directives for Catholic Health Care Services* (ERDs).[77] Their position acknowledges the sanctity of life "from the moment of conception until death." Furthermore, abortion is defined in ERD 45 as "the directly intended termination of pregnancy before viability or the directly intended destruction of a viable fetus." This directive states that "every procedure whose sole immediate effect is the termination before viability is an abortion, which, in its moral context, includes the interval between conception and implantation of an embryo."[78]

One possible consequence of overturning *Roe v. Wade* is the rise of medical abortions, which have been available since the year 2000.[79] Especially in states with stringent restrictions on abortion, these medications provide a nonsurgical alternative. Emergency contraception (EC), as it is sometimes called, can prevent an unwanted pregnancy when taken after unprotected intercourse. Often, this treatment is used in the emergency department with rape victims. Studies show that the available methods of EC are safe and effective. However, unfortunately, it has not been possible to demonstrate a clear public health benefit of EC in that it has not been shown to decrease rates of abortion. Of course, this could change with our current situation. Although availability from pharmacies and an advanced supply of EC undoubtedly make access more accessible for women who wish to use EC, such approaches risk reducing the use of more effective contraceptive methods.[80] Nevertheless, although they are safe, there is debate on how these medications work.

While most evidence demonstrates that ECs work by preventing ovulation and are ineffective after that, some researchers contend that ECs prevent implantation. At one point, Catholic hospitals urged to be excused from a bill that required all hospitals to provide emergency contraception to victims of rape. Instead, the Catholic hospitals favored providing emergency contraception to victims of rape but only following a negative ovulation test.[81] They reasoned that if the ovulation test was negative, the EC provided contraception; however, if it were positive, the EC would provide a medical abortion. Technically, that is incorrect, as the EC pill can prevent fertilization and not just ovulation. However, even if the Catholic Hospital cannot prescribe EC, there are still ways to obtain it. Although the Supreme Court decision has limited access to abortion pills in the United States, some patients will drive across state lines for telehealth appointments to access the drugs where they are still legal. Abortion pills were utilized in the majority of abortions in the US as of 2020, according to information from the Guttmacher Institute, a research organization that supports abortion rights. Nevertheless, the confusion over abortion pills has intensified concerns about EC, even though ECs are not related to abortion—they are taken to prevent a pregnancy rather than to end one.[82]

It should be noted that the Catholic Church also restricts contraception. According to the Catholic teaching declared by Pope Pius XI in his 1930 encyclical Casti Connubii (Chaste Marriage), intentional contraception is contrary to natural law because this act frustrates "the conjugal act," which is "destined primarily by nature for the begetting of children." Therefore, Pius XI reasons that deliberately "frustrating the marriage act … is an offense against the law of God and nature."[83] The ERD for this states that in the Catholic moral tradition, human sexuality is a gift from God and therefore virtuous, with an affirmation of marriage and its sexual expression, but warns of "medical practices that undermine the biological, psychological, and moral bonds on which the strength of marriage and the family depends."[84] However, many Catholic families use artificial contraception rather than natural practices such as the rhythm method.[85] It is clear that even though the Catholic Church restricts oral contraception, it takes a more robust view on outlawing abortion.

To conclude this section, EC is considered lawful by the Catholic Church under certain circumstances and can be seen as compatible with PDE. Deciding to prevent a pregnancy is distinctly different from ending a pregnancy and can be allowed in Catholic hospitals and states where abortion is prohibited. Therefore, there is a problematic relationship between EC and abortion. Even if hormonal contraception causes a medical abortion, its use is not morally identical to procuring an early surgical abortion.[86] For example, a woman who obtains a surgical abortion directly intends to cause the death of the fetus. However, someone who uses EC does not intend to cause the death of any particular fetus. What she may intend to do, and what EC does do in the vast majority of cases, is prevent the conception of a fetus.[87] Because of this, the use of EC is compatible with PDE. In the following section, surgical abortions will be studied, specifically when the mother's health is in question.

It may be surprising to read that the Catholic Church allows abortion under certain circumstances. For example, ERD 47 describes a situation when a pregnant woman is diagnosed with uterine cancer. Since the mother's life is also considered sacred, any clinical discussion must include the stage of her cancer and pregnancy. Indeed, after discussing this with her clinicians, she may make the courageous decision to postpone her treatment until after she delivers.[88] Remarkably, a woman was made a saint by the Catholic Church for refusing treatment until after she delivered. Gianna Beretta Molla, a pediatrician, died in 1962 because she refused medical treatment that would have caused her to abort her pregnancy. Gianna was diagnosed with uterine fibroma or fibroid during the second month of her pregnancy. Although, as a physician, she was aware of the risks involved, she chose to prioritize her unborn child's life. Consequently, instead of the total removal of the uterus recommended by doctors, Gianna decided to remove only the fibroma so that she could continue the pregnancy. On April 20, 1962, she gave birth to a healthy baby girl, her fourth daughter. Sadly, however, a week later, Gianna died of septic peritonitis, a severe abdomen infection. She was forty years old. Molla was proclaimed a saint of the Roman Catholic Church in Saint Peter's Square on May 16, 2004.[89] She knew the danger but did not want to end her pregnancy, even if it meant losing her life. Nevertheless, she went against the advice of her physicians and chose to pay the ultimate price to save her baby. Although the Catholic Church canonized Gianna, her decision should not be considered normative. In fact, ERD 47 describes another pathway.

The directive states that under her physicians' advice, a woman may accept treatment even if that treatment cannot be safely postponed until fetal viability. It further says that such treatment could include a hysterectomy, which would obviously result in fetal loss. Fetal death, in this case, does not fit the definition of ERD for abortion, which is "directly intended termination" in a procedure "whose sole immediate effect" is termination.[90] This discussion regarding lawful termination of pregnancy will continue later with two other cases, one from Phoenix and one from Ireland, but first, some information regarding direct and indirect abortions.

Referring back to ERDs, the US Conference of Catholic Bishops has defined the evil of direct abortion as opposed to the valid, although tragic, situation in which a procedure or medication aimed at treating a serious medical condition results secondarily in the death of the unborn child. This reasoning would seem consistent with PDE, where the death of the fetus is not intended but foreseen. While the ethical principles of these directives seem straightforward, Catholic moral theologians are divided on how these directives should be interpreted. The first interpretation is the traditional natural law (TNL) theory, which holds that the moral object in an indirect abortion involves not only that the abortion is unintended by the subject but also indirectly caused. The second interpretation, referred to as the new natural law (NNL) theory, is that an indirect abortion refers only to abortions that the acting person does not intend, whether or not the action directly causes an abortion to occur.[91] This first interpretation looks at the intention and the action, while the second looks only at the intention. In the following two cases, it will be apparent why these two interpretations can be tricky. In both scenarios, the actions proposed were intended to save the mother's life. However, details about the actual procedures used or offered became provocative, and the applicability of PDE will be questioned.

A case in Phoenix, Arizona, dramatically illustrates this problem. A pregnant woman was admitted in critical condition to St. Joseph's Hospital and Medical Center in Phoenix. She suffered from severe pulmonary hypertension as a pregnancy complication, and her doctor felt that terminating her pregnancy was the only way to save the mother's life. The unborn child was not viable; therefore, if the mother died, so would the child.[92] Pulmonary hypertension (PH) in pregnancy is among the most severe challenges in medicine. Despite advances in medical therapy and care for high-risk pregnancies, PH during gestation remains a dangerous clinical scenario requiring a comprehensive multidisciplinary management strategy to optimize outcomes.[93] Reported outcomes are variable depending on the population studied, inclusion criteria, and duration of follow-up. Historically, maternal mortality rates have been as high as 30–56% in PH, although more recent studies report mortality in the 9–25% range. The causes of death are primarily right heart failure, life-threatening arrhythmias, sudden death, and blood clots. The overwhelming majority of deaths occur during the peripartum and early post-partum periods.[94]

Termination of the pregnancy is usually the safest option, and clinically, it should be offered to all pregnant women with PH. While a successful outcome is possible and, in many cases, probable, those with profound derangements, as in the Phoenix case, are at extremely high risk. Since most deaths occur post-partum, these patients and family members need to be advised regarding the possibility of a new baby without a mother. Most series suggest pregnancy termination may be accomplished with minimal risk of maternal mortality.[95]

The procedure was performed at the hospital with the patient's consent, and the woman survived. However, the case does not end here. Sr. Margaret McBride, a Catholic nun and a member of the hospital's ethics committee, was excommunicated and reassigned for her role in allowing an abortion at the hospital, according to the Pheonix Archdiocese. The decision to terminate the pregnancy drew a sharp rebuke from Bishop Thomas J. Olmsted, head of the

Phoenix diocese. He said abortion is not permissible under any circumstances. In a statement announcing his decision, Olmsted said McBride was excommunicated because she "gave her consent that the abortion was morally good and allowable under church teaching." Olmsted further declared as excommunicated anyone "who gave their consent, encouraged the abortion" or "who participated in the action, including doctors and nurses." The hospital also lost its Catholic designation.[96]

This problematic case demonstrates two directives in the ERDs for Catholic Health Care Services that were used as guidance by Sr. Margaret and the hospital officials. ERD 45 states that abortion is the directly intended termination of pregnancy and is not permitted under any circumstances. However, ERD 47 allows conditions other than the pregnancy to be treated, even if it results in the termination of the pregnancy. As stated previously, the example given for this directive is uterine cancer. PDE asserts that pursuing an act with the intent of a good end is permissible even when one knows it will have bad results. One theologian who disagrees with Bishop Olmstead is Germain Grisez, who teaches Christian ethics at Mount St. Mary College and Seminary in Emmetsburg, Maryland. In his three-volume book *The Way of the Lord Jesus*, Grisez outlines four conditions essential in holding that "a baby's death may be accepted to save the mother": some pathology that threatens the lives of both a pregnant woman and her child; it is not safe to wait, or waiting will result in the death of both; there is no way to save the child; an operation that can save the mother's life will result in the child's death."[97] This case would appear to meet these conditions.

Another esteemed Catholic ethicist also disputed that the woman's treatment violated Church teachings. Dr. Gerard Magill, an ethics professor at Duquesne University in Pittsburgh, PA, wrote:

> *[The] procedure to remove the placenta appears to constitute a directly intended moral action that was necessarily undertaken to resolve the pathological condition of the mother. Removing the placenta could occur only by removing the amniotic membranes containing the fetus. However, causing the death of this nonviable fetus (destined to die, whatever transpired) while avoiding a direct physical assault on it can be construed as being an indirect and unintended side effect of the justified moral action.*

Magill further states that while the deliberate killing of innocent human life is wrong, in this case, the action was justified to save the mother's life, which concurs with ERD 47.[98]

Finally, Rev. John F. Tuohey, the Endowed Chair of Applied Health Care Ethics and regional director of the Providence Center for Health Care Ethics for Providence Health & Services in Oregon, wrote this opinion about the case. He argues that Catholic Healthcare in this country provides a public service and must take responsible action when "the potential for religious freedom comes into sharp conflict with the physical welfare of certain pregnant women." He further asks whether the Catholic Church's exercise of its own religious liberty justifies allowing a patient to die because of the application of their self-imposed directives. Father Touhey concludes that the "Catholic identity in health care requires not merely following moral precepts to their logical conclusion, but also having the wisdom to discern when not to."[99]

For the record, some theologians did agree with Bishop Olmstead. For example, John Paul Slosar, director of ethics for Ascension Health, argues in a 2010 article:

> *In the Phoenix case, neither the child nor the placenta were pathological. However, because the placenta was causing increased blood flow to the heart, its normal function during pregnancy, the moral object was removing the baby and its maternal environment to save her life. While the intention is understandable, the means used amounted to a direct abortion.*[100]

By calling the action a direct abortion, he affirms Bishop Olmstead's conclusion that the procedure should not have happened. However, if the hospital had not done the procedure, the mother and the child would have likely died. While it is difficult to speculate what would have happened if the action had not been performed and the mother died, a similar case in Ireland may shed some light.

In October 2012, a comparable case occurred in Ireland. A 31-year-old Hindu woman living in Ireland died from a severe infection following surgery to remove the remains of the fetus she had been carrying. Savita Halappanavar, a dentist from a privileged background in India, had complications from a very wanted pregnancy and died in the maternity ward of a hospital in Ireland, a country with a very low maternal death ratio.[101] According to media reports, she had been repeatedly refused an abortion, despite her and her husband's pleas to perform this, because they believed the continued pregnancy represented a grave and growing risk to Savita's life. Savita had been admitted to the hospital, 17 weeks pregnant, a few days beforehand. When she asked to have her pregnancy terminated to save her life, she was apparently told, "This is a Catholic country."[102]

Part of the treatment required to save Savita's life, which should have been carried out without delay, was the evacuation of her uterus to terminate the pregnancy.

Because her cervix was fully dilated on admission to the hospital, the pregnancy was no longer viable; there was no treatment or way to make it possible at 17 weeks for the pregnancy to continue long enough for the baby to survive. The standard of care for intrauterine sepsis is pregnancy termination to remove the infected material.[103] However, based on what was reported, the termination of the pregnancy appears to have been delayed because there was still a fetal heartbeat.[104] As with the Phoenix case, Savita Halappanavar's death asks whether refusing to terminate a nonviable pregnancy is unethical when the woman's life may be at risk. In Catholic maternity services, this decision intersects with health professionals' interpretation of Catholic health policy on the treatment of miscarriage and the law on abortion.[105]

John Paul Slosar, who agreed with Bishop Olmstead that the Phoenix abortion was illicit, by contrast, had this to say about the Irish case. He states:

> *[A] pregnant woman with preterm rupture of membranes causing leakage of amniotic fluid puts the life of the preterm fetus at severe risk and puts the mother at risk for a life-threatening infection. To eliminate the infection source, the patient and her physician propose ending her pregnancy. Therefore, the direct intention [the moral object] is to evacuate the infection, which can only be treated by removing the contents of the uterus.*[106]

In this case, ERD no. 47 correctly applies because the intention is to eliminate an infection threatening the mother's life. The baby's death is a "foreseen but unintended consequence."[107] He distinguishes between the two cases based on the health of the uterus and fetus; in the Phoenix case, both were healthy, but in the Irish case, they were infected.

Publicity regarding Savita's death was a critical event leading to a referendum on May 25, 2018, when the Irish voters repealed the Constitution's Eighth Amendment, removing the constitutional abortion ban. The name Savita in Ireland has become indelibly linked to the changing course of abortion politics.[108] One can only guess what would occur in this country if the Phoenix mother had died, like Sativa. Perhaps, like in Ireland, the legislature would have passed laws that better define abortions to save a woman's life. This consequence could have drastically changed the impact of the *Roe v. Wade* decision some 12 years later.

To conclude this section, it should be noted that on December 8, 2010, St. Joseph's Hospital released a statement that said Sister Margaret has since "met the requirements for reinstatement with the Church, and she is no longer excommunicated. She continues to be a member in good standing with the Sisters of

Mercy and is a valued member of the St. Joseph's executive team."[109] Nevertheless, the Phoenix case illustrates ethics committees' difficulties when dealing with serious, life-and-death situations. It appears they thoughtfully looked at the ERDs and considered the PDE when deciding. However, after reviewing the case, Bishop Olmstead and multiple theologians and ethicists came to different conclusions. Remember that these distinguished experts also had the luxury of time, whereas the St. Joseph's Hospital ethics committee had to make a quick decision; otherwise, they would have dealt with two deaths. So, who was right in this case? When faced with two outcomes, it seems reasonable that the ethics committee made a less evil decision: the death of one life rather than two. This judgment appears to be the most closely aligned with the ethical principle of nonmaleficence.

The Principle of Double Effect and End-of-Life Issues

In bioethics, the PDE has been a practical, normative argument for a long time, and it can be used to determine the validity of actions that contain both good and bad outcomes. As with beginning-of-life issues, the PDE is exceptionally useful in end-of-life care because many decisions inherently have good and bad consequences. For example, the PDE can be used to make both practical and moral distinctions between euthanasia, PAS, palliative sedation, aggressive pain control, and the withholding and withdrawal of life-sustaining treatment. These decisions can be classified as either unjustified acts of killing or justifiable acts of allowing others to die. This section will explore PDE under these circumstances to help clarify the ethical principles involved.[110]

This concept will begin with a discussion of euthanasia. Like abortion at the beginning of life, euthanasia has been the most significant bioethical issue at the end of life. In addition, medical advances have brought numerous end-of-life options, which have significant consequences in both bioethics and law. The media had also presented and, in some cases exploited, the tragic stories of Karen Ann Quinlan (1976), Nancy Cruzan (1990), Terri Schiavo (2005), and Brittany Maynard (2014) when tough decisions were made. Nevertheless, the practical differences between end-of-life practices such as euthanasia and PAS have not always been apparent. Even the experts find the line between these issues somewhat hazy.

The dictionary definition of euthanasia is "the act or practice of killing or permitting the death of hopelessly sick or injured individuals in a relatively painless way for reasons of mercy." It comes from the Greek *euthanatos*, which means "easy or good death."[111] Euthanasia is then divided into active and passive. Active euthanasia causes death intentionally by medical means, whereas passive euthanasia refers to the withholding or withdrawing of life-sustaining treatment.[112]

Euthanasia is further divided into voluntary, nonvoluntary, and involuntary. Voluntary euthanasia is taking a person's life at that person's request. Nonvoluntary euthanasia is the act without such a request and is usually used in the context of incompetent persons. Finally, involuntary euthanasia is killing a person who rejects this action.[113] This latter distinction, active involuntary euthanasia, was once justified to save money spent on the ill and disabled for other more critical societal needs. However, visions of Nazi atrocities in the Holocaust come to mind, and this practice is universally considered murder; it will not be discussed further—nevertheless, other types of euthanasia need examination.[114] For example, although passive euthanasia, which is simply the process of allowing a patient to die, is generally accepted as ethical, many people confuse it with active euthanasia, which is the willful killing of a patient. Euphemizing it by calling it "mercy-killing" only adds to the confusion.[115]

Nonvoluntary, active euthanasia (NAE) also needs further discussion. Although illegal in most countries, there has been some discussion about it in Belgium and the Netherlands. In 2014, the Belgian Society of Intensive Care Medicine advocated the administration of sedatives with the direct intention of shortening the lives of terminal patients with no prospect of a meaningful recovery. They further state that administering sedatives beyond what is needed for patient comfort can be not only acceptable but, in many cases, desirable.[116] In Belgium, ending patients' lives without request is more common than other types of euthanasia.[117] One Belgian study found that in 17.0% of these cases, physicians injected lethal drugs even though this had not been discussed with the patient because the decision was felt to be in the patient's best interest or, in 8.2% of cases because they felt that the discussion would have been harmful. Some authors think these are probably acts of compassionate murder, or in the true sense, mercy killing or murderous paternalism.[118] While these acts are not explicitly acknowledged in the US, this discussion will continue later in this chapter with a discussion of palliative sedation and pain control.

The last type of active euthanasia is voluntary when a patient requests that their life be terminated. One notable proponent of this action was Jack Kevorkian, an American pathologist known to have assisted at least 130 patients with dying and consequently spent eight years in prison for this.[119] At about the same time he was imprisoned in 1998, PAS became legal in Oregon. It stated that if a patient has less than six months to live and is mentally competent, they can request that a physician prescribe drugs (oral barbiturates) that will cause a quick and painless death.[120] Currently, nine states allow terminally ill, mentally competent individuals to request a life-ending prescription from a physician. (California, Colorado, District of Columbia, Hawaii, Maine, New Jersey, New Mexico, and Oregon.)[121]

Interest in PAS increased in 2014 when 29-year-old Brittany Maynard, diagnosed with terminal brain cancer, moved from California (where PAS was not yet legal) to Oregon, where PAS was legal. The right-to-die advocacy group Compassion & Choices and others assisted Maynard in making her choice public through multiple outlets, including *People Magazine*, and her widower and mother continued to advocate for options in end-of-life care after her death. In addition, California lawmakers cited Maynard's death as the incentive for instituting the End-of-Life Options Act, which passed in 2015 and took effect in 2016.[122] Indeed, it was nearly impossible not to be sympathetic to Maynard, a beautiful young woman with an incurable, terminal illness; her openness to request PAS led many to ask why it was wrong.

When PAS is analyzed using the PDE, it is ethically unjustifiable. This conclusion is because PAS fails the same conditions as other forms of euthanasia. It fails to meet the first condition because the action, killing, is a morally evil act in itself, and it fails to meet the second condition because the evil effect of the action, the death of the patient, is what causes the good effect of the action, the relief of the patient's suffering.[123] As with euthanasia, PAS supports the intentional termination of life to relieve suffering. In addition, the medical procedure utilized is proscribing an overdose of a sedative that will directly cause the patient to stop breathing and die. Advancements in pain and symptom control have led many PAS opponents to believe it is much less necessary to relieve physical suffering. However, it is undoubtedly true that the existential anxiety that comes with the dying process is problematic. Nevertheless, even neuropsychological or existential suffering can be lessened with the promise of better pain management and the compassionate care of clinicians, family members, and others. Patients can reject PAS and allow palliative care to provide them with the comfort they need and deserve.[124]

According to Catholic tradition, the direct killing of an innocent person is never morally right, but allowing a person to die can be ethically correct—sometimes.[125] In this section, that concept will be examined using the PDE. As previously stated, passive euthanasia refers to withholding or withdrawing life-sustaining treatment.[126] Withholding refers to not starting a treatment, whereas withdrawing refers to removing a treatment once it has begun. Even though withdrawing treatment is commonly viewed as an active, different, and often more emotionally challenging action than withholding treatment, there is no moral distinction between the two. This distinction allows a treatment to be removed when it is no longer considered medically effective. It also allows patients or their families to agree to a treatment, knowing that it could be morally discontinued if it is no longer deemed beneficial to the patient. [127] Not starting or stopping a medical treatment fulfills the first condition of PDE, that the act must be good or indifferent; people stop or refuse treatments all the time for multiple reasons. Therefore, this makes the act different from active euthanasia, which always involves killing.[128]

For example, a terminally ill patient may decide on comfort measures only. In this case, the intent is not death but the relief of suffering. The patient may decide that they do not want to be placed on life support. If, for some reason, the person was placed on life support, the patient or their family could request its removal to fulfill the goal of comfort. However, the action is not meant to cause death but to remove the patient from a distressing situation. Allowing comfort and for the patient to have a dignified death outweighs the possibility of an earlier death in a dying patient; therefore, the conditions for PDE are met.[129] Alas, there are times when the removal of life support is problematic, and the following cases will examine this.

The decision to forgo life-sustaining treatment (DFLST) made by a dying patient or the patient's family (if the patient cannot make a decision) can decide not to use specific medical treatments, such as a ventilator if that treatment would only prolong the dying process. Not using extraordinary procedures where the burdens outweigh the benefits is typical in the US and consistent with Catholic moral tradition. However, sometimes clinicians, patients, and families have issues with removing life support once it has been started. David Kelly, in his book *Medical Care at the End of Life: A Catholic Perspective*, states it very clearly: "if it is morally right and legal to withhold treatment X in circumstances ABC, then it is morally right and legal to withdraw treatment X in the same circumstances."[130] Therefore, legally or ethically, there is no difference between withholding (not starting) or withdrawing (stopping) treatment. This reasoning allows patients to try a treatment but not be stuck to it if it is not helpful; without this, patients may hesitate to take a chance. Therefore, this view of withholding and withdrawing, which originates in Catholic ethics, illustrates good ethics, law, and medicine. Unfortunately, this concept is not universal.

Piergiorgio Welby (1945–2006) was an Italian poet and artist who was diagnosed with muscular dystrophy as a teenager in Rome. In 1997, he developed respiratory failure and was placed on a ventilator. From then on, Welby could never breathe independently and required artificial feeding. In 2006, he requested that the ventilator be withdrawn. As previously stated, this would be legal in the US and be considered voluntary passive euthanasia. However, the government of Italy and the Catholic Church both opposed his request. Although Welby advocated for legalizing euthanasia in Italy, in his case, he was just asking to be removed from a medical treatment that he no longer wanted.[131]

Additionally, it was proposed that if the healthcare team removed him from the ventilator, they would be prosecuted for his death. Piergiorgio also asked for his tube feedings to be stopped. (Later in this chapter, we will examine how the Church differentiates between extraordinary treatments like mechanical ventilation and artificial nutrition and hydration.) In this case, however, the Church was torn between its opposition to aggressive medical treatment and euthanasia. Eventually, the Italian courts allowed Piergiorgio Welby to be removed from the ventilator without prosecuting the physicians involved. He died on December 20, 2006.

The Catholic Church, however, would not permit a religious funeral, stating that "Welby had repeatedly and publicly affirmed his desire to end his own life, which is against Catholic doctrine."[132] As a Catholic palliative care physician, I find this decision by the Church both troubling and confusing. Sadly, this controversy will most likely never be resolved.

Welby's writings did advocate for euthanasia, but in his case, he only wanted his ventilator removed. While on the machine, he even wrote a book, Let Me Die. He stated that he is not seeking to commit suicide but to remove himself from medical treatment he does not want, and wrote, "It is an unbearable torture."[133]

The Brittany Maynard and Piergiorgio Welby stories showcase two issues with dying patients: overemphasizing dignity and sanctity. The Oregon Death with Dignity Act is an essential example of a legal policy implemented to ensure patient autonomy in the dying process, thereby promoting dignity. Although the act began as the pursuit of patient empowerment in end-of-life situations, it soon dissolved into merely an attempt to end suffering quickly and to avoid challenging circumstances that would not necessarily lead to immediate death. This act, called Measure 16, was ultimately an affirmation "of the ideology of patient control and self-determination."[134] Sadly, Ms. Maynard and many others choose this path.

On the other side of the spectrum is the elevation of autonomy in living, which wrongfully prioritizes life's sanctity over dignity. This practice is commonly seen in the use of extensive medical efforts in an attempt to do "everything" possible. Unfortunately, these attempts at prolonging life can quickly turn into dragging out an inevitable death. When death seems the alternative, we will often spend immense amounts of money and resources to buy time at the end of life for the patient or their loved ones.[135] Sometimes, the patient has asked for this type of treatment, but their family often states that their loved one would have wanted this. Ultimately, a patient like Mr. Welby and the medical team are forced to choose between what the patient wants (autonomy) and what the law or the Church dictates.

In most cases, The Roman Catholic tradition has called life-sustaining treatments that go beyond what a person can be required to endure "extraordinary" means of care. Although Catholics respect human life, we do not worship it. For patients like Mr. Welby, one cannot make death their aim, but they should be able to forgo measures knowing that this could lead to death as a consequence. Requiring a person to stay alive at all costs is inconsistent with respecting dignity. Therefore, withholding or withdrawing life-sustaining futile, costly, or burdensome treatments is consistent with respect for the intrinsic dignity of the human. Overall, the Catholic Church has taught us to value the sanctity of life but not to cling vainly to it, which opposes dignity.[136] Assessing the thin line between sanctity and dignity in some cases can be challenging.

The next three cases involve young women who tragically were left in a persistent vegetative state (PVS). By definition, a person in PVS has no higher cognitive function, resulting in a lack of awareness of self and their surroundings. However, the brainstem still functions, allowing the patient's autonomic functions, such as breathing, digestion, maintenance of body temperature, and blood circulation, to continue. Unfortunately, the patient is incapable of voluntary or purposeful acts and only responds reflexively to painful stimuli. Although alive, the PVS patient is not terminally ill but will remain unconscious. Depending on the condition's cause, medical or traumatic, the condition will be referred to as a permanent vegetative state after a determined period of time elapses. At this point, there is no chance of recovery.[137]

Karen Quinlan suffered permanent brain damage in April 1975.[138] When it became clear that she would not recover, her family requested that she be removed from the ventilator. After a prolonged legal battle, the Supreme Court of New Jersey allowed her to be removed from life support in May 1976. However, maintained by a feeding tube, she lived for another nine years. Decades later, two other women, Nancy Cruzan and Terri Schiavo, found themselves in a similar state. Their legal cases concerned whether families could request that artificial nutrition and hydration (ANH) be legally and morally stopped in people with PVS.[139] So, is there a difference between taking someone off a ventilator versus stopping ANH?

What is the same in all cases of PVS is the assertion that although seriously debilitated, they are still human beings. This leading viewpoint is manifested in judicial opinions and the writings of scholars, ethicists, religious leaders, and others.[140] Next, while mechanical ventilation is undoubtedly medical treatment, AHN is considered basic or ordinary care. Finally, the withdrawal of AHN introduces a new cause of death, namely, dehydration and malnutrition, which ultimately cause the patient's death. In contrast, the withdrawal of mechanical ventilation allows the patient to die from their underlying disease.[141] Therefore, the PDE cannot validate the removal of AHN. Although the procedure itself is neutral, the intent is to cause a condition that will ultimately cause the patient to die.

Nevertheless, this does not mean that stopping ANH is never just justified. Indeed, it is permitted to stop ANH in patients where it is medically ineffective or causes a burden. ANH is not indicated in patients with dementia because of the burden it causes and because it has been found to shorten life expectancy.[142] Second, patients with dementia who are tube-fed often need to be physically or chemically restrained to prevent them from pulling out the tube. Chemically restraining a patient is a euphemism for "drugging" the patient to the point that they are not conscious enough to remove the feeding tube. Another reality with tube-fed dementia patients is that they are more likely to develop bed sores as the result of frequent loose stools that are often present with the nutritional liquids given.

Third, dementia patients who receive tube feedings lose the experience of being hand-fed. It is not just the sensory experience of receiving food but also the care involved with having another person interact with you by carefully offering you a meal. Assisted feeding, as it is called, is a far more compassionate and peaceful way of caring for a patient who is dying from dementia. Assisted feeding should be differentiated from forced feeding, where the patient's dignity and comfort are superseded by the goal of getting as much food in as possible, regardless of the patient's condition. Assisted feeding, when done correctly, shows the beauty of caring for another human being, not unlike a mother feeding her baby. This humane treatment is stopped regularly once artificial nutrition is started, leading to increased patient suffering. Fourth, suppose a patient has completed an advance directive stating they would not want ANH at all or under certain conditions. In that case, the principle of autonomy should be respected.[143] Finally, most State laws allow families to make this decision if there are no advance directives if the patient has a terminal condition or is permanently unconscious.[144]

Patients with advanced cancer frequently lose weight and become cachectic. This condition is also seen in patients with end-stage heart or lung disease for reasons that are not medically clearly understood. The goals of ANH for these people would be to improve their equality of life and prolong their lives. For patients with esophageal or head and neck cancer who physically cannot eat, this makes sense because the tumors prevent the food from passing from the mouth to the stomach, making normal eating impossible.[145] Yet, even patients without an obstructive lesion often cannot eat or have no desire to eat. The same goals would be achieved for those patients: to provide comfort and extend their lives. However, placing a feeding tube in these patients is rarely done, essentially because this treatment has failed to show a comfort or survival benefit. In addition, adding ANH to dying patients has been shown to increase secretions, dyspnea, nausea, and vomiting without any real benefit. Therefore, patients and their families should not be persuaded by medical personnel to allow this treatment, which provides far more burdens than benefits.[146] From a Catholic perspective, the ERDs state that if a treatment is offered and it does not "offer a reasonable hope of benefit or entail an excessive burden, or impose excessive expense on the family or the community,"[147] there is no obligation to ask or accept it. Nevertheless, the Church's stance on the Terri Schiavo case has raised questions about when ANH is considered obligatory.

Chapter 1 of this book looked at the tragic story of Terri Schiavo and the dispute between her husband and her parents regarding the continuation of her artificial nutrition through a percutaneous (through the skin) stomach catheter. Unlike the case with Nancy Cruzan, where her parents petitioned the courts to have her tube feedings stopped, Terri's parents, the Schindlers, wanted her tube feedings to continue, against the wishes of her husband, Michael. Her tube was eventually removed, and she died on March 31, 2005, but not before the state and federal courts got involved. Multiple parties weighed in on this decision, including antiabortion and disability rights groups. Ultimately, even the Pope got involved.

Most states allow for families to remove life support, including ANH, if the patient has an end-stage medical condition or is permanently unconscious. As we stated above, there is no obligation to provide this treatment for dying patients or patients so sick that they are so ill that they are no longer awake. Nevertheless, in the Terri Schiavo case, Pope John Paul II absolutely took exception about removing ANH in a person in a PVS. For Catholics and other ethicists, this requires further discussion.

CATHOLICS AND ARTIFICIAL NUTRITION AND HYDRATION

Catholic directives on withholding or withdrawing life-sustaining treatment have provided practical guidelines for end-of-life decisions for Catholic patients, families, professionals, and their healthcare institutions for at least five hundred years. However, on the surface, Pope John Paul II's 2004 "Life-Sustaining Treatments and the Vegetative State," along with statements from religious committees and the Congregation for the Doctrine of the Faith (CDF) regarding providing ANH to PVS patients, have seemingly reversed their previous position. The Pope now states that providing ANH to these patients is considered "ordinary care" and, therefore, is "in principle" obligatory.[148] Many Catholic Advance Directives now state the following in one way or another:

> *I wish to receive nutrition and hydration, even if its supply is medically assisted, as long as it effectively sustains my life. Even if I am permanently unconscious, medically assisted nutrition and hydration should be continued until it is deemed futile (i.e. no longer able to sustain my life) or it imposes disproportionate burdens on me (i.e. serious risk, excessive pain, excessive expense on my family or the community). If my death is truly imminent, or if my body is unable to assimilate foods and fluids, or if there is some other serious medical problem preventing nourishment, the medically assisted supply of nutrition and hydration may be considered unnecessary and discontinued.*[149]

So, is this really a change? Let's look into this further. First, is a person in PVS still a person? One of the problems that the Church sees is the dehumanization of people for many reasons in today's society. Even the name Permanent Vegetative State seems to imply that someone with this condition is less than human. Pope John Paul II wrote:

> *No matter what the concrete circumstances of his or her life, a man, even if seriously ill or disabled in the exercise of his highest functions, is and always will be a man, and he will never become a vegetable or an animal. Even our brothers and sisters who find themselves in the clinical situation of a vegetative state retain their human dignity in all its fullness. The loving gaze of God the Father continues to fall upon them, acknowledging them as his sons and daughters, especially in need of help.*[150]

Clearly, the pontiff wished to emphasize that human life unconditionally has value. The term PVS is demeaning, and many clinicians have suggested changing the name of this condition to unresponsive wakefulness syndrome (UWS), which is more descriptive and less derogatory. From here on, this book will preferentially use UWS.

Second, do patients with UWS suffer? Both sides seemed confused about this, and the short answer is no. Tube feedings did not cause Ms. Schiavo to suffer by having to remain in such a state, nor did removing it and starving her to death.

This inaccuracy must be stated as it does not add anything to the argument but emotional responses. Third, does this directive change the way the Catholic Church feels about ANH for other medical problems? Probably not; these directives appear only to target people with UWS. Mandating ANH in patients with advanced dementia was not the purpose of the Pope's statements. Alzheimer's disease and other dementias are terminal illnesses, and people afflicted with these diseases will die despite treatment. Also, ANH most likely will increase the patient's suffering. Is UWS a terminal illness? Not by objective standards; both Karen Quinlan (9 years) and Terri Schiavo (15 years) showed that young and otherwise healthy patients receiving ANH could live for quite some time.[151]

Finally, is providing ANH to patients with UWS obligatory until the person's death? The answer is no. Pope John Paul II stated that supplying UWS patients with ANH was obligatory "in principle." By expressing it that way, the Pope recognized that there could be exceptions. The revised ERD #58 now states, "Medically assisted nutrition and hydration become morally optional when they cannot reasonably be expected to prolong life or when they would be "excessively burdensome for the patient or [would] cause significant physical discomfort, for example resulting from complications in the use of the means employed."[152]

These statements show multiple scenarios for ANH to be stopped in these individuals. Although proving that it is causing the patient to suffer may be challenging, other valid reasons exist. Some examples of that would be that the patient is dying from something else, or they begin to aspirate, causing pneumonia, or the tube comes out and cannot be replaced, or the tube repeatedly gets infected. Another reason that would allow ANH to be stopped would be if the treatment is overly burdensome to the family.[153] Generally, the care for these patients is not costly, but what would be considered excessively difficult for a family or community would need to be looked at individually.

AGGRESSIVE END-OF-LIFE SYMPTOM MANAGEMENT

The final topic in this chapter deals with PDE and aggressive symptom control at the end of life. This matter includes aggressive pain management and palliative sedation. Very few people want to be uncomfortable when they are dying, nor do they want to see their family members suffer either. Healthcare professionals are often conflicted by the challenge of treating suffering patients with potent medications that could potentially kill them. Under PDE, intentionally killing an innocent person is wrong; however, this outcome could occur to relieve suffering by prescribing large doses of pain medications. The intent is to provide relief of pain by using potent analgesics and not by the patient's death, although that possibility is foreseen. Nevertheless, relief from suffering, especially with a dying patient, is a good thing, and tough treatment decisions are often made reluctantly by the clinician, hoping that the right choice is made.[154]

In November 2018, an Ohio physician was charged with murder, accused of prescribing lethal doses of fentanyl to critically ill patients. William Husel, 43, turned himself in. He faced 25 charges of second-degree murder, each with a maximum penalty of life imprisonment. Husel, an intensive care physician, prescribed an opioid, fentanyl when doing a palliative wean from a ventilator. This practice is done when a patient cannot be weaned conventionally from the breathing machine because the clinicians believe the patient is too ill to breathe without mechanical assistance. Medications like fentanyl or morphine are often prescribed to relieve suffering and prevent "air hunger" during this process. However, Husel used very high doses of fentanyl (500 to 2000 micrograms), which the prosecutors stated was meant to purposely cause the death of the patients rather than provide comfort.[155] Husel's attorney told the Columbus Dispatch that his client sought only to give "comfort care" to patients near death and never intended to harm or euthanize them.[156]

Prosecutors in Ohio alleged that Dr. William Husel intentionally prescribed lethal amounts of painkillers, mainly the synthetic opioid fentanyl, to 29 patients aged 37 to 85 between 2014 and 2018, resulting in all but four deaths. Many of the patients who died had been on ventilators and were receiving palliative care. Becky McNeil, a former clinical educator at Mount Carmel, said patients "kept alive by ventilators and other life support measures were evaluated differently. If life support was being withdrawn, she said, those patients might require higher doses of fentanyl than would patients who did not have minutes left to live."[157] Several ICU nurses stated that Husel gave high but "appropriate doses of fentanyl" to patients who were being removed from life support. They maintain that no one was trying to hasten those patients' deaths with pain medication or euthanize them, which is illegal in Ohio and all fifty states.[158]

The perception of suffering after DFLST in an unconscious patient is perplexing. By definition, if the person is unconscious, they cannot tell how they feel. An order that states "titrate the opioid to comfort" is, therefore, at best, inadequate. There is at least one assessment tool available that could have been utilized. The Respiratory Distress Observation Scale (RDOS) is a solution to recognizing respiratory distress when the patient cannot provide a dyspnea report. The RDOS was initially developed in an observation study of mechanically ventilated patients undergoing a ventilator weaning trial.[159] This scale was developed from a biobehavioral framework by Dr. Margaret L. Campbell and uses clinical and observational data (heart rate, respiratory rate, use of accessory muscles, etc.) to give a numerical dyspnea assessment.[160] This assessment tool and documentation of specific indications for opioid titration are recommended to prevent litigation. Because most clinicians do not wish to engage in actively shortening life with opioids or even appear to be doing so, it would be prudent to be diligent in documenting intent to palliate when using high doses of opioids.[161]

The Columbus-area Mount Carmel Health System fired Husel in December 2018. He pleaded not guilty after turning himself into the police in June 2019. A judge set bail at $1 million.[162] On October 21, 2020, his attorneys motioned that the 25 murder charges be dismissed.[163] Although he was acquitted of all charges, he had to surrender his medical license in Ohio and faced multiple wrongful-death civil suits.[164] Even though the physician claims that his goal was comfort and not killing, this case raises the question, when do aggressive pain and symptom control become euthanasia?

Criminal prosecution of physicians prescribing opioids is very rare. However, in February 2016, a physician in California, Dr. Hsiu-Ying Tseng, was sentenced to 30 years to life in prison after a jury found her guilty of second-degree murder for three patient drug overdose deaths. For the first time in American history, a physician was held criminally liable for the murder of a patient using extreme recklessness in opioid prescribing.[165] The outcome of the Husel case is unknown. Still, it does suggest some vulnerability of physicians to the legal system when prescribing opioids for DFLST. However, straightforward documentation of intent and a rationale for the opioid doses should prevent criminal prosecution.

For clinicians who believe in an absolute prohibition against actions that intentionally cause death, the rule of double effect may be helpful as a way of explaining adequate pain relief and other palliative measures for dying patients.[166] However, others contend that PDE is unnecessary because death does not necessarily have a bad effect. These authors point to Aquinas and his original PDE beliefs, calling their applicability in a multicultural society into question. Comparable discussions surrounding PAS reveal that, for many, there are fates worse than death, such as unrelieved physical or emotional suffering.[167] Nevertheless, a study showed that even though 60% of US physicians believe that PAS should be legalized, only 9% of respondents indicated that they would unequivocally perform PAS if it were legal.[168] Therefore, even if clinicians accept that death may not necessarily be a bad outcome, they still might be reluctant to prescribe analgesics that could cause death.

Another criticism of PDE with potent analgesics at the end of life is that there is little evidence that these agents shorten life. An excellent study in the pharmacy literature from 2021 concluded that there was no impact on the time of death with opioid dose escalation in comfort measures only (CMO) patients. The study also found that patients who were seen by the palliative care team in the hospital survived an average of 20.1 hours longer than those who did not receive a consult during their final hospital visit. Furthermore, patients receiving a consult survived longer even when receiving higher opioid dose escalation.[169] Therefore, some palliative physicians conclude that prescribing analgesics in appropriate doses does not shorten life but only relieves suffering; there is no need to resort to PDE to justify the prescribing practice, whatever inherent merits or challenges the doctrine may possess. Since PDE implies that there could be a bad effect, such as the patient's death, when prescribing analgesics, why should PDE be used if that bad effect has not been shown to occur? PDE could be seen as a hindrance to adequate pain control, implying a negative that most likely occurs only rarely.[170]

The final critique of PDE to be discussed here concerns intent. PDE in this scenario implies that the clinician only wants to relieve the patient's suffering through the proper use of analgesics and not to hasten death. However, some have argued that PDE cannot reasonably be utilized since it relies on the clinician's intention while treating a patient. These critics claim that human intention is complicated; therefore, arguing that a possible bad outcome can be entirely unintended is impractical. For example, what happens if a clinician's primary intention is to comfort a dying patient, and the patient dies peacefully?[171] Although William Husel argued that he just wanted to keep his patients comfortable, does this conform with PDE?

Many of the same arguments for and against aggressive pain management can also be made for palliative sedation. Palliative sedation (PS) is used when terminally ill patients experience intolerable symptoms that cannot be relieved by conventional means. It involves the administration of sedatives to induce unconsciousness as a last resort to ease suffering.[172] PS is used when clinicians intentionally sedate and lower a patient's consciousness level to a sufficient level to address otherwise refractory symptoms at the end of life. The symptoms that are most frequently responsible for a refractory state requiring PS are delirium (55–65%), dyspnea (26–27%), pain (14–18%), and vomiting (4%).[173] As with the use of strong analgesics, the potential of PS hastening death by depressing patients' respiratory drive is widely accepted and can be justified by PDE in that this action has both good and bad consequences.[174] In the classic case, the PS passes the first two conditions of PDE because sedation is morally neutral. The bad result, the possible hastening of death, does not cause or bring about the good consequence, the relief of suffering. The action also passes the latter two conditions because the clinician intends to relieve the patient's suffering and not to hasten the patient's death, as well as the value of the relief of suffering is proportional to the possible hastening of death in an already dying patient.[175]

Nevertheless, PS is controversial, and some opponents state that it is only superficially different from euthanasia and, therefore, cannot use PDE or other moral arguments for its justification. Other critics of using PDE to justify PS will state that this act does not hasten death. One study examined PS use in over 500 hospice patients. The median survival of the unsedated group from the time of admission to the hospice was nine days. In comparison, the sedated cohort was twelve days.[176] Therefore, if PS does not hasten death, why invoke PDE at all? Another criticism of PDE deals with intent. In considering physicians' intentions in end-of-life care, one noted palliative care physician, Dr. Timothy Quill, stated, "We would do well to look beneath the idealized, sanitized intentions espoused by many medical ethicists to the actual experience of doctors and patients." Quill suggests that physicians and nurses involved in the treatment of terminal patients may intend to bring about the death of their patients to alleviate their suffering. However, interpreting what nurses and clinicians say, think, and do under these challenging circumstances can be difficult.[177]

Although there are criticisms of using PDE to justify PS, it remains a valuable tool to help clinicians make moral decisions. For instance, knowing the difference between euthanasia and PS PDE can help decide whether this action is appropriate. The individuals involved, including the patient, the family, and the clinicians, would be assured that PS is not intrinsically evil and that the patient's death would not be the means to relieve suffering if the medication were titrated correctly. Furthermore, by examining the details of the situation, the individuals involved could decide whether the intent was for relief of suffering and not for death and whether the severity of the suffering the patient is experiencing is proportionate to the risk of death.[178] PDE may also be useful when making PS and other end-of-life decisions, such as withdrawing life-sustaining mechanical ventilation and compassionate extubation.[179]

One final word about analgesics and PS at the end of life is the need for better clinician education on the appropriate use of the medications and procedures involved. In addition, expertise is needed to titrate these medications to achieve comfort. However, knowing that these drugs can depress respirations and how to titrate to comfort and not death is essential. Finally, if PS is used in a hospital setting, protocols need to be established along with training of the nursing staff to ensure that the goals are clear to all involved with the patient's care.[180] Although we may never know his intent, perhaps Dr. Husel's true crime was not knowing how to use fentanyl in a way that more clearly provided comfort and not death to the patients in his care.

CONCLUSION

This chapter looked to explain the ethical principle of nonmaleficence clinically. First, the origin of the phrase *primum non nocere* and how it is utilized in medicine today was discussed. Nonmaleficence was then addressed, and how it fits in with the other ethical principles by Beauchamp and Childress. Finally, nonmaleficence was explored along with the contemporary model of patient safety that is so prevalent in healthcare today.

The subsequent section explored nonmaleficence using the PDE. First, the theologian Thomas Aquinas was presented, along with this principle and how it was used to justify homicide. Next, this idea was raised in a way that helped clinicians understand how to approach complex decisions in both beginning-of-life and end-of-life circumstances. The goal was to explain nonmaleficence in a manner that benefits professionals faced with ethical dilemmas and emphasizes practical, everyday aspects of this vital concept.

TAKE-HOME POINTS

- Nonmaleficence is an obligation not to harm others and is often linked to the adage *primum non nocere*.
- Nonmaleficence's most significant importance is as a balance to a clinician's primary obligation to do good for their patients, recognizing that all treatments have some potential for harm.
- Patient safety is essential to nonmaleficence as health systems devise methods to protect patients from accidental injuries. The emphasis must be on systemic solutions and not blaming people for mistakes.
- The principle of double effect (PDE) integrates a critical distinction between intended and merely foreseen effects, where effects are consequences of actions. It serves as a guide to help clinicians with difficult treatment decisions.
- Although it is difficult to establish whether an outcome is intended or foreseen, PDE also looks at the action itself when judging appropriateness.
- PDE allows for taking one life to protect another under some very rigorous conditions. With beginning-of-life issues, this often comes down to whether there is a need to sacrifice the unborn child's life to save the mother.
- The Catholic Church's position on beginning-of-life issues is stated by the National Conference of Catholic Bishop's document known as the *Ethical and Religious Directives for Catholic Health Care Services* (ERDs).

- The Catholic Church allows abortion under certain circumstances. ERD 47 describes a situation when a pregnant woman is diagnosed with uterine cancer, and a hysterectomy may be performed to save the mother's life.
- PDE can be used to make both practical and moral distinctions between euthanasia, medical aid in dying, palliative sedation, aggressive pain control, and the withholding and withdrawal of life-sustaining treatment.
- The Catholic Church makes a distinction between ordinary and extraordinary means of care. It states that the former should be continued while allowing the removal of the latter in dying patients.

NOTES

1 Vittorio Bufacchi, "Justice as Non-Maleficence," *Theoria* 67, no. 1 (March 1, 2020): 1, https://doi.org/10.3167/th.2020.6716201, page 2.

2 Merriam-Webster, *Merriam-Webster's Intermediate Dictionary* (Springfield, MA: Merriam-Webster, 2020).

3 Tom L. Beauchamp and James F. Childress, *Principles of Biomedical Ethics*, eighth edition (New York: Oxford University Press, 2019), page 157.

4 Tom L. Beauchamp and James F. Childress, *Principles of Biomedical Ethics*, eighth edition (New York: Oxford University Press, 2019), page 155.

5 Raanan Gillon, "'Primum Non Nocere' and the Principle of Non-Maleficence," *British Medical Journal (Clinical Research Edition)* 291, no. 6488 (July 13, 1985): 130–131, page 130.

6 Paul A. Baker, Britta S. Ungern-Sternberg, and Thomas Engelhardt, "Primum Non Nocere ('first Do No Harm') with Oxygen Therapy," *Pediatric Anesthesia* 32, no. 2 (February 1, 2022): 101, https://doi.org/10.1111/pan.14367, page 101.

7 Majid Bassuni and Ahmed-Hazem Helmy, "'Primum Non Nocere'—First Do No Harm—in the Time of SARS-CoV-2/COVID-19 Pandemic.," *Egyptian Journal of Surgery* 39, no. 3 (July 2020): 513–514, page 513.

8 Marco T. Medina and Sir Salvador Moncada, "Hydroxychloroquine/ Chloroquine as a Treatment Choice or Prophylaxis for Covid-19 at the Primary Care Level in Developing Countries: A Primum Non Nocere Dilemma," *Journal of the Neurological Sciences* 415 (August 15, 2020), page 1.

9 Miquel Vives-Borràs and Alessandro Sionis, "Elderly Patients with Comorbidities and Acute Coronary Syndrome: Primum Non Nocere?," *REC: Interventional Cardiology (English Ed.)* 3, no. 1 (February 1, 2021): 3–4, https://doi.org/10.24875/RECICE.M20000167, page 3.

10 Gregorio Stratta et al., "Multidisciplinary Management of Breast Cancer in a 103 Years Old Patient: The Ultimate 'Primum Non Nocere' Challenge," *Aging and Health Research* 1, no. 4 (December 1, 2021), page 1.

11 Philippe Hernigou, "Primum Non Nocere: Is It Really True with Corticosteroid Hip Injections?: Commentary on an Article by Kanu Okike, MD, MPH, et al.: 'Rapidly Destructive Hip Disease Following Intra-Articular Corticosteroid Injection of the Hip'," *Journal of Bone & Joint Surgery, American Volume* 103, no. 22 (November 17, 2021): e92.

12 Mike van der Have and Jeroen Maljaars, "Editorial: Opioids in Inflammatory Bowel Disease-Primum Non Nocere.," *Alimentary Pharmacology & Therapeutics* 53, no. 7 (April 2021): 844–845, https://doi.org/10.1111/apt.16286, page 844.

13 Raanan Gillon, "'Primum Non Nocere' and the Principle of Non-Maleficence," *British Medical Journal (Clinical Research Edition)* 291, no. 6488 (July 13, 1985): 130–131, page 131.

14 Eli A. Gordin et al., "Care in the Time of Coronavirus: Ethical Considerations in Head and Neck Oncology," *Head & Neck* 42, no. 7 (July 2020): 1519–1525, https://doi.org/10.1002/hed.26272, page 1521.

15 Maria Cherba et al., "Framing Concerns about Body Image during Pre- and Post-Surgical Consultations for Head and Neck Cancer: A Qualitative Study of Patient–Physician Interactions," *Current Oncology* 29, no. 5 (May 5, 2022): 3341–3363, https://doi.org/10.3390/curroncol29050272, page 3342.

16 Vittorio Bufacchi, "Justice as Non-Maleficence," *Theoria* 67, no. 1 (March 1, 2020): 1, https://doi.org/10.3167/th.2020.6716201, page 6.

17 Olivia Olson, Corinne Berry, and Nirbhay Kumar, "Addressing Parental Vaccine Hesitancy towards Childhood Vaccines in the United States: A Systematic Literature Review of Communication Interventions and Strategies," 2020, https://hsrc.himmelfarb.gwu.edu/sphhs_global_facpubs/543.

18 Nirbachita Biswas et al., "The Nature and Extent of COVID-19 Vaccination Hesitancy in Healthcare Workers," *Journal of Community Health* 46, no. 6 (December 2021): 1244–1251, https://doi.org/10.1007/s10900-021-00984-3, page 1244.

19 Nirbachita Biswas et al., "The Nature and Extent of COVID-19 Vaccination Hesitancy in Healthcare Workers," *Journal of Community Health* 46, no. 6 (December 2021): 1244–1251, https://doi.org/10.1007/s10900-021-00984-3, page 1250.

20 Daniel Sokol, "Covid-19 Vaccination Should Be Mandatory for Healthcare Workers," *BMJ*, November 2, 2021, n2670, https://doi.org/10.1136/bmj.n2670, page 1.

21 Ezekiel J. Emanuel and David J. Skorton, "Mandating COVID-19 Vaccination for Health Care Workers.," *Annals of Internal Medicine* 174, no. 9 (September 2021): 1308–1310, https://doi.org/10.7326/M21–3150, page 1310.

22 Ezekiel J. Emanuel and David J. Skorton, "Mandating COVID-19 Vaccination for Health Care Workers.," *Annals of Internal Medicine* 174, no. 9 (September 2021): 1308–1310, https://doi.org/10.7326/M21–3150, page 1308.

23 Philipp Sprengholz et al., "Vaccination Policy Reactance: Predictors, Consequences, and Countermeasures," *Journal of Health Psychology* 27, no. 6 (May 2022): 1394–1407, https://doi.org/10.1177/13591053211044535, page 1405.

24 Samuel J. Skidmore and Sharon E. Robinson Kurpius, "Euthanasia in an Aging America: An Ethical Challenge for Mental Health Counselors," *Journal of Mental Health Counseling* 43, no. 2 (April 1, 2021): 125–138, https://doi.org/10.17744/mehc.43.2.03, page 125.

25 David F. Kelly, Gerard Magill, and H. ten Have, *Contemporary Catholic Health Care Ethics*, 2nd ed (Washington, DC: Georgetown University Press, 2013), page 64.

26 Vittorio Bufacchi, "Justice as Non-Maleficence," *Theoria* 67, no. 1 (March 1, 2020): 1, https://doi.org/10.3167/th.2020.6716201, page 11.

27 Vittorio Bufacchi, "Justice as Non-Maleficence," *Theoria* 67, no. 1 (March 1, 2020): 1, https://doi.org/10.3167/th.2020.6716201, page 15.

28 Talia K. Ben-Jacob and Lars-Kristofer N. Peterson, "Drastic Changes in the Practice of End-of-Life Care during the COVID-19 Pandemic," *Journal of Critical Care* 67 (February 1, 2022): 195–197.

29 Linda T. Kohn, Janet Corrigan, and Molla S. Donaldson, *To Err Is Human: Building a Safer Health System*, 2000, http://site.ebrary.com/id/10038653, page ix.

30 Viessman, Sara S, "New CME Requirements for Pennsylvania Physicians," *Lehigh Valley Medical Staff Progress Notes* 18, no. 11 (November 2004): 1.

31 J. Bauer Horton, Jeffrey E. Janis, and Rod J. Rohrich, "MOC-PS(SM) CME Article: Patient Safety in the Office-Based Setting:," *Plastic and Reconstructive Surgery* 122, no. Supplement (September 2008): 1–21, https://doi.org/10.1097/PRS.0b013e318183c118, page 1.

32 Harris Meyer, "Hospitals Fall Short of Patient-Safety Goals 20 Years after 'To Err Is Human,'" *Modern Healthcare*, November 11, 2019.

33 Dalia Sofer, "Is a Medical Mistake an Error or a Crime?," *AJN American Journal of Nursing* 119, no. 5 (May 2019): 12.

34 Alan C. Horowitz, "Medication Errors and Homicide: When Law and Medicine Collide," *Caring for the Ages* 23, no. 5 (June 2022): 1–3, https://doi.org/10.1016/j.carage.2022.04.033.

35 Dalia Sofer, "Is a Medical Mistake an Error or a Crime?," *AJN American Journal of Nursing* 119, no. 5 (May 2019): 12.

36 Linda Laskowski-Jones, "Fatal Flaws.," *Nursing*, June 2022, 6.

37 Linda Laskowski-Jones, "Fatal Flaws.," *Nursing*, June 2022, 6.

38 Brett Kelman and Hannah Norman, "Why Nurses Are Raging and Quitting After the RaDonda Vaught Verdict.," *Biomedical Safety & Standards*, June 15, 2022, 81–83.

39 Alan C. Horowitz, "Medication Errors and Homicide: When Law and Medicine Collide," *Caring for the Ages* 23, no. 5 (June 2022): 1–3, https://doi.org/10.1016/j.carage.2022.04.033.

40 Brett Kelman and Hannah Norman, "Why Nurses Are Raging and Quitting After the RaDonda Vaught Verdict.," *Biomedical Safety & Standards*, June 15, 2022, 81–83.

41 Ann E. Marimow, "Supreme Court Sides with Doctors Convicted of Overprescribing Opioids," *The Washington Post*, June 28, 2022.

42 Craig S. Webster, "Existing Knowledge of Medication Error Must Be Better Translated Into Improved Patient Safety," *Frontiers in Medicine* 9 (2022): 870587, https://doi.org/10.3389/fmed.2022.870587.

43 Melissa D. McCradden et al., "Patient Safety and Quality Improvement: Ethical Principles for a Regulatory Approach to Bias in Healthcare Machine Learning.," *Journal of the American Medical Informatics Association* 27, no. 12 (December 2020): 2024–2027, page 2025.

44 Harris Meyer, "Hospitals Fall Short of Patient-Safety Goals 20 Years after 'To Err Is Human,'" *Modern Healthcare*, November 11, 2019.

45 Sonal Arora et al, "Patient Safety Education 20 Years After the Institute of Medicine Report: Results From a Cross-Sectional National Survey," *Journal of Patient Safety* 17, no. 8 (December 2021): 1884–1888, page 1885.

46 Charles Vincent, *Patient Safety*, second edition (Chichester: Wiley-Blackwell, 2010).

47 Linda T. Kohn, Janet Corrigan, and Molla S. Donaldson, *To Err Is Human: Building a Safer Health System*, 2000, http://site.ebrary.com/id/10038653, page 36.

48 Rebecca L. Jessup and Rachelle Buchbinder, "What If I Cannot Choose Wisely? Addressing Suboptimal Health Literacy in Our Patients to Reduce over-Diagnosis and Overtreatment:

Health Literacy and Too Much Medicine," *Internal Medicine Journal* 48, no. 9 (September 2018): 1154–1157, https://doi.org/10.1111/imj.14025.page 1156.

49 Christopher Moriates et al., "The Value in the Evidence: Teaching Residents to 'Choose Wisely,'" *JAMA Internal Medicine* 173, no. 4 (February 25, 2013), https://doi.org/10.1001/jamainternmed.2013.2286, page 308.

50 Linda T. Kohn, Janet Corrigan, and Molla S. Donaldson, *To Err Is Human: Building a Safer Health System*, 2000, http://site.ebrary.com/id/10038653, page 132.

51 Agani Afaya, Kennedy Diema Konlan, and Hyunok Kim Do, "Improving Patient Safety through Identifying Barriers to Reporting Medication Administration Errors among Nurses: An Integrative Review," *BMC Health Services Research* 21, no. 1 (December 1, 2021), https://doi.org/10.1186/s12913-021-07187-5, page 2.

52 Jennifer L. Cole, "Why the USA Should 'Drop the Pounds' to Improve Patient Safety in Adults," *Drugs & Therapy Perspectives* 36, no. 2 (February 1, 2020): 67–68, https://doi.org/10.1007/s40267-019-00703-y, page 68.

53 Yujeong Kim and Eunmi Lee, "The Relationship between the Perception of Open Disclosure of Patient Safety Incidents, Perception of Patient Safety Culture, and Ethical Awareness in Nurses," *BMC Medical Ethics* 21, no. 1 (October 27, 2020), https://doi.org/10.1186/s12910-020-00546-7, page 8.

54 Ranielle de Lima Silva Nunes et al., "Factors Influencing the Patient Safety Climate in Intensive Care Units: Cross-Sectional Study," *BMC Nursing* 20, no. 1 (December 1, 2021), https://doi.org/10.1186/s12912-021-00643-x, page 7.

55 Linda Laskowski-Jones, "Fatal Flaws.," *Nursing*, June 2022, 6.

56 Amrita Shenoy, "Patient Safety from the Perspective of Quality Management Frameworks: A Review," *Patient Safety in Surgery* 15, no. 1 (December 1, 2021), https://doi.org/10.1186/s13037-021-00286-6, page 8.

57 J. Bauer Horton, Jeffrey E. Janis, and Rod J. Rohrich, "MOC-PS(SM) CME Article: Patient Safety in the Office-Based Setting:," *Plastic and Reconstructive Surgery* 122, no. Supplement (September 2008): 1–21, https://doi.org/10.1097/PRS.0b013e318183c118, pages 1–21.

58 Pius Cavanaugh, *The Life of the Angelic Doctor St. Thomas Aquinas* (New York: P.J. Kenedy and Sons, 1881).

59 Anna Bogatyńska-Kucharska, "The Doctrine of Double Effect: A Comparison of the Version of Thomas Aquinas and Contemporary Accounts as Formulated by Joseph Mangan and Joseph Boyle," *Forum Philosophicum* 25, no. 2 (December 4, 2020): 273–292, https://doi.org/10.35765/forphil.2020.2502.18, page 275.

60 Raanan Gillon, "The Principle of Double Effect and Medical Ethics," *BMJ* 292, no. 6514 (January 18, 1986): 193–194, https://doi.org/10.1136/bmj.292.6514.193, page 193.

61 Bernard G. Prusak, "Double Effect, All over Again: The Case of Sister Margaret McBride," *Theoretical Medicine and Bioethics* 32, no. 4 (August 2011): 271–283, https://doi.org/10.1007/s11017-011-9183-z, page 275.

62 James F. Keenan, "The Function of the Principle of Double Effect," *Theological Studies* 54, no. 2 (June 1993): 294–315, page 300.

63 Albert R. Jonsen, *A Short History of Medical Ethics* (New York: Oxford University Press, 2000), page 49.

64 Anna Bogatyńska-Kucharska, "The Doctrine of Double Effect: A Comparison of the Version of Thomas Aquinas and Contemporary Accounts as Formulated by Joseph Mangan and Joseph Boyle," *Forum Philosophicum* 25, no. 2 (December 4, 2020): 273–292, https://doi.org/10.35765/forphil.2020.2502.18, page 274.

65 Tom L. Beauchamp and James F. Childress, *Principles of Biomedical Ethics*, eighth edition (New York: Oxford University Press, 2019), page 170.

66 Raanan Gillon, "The Principle of Double Effect and Medical Ethics," *BMJ* 292, no. 6514 (January 18, 1986): 193–194, https://doi.org/10.1136/bmj.292.6514.193, page 193.

67 P. A. Reed, "The Danger of Double Effect," *Christian Bioethics* 18, no. 3 (December 1, 2012): 287–300, https://doi.org/10.1093/cb/cbs021, page 290.

68 Daniel F Montaldi, "A Defense of St Thomas and the Principle of Double Effect," *Journal of Religious Ethics* 14, no. 2 (1986): 296–332, page 322.

69 Albert R. Jonsen, *A Short History of Medical Ethics* (New York: Oxford University Press, 2000), pages 49–50.

70 Nina Totenberg and Sarah McCammon, "Supreme Court Overturns Roe v. Wade, Ending Right to Abortion Upheld for Decades," *NPR*, June 24, 2022, sec. *Roe v. Wade* and the future of reproductive rights in America, www.npr.org/2022/06/24/1102305878/supreme-court-abortion-roe-v-wade-decision-overturn.

71 United States Conference of Catholic Bishops, *Ethical and Religious Directives for Catholic Health Care Services*, sixth edition (Washington, DC: United States Conference of Catholic Bishops, June 2018).

72 Amrita Shenoy, Gopinath N. Shenoy, and Gayatri G. Shenoy, "The Impact of EMTALA on Medical Malpractice Framework Models: A Review," *Patient Safety in Surgery* 16, no. 1 (December 2022): 21, https://doi.org/10.1186/s13037-022-00325-w, page 1.

73 Stephen R. Latham, "US Lawsuit Claims Federal Law Can Require Emergency Abortions," *Hastings Center Report* 52, no. 5 (September 2022): 4–5, https://doi.org/10.1002/hast.1414, page 4.

74 Raanan Gillon, "The Principle of Double Effect and Medical Ethics," *BMJ* 292, no. 6514 (January 18, 1986): 193–194, https://doi.org/10.1136/bmj.292.6514.193.

75 C. S. Lewis, "Beyond Personality—Mere Men," BBC Home Service radio broadcast, March 21, 1944.

76 Rita Rubin et al., "How Caring for Patients Could Change in a Post-*Roe v Wade* US," *JAMA* 327, no. 21 (June 7, 2022): 2060–2062.

77 United States Conference of Catholic Bishops, *Ethical and Religious Directives for Catholic Health Care Services*, sixth edition (Washington, DC: United States Conference of Catholic Bishops, June 2018).

78 Joseph J. Piccione, "An Exploration of the ERD, Fourth Edition Ethical and Religious Directives for Catholic Health Care Services," *The Journal of the Association of Professional Chaplains* 17, no. 1 (Summer 2001): 22–34, page 10.

79 Rita Rubin et al., "How Caring for Patients Could Change in a Post-*Roe v Wade* US," *JAMA* 327, no. 21 (June 7, 2022): 2060–2062.

80 Anna Glasier, "Emergency Contraception: Clinical Outcomes," *Contraception* 87, no. 3 (March 2013): 309–313, https://doi.org/10.1016/j.contraception.2012.08.027, page 309.

81 Rebecca Stangl, "Plan B and the Doctrine of Double Effect," *Hastings Center Report* 39, no. 4 (2009): 21–25, https://doi.org/10.1353/hcr.0.0162, page 24.

82 Praveena Somasundaram, "Explainer: What's next for Abortion Pills after the Fall of Roe.," *The Washington Post*, July 9, 2022.

83 Murray Joseph Casey and Todd A. Salzman, "Therapeutic, Prophylactic, Untoward, and Contraceptive Effects of Combined Oral Contraceptives: Catholic Teaching, Natural Law, and the Principle of Double Effect When Deciding to Prescribe and Use," *American Journal of Bioethics* 14, no. 7 (July 1, 2014): 20–34, page 26.

84 Joseph J. Piccione, "An Exploration of the ERD, Fourth Edition Ethical and Religious Directives for Catholic Health Care Services," *The Journal of the Association of Professional Chaplains* 17, no. 1 (Summer 2001): 22–34.

85 Glenn Kessler, "The Claim That 98 Percent of Catholic Women Use Contraception: A Media Foul," *The Washington Post*, February 17, 2012.

86 Rebecca Stangl, "Plan B and the Doctrine of Double Effect," *Hastings Center Report* 39, no. 4 (2009): 21–25, https://doi.org/10.1353/hcr.0.0162, page 24.

87 Rebecca Stangl, "Plan B and the Doctrine of Double Effect," *Hastings Center Report* 39, no. 4 (2009): 21–25, https://doi.org/10.1353/hcr.0.0162, page 23.

88 Joseph J. Piccione, "An Exploration of the ERD, Fourth Edition Ethical and Religious Directives for Catholic Health Care Services," *The Journal of the Association of Professional Chaplains* 17, no. 1 (Summer 2001): 22–34.

89 Jenny Ponzo, "Motherhood and Personhood: The Canonization of Gianna Beretta Molla and the Figurativization of Catholic Norms," *International Journal for the Semiotics of Law—Revue Internationale de Sémiotique Juridique*, February 5, 2021, https://doi.org/10.1007/s11196-020-09813-7, page 72.

90 Joseph J. Piccione, "An Exploration of the ERD, Fourth Edition: Ethical and Religious Directives for Catholic Health Care Services," *Chaplaincy Today* 17, no. 1 (2001): 22–34.

91 Irene Alexander, "Redefining Direct and Indirect Abortions through 'The Perspective of the Acting Person': A Misreading of *Veritatis Splendor*," *The Linacre Quarterly* 86, no. 1 (February 2019): 28–46, https://doi.org/10.1177/0024363919838852, page 29.

92 Michael Clancy, "Bishop Says Nun Excommunicated for Allowing Abortion," *National Catholic Reporter* 46, no. 16 (May 28, 2010): 1, 12.

93 Sheila Krishnan et al., "Pulmonary Hypertension Complicating Pregnancy," *Current Pulmonology Reports* 10, no. 2 (June 1, 2021): 71–83, https://doi.org/10.1007/s13665-021-00275-1, page 71.

94 Sheila Krishnan et al., "Pulmonary Hypertension Complicating Pregnancy," *Current Pulmonology Reports* 10, no. 2 (June 1, 2021): 71–83, https://doi.org/10.1007/s13665-021-00275-1, page 75.

95 Stephanie R. Martin and Alexandra Edwards, "Pulmonary Hypertension and Pregnancy.," *Obstetrics & Gynecology* 134, no. 5 (November 2019): 974–987, pages 982–983.

96 Michael Clancy, "Bishop Says Nun Excommunicated for Allowing Abortion," *National Catholic Reporter* 46, no. 16 (May 28, 2010): 1, 12.

97 Tom Roberts, "Ethicists Fault Bishop's Action in Phoenix Abortion Case," *National Catholic Reporter* 46, no. 17 (n.d.): 1, 12–13.

98 Gerard Magill, "Threat of Imminent Death in Pregnancy: A Role for Double-Effect Reasoning," *Theological Studies* 72, no. 4 (December 2011): 848–878, page 878.

99 John F. Tuohey, "A Fatal Conflict: Can Catholic Hospitals Refuse to Save Lives?," *Commonweal* 138 (January 28, 2011), page 10.

100 J. P. Slosar, "Pregnancy Complications Can Bring on Complex Ethical Questions," *Catholic Health World* 26, no. 21 (2010).

101 Marge Berer, "Termination of Pregnancy as Emergency Obstetric Care: The Interpretation of Catholic Health Policy and the Consequences for Pregnant Women: *An Analysis of the Death of Savita Halappanavar in Ireland and Similar Cases*," *Reproductive Health Matters* 21, no. 41 (January 2013): 9–17, https://doi.org/10.1016/S0968–8080(13)41711-1.

102 C. A. Gearty, "Could Ireland Have Saved Savita?," *The Tablet* 266, no. 8974 (November 24, 2012): 12–13.

103 María Fernanda Escobar et al., "Maternal Sepsis," *American Journal of Obstetrics & Gynecology MFM* 2, no. 3 (August 2020): 100149, https://doi.org/10.1016/j.ajogmf.2020.100149.

104 Marge Berer, "Termination of Pregnancy as Emergency Obstetric Care: The Interpretation of Catholic Health Policy and the Consequences for Pregnant Women: *An Analysis of the Death of Savita Halappanavar in Ireland and Similar Cases*," *Reproductive Health Matters* 21, no. 41 (January 2013): 9–17, https://doi.org/10.1016/S0968–8080(13)41711-1.

105 Marge Berer, "Termination of Pregnancy as Emergency Obstetric Care: The Interpretation of Catholic Health Policy and the Consequences for Pregnant Women: *An Analysis of the Death of Savita Halappanavar in Ireland and Similar Cases*," *Reproductive Health Matters* 21, no. 41 (January 2013): 9–17, https://doi.org/10.1016/S0968–8080(13)41711-1.

106 J. P. Slosar, "Pregnancy Complications Can Bring on Complex Ethical Questions," *Catholic Health World* 26, no. 21 (2010).

107 Gerald D. Coleman S. S., "Direct and Indirect Abortion in the Roman Catholic Tradition: A Review of the Phoenix Case," *HEC Forum: HealthCare Ethics Committee Forum: An Interprofessional Journal on Healthcare Institutions' Ethical and Legal Issues* 25, no. 2 (June 1, 2013): 127–143, https://doi.org/10.1007/s10730-013-9211–7, page 142.

108 Orla McDonnell and Padraig Murphy, "Mediating Abortion Politics in Ireland: Media Framing of the Death of Savita Halappanavar," *Critical Discourse Studies* 16, no. 1 (January 2019): 1–20, https://doi.org/10.1080/17405904.2018.1521858.

109 Lisa Zilinski, "Sister Margaret McBride," *Carnegie Mellon University Research Showcase*, January 2013.

110 Jordan G. Potter, "The Principle of Double Effect in End-of-Life Care," *The National Catholic Bioethics Quarterly* 15, no. 3 (2015): 515–529, page 515.

111 Merriam-Webster, *Merriam-Webster's Intermediate Dictionary* (Springfield, MA: Merriam-Webster, 2020).

112 Jordan G. Potter, "The Principle of Double Effect in End-of-Life Care," *The National Catholic Bioethics Quarterly* 15, no. 3 (2015): 515–529, page 519

113 David F. Kelly, Gerard Magill, and H. ten Have, *Contemporary Catholic Health Care Ethics.*, Second edition. (Georgetown University Press, 2013), page 213

114 Ajay Kumar et al., "Euthanasia: A Debate—For and Against," *Journal of Postgraduate Medicine, Education and Research,* 55, no. 2 (June 2021): 91–96.

115 Jordan G. Potter, "The Principle of Double Effect in End-of-Life Care," *The National Catholic Bioethics Quarterly* 15, no. 3 (2015): 515–529.

116 Raphael Cohen-Almagor, "First Do No Harm: Intentionally Shortening Lives of Patients without Their Explicit Request in Belgium," *Journal of Medical Ethics* 41, no. 8 (August 2015): 625–629, https://doi.org/10.1136/medethics-2014–102387, page 626.

117 Raphael Cohen-Almagor, "First Do No Harm: Intentionally Shortening Lives of Patients without Their Explicit Request in Belgium," *Journal of Medical Ethics* 41, no. 8 (August 2015): 625–629, https://doi.org/10.1136/medethics-2014–102387, page 628.

118 Lars Johan Materstvedt and Morten Magelssen, "Medical Murder in Belgium and the Netherlands," *Journal of Medical Ethics* 42, no. 9 (September 2016), page 622.

119 Samuel J. Skidmore and Sharon E. Robinson Kurpius, "Euthanasia in an Aging America: An Ethical Challenge for Mental Health Counselors," *Journal of Mental Health Counseling* 43, no. 2 (April 1, 2021): 125–138, https://doi.org/10.17744/mehc.43.2.03, page 128.

120 Michael B. Gill, "A Moral Defense of Oregon's Physician-Assisted Suicide Law.," *Mortality* 10, no. 1 (February 2005): 53–67, page 53.

121 Patients Rights Council, "Assisted Suicide Laws in the United States," accessed August 22, 2022, www.patientsrightscouncil.org/site/assisted-suicide-state-laws.

122 Sean Baker and Kimberly A. Lauffer, "DC-Based Religious and Secular Media Coverage of the District's Death with Dignity Act," *Journal of Media and Religion* 18, no. 3 (July 3, 2019): 75–84, https://doi.org/10.1080/15348423.2019.1678944, page 76.

123 Jordan G. Potter, "The Principle of Double Effect in End-of-Life Care," *The National Catholic Bioethics Quarterly* 15, no. 3 (2015): 515–529, page 520.

124 Peter A. DePergola, "Euthanasia, Assisted-Suicide, and Palliative Sedation: A Brief Clarification and Reinforcement of the Moral Logic," *Online Journal of Health Ethics* 14, no. 2 (November 1, 2018), https://doi.org/10.18785/ojhe.1402.04, page 6.

125 David F. Kelly, *Medical Care at the End of Life : A Catholic Perspective*, 1st ed. (Georgetown University Press, 2006), page 22.

126 Jordan G. Potter, "The Principle of Double Effect in End-of-Life Care," *The National Catholic Bioethics Quarterly* 15, no. 3 (2015): 515–529, page 519.

127 Jordan G. Potter, "The Principle of Double Effect in End-of-Life Care," *The National Catholic Bioethics Quarterly* 15, no. 3 (2015): 515–529, page 523.

128 James F. Childress, "Non-Heart-Beating Donors of Organs: Are the Distinctions Between Direct and Indirect Effects & Between Killing and Letting Die Relevant and Helpful?," *Kennedy Institute of Ethics Journal* 3, no. 2 (1993): 203–216, https://doi.org/10.1353/ken.0.0014, page 205.

129 David F. Kelly, *Medical Care at the End of Life : A Catholic Perspective*, 1st ed. (Georgetown University Press, 2006), page 13.

130 David F. Kelly, *Medical Care at the End of Life : A Catholic Perspective*, 1st ed. (Georgetown University Press, 2006).

131 Ian Fisher, "A Poet Crusades for the Right to Die His Way," *The New York Times*, December 20, 2006.

132 Wikipedia, "Piergiorgio Welby," accessed April 7, 2024, https://en.wikipedia.org/wiki/Piergiorgio_Welby.

133 Ian Fisher, "A Poet Crusades for the Right to Die His Way," *The New York Times*, December 20, 2006.

134 Hannah B. Martin and Daryl F. Sas, "Autonomy vs. Selflessness at the End of Life," *Ethics & Medicine: An International Journal of Bioethics* 31, no. 2 (June 22, 2015): 109.

135 Hannah B. Martin and Daryl F. Sas, "Autonomy vs. Selflessness at the End of Life," *Ethics & Medicine: An International Journal of Bioethics* 31, no. 2 (June 22, 2015): 109.

136 Daniel P. Sulmasy, "Death and Dignity in Catholic Christian Thought," *Medicine, Health Care and Philosophy* 20, no. 4 (December 2017): 537–543, https://doi.org/10.1007/s11019-016-9690–9.

137 Maura A. Flood, "Treatment of the Vegetative Patient: The Legacies of Karen Quinlan, Nancy Cruzan and Terri Schiavo," *J. Health & Biomedical L. 1 (2005) / Journal of Health & Biomedical Law* 1, no. 2 (2005): 1–48, page 10.

138 Norman N. Cantor, "'In the Matter of Karen Quinlan': A Comment," *BioScience* 26, no. 4 (April 1, 1976): 257–259, https://doi.org/10.2307/1297348.

139 Maura A. Flood, "Treatment of the Vegetative Patient: The Legacies of Karen Quinlan, Nancy Cruzan and Terri Schiavo," *J. Health & Biomedical L. 1 (2005) / Journal of Health & Biomedical Law* 1, no. 2 (2005): 1–48, pages 12–14.

140 Maura A. Flood, "Treatment of the Vegetative Patient: The Legacies of Karen Quinlan, Nancy Cruzan and Terri Schiavo," *J. Health & Biomedical L. 1 (2005) / Journal of Health & Biomedical Law* 1, no. 2 (2005): 1–48, page 14–15.

141 Michael A. Vaccari, "Artificial Respiration and AHN: Some Similarities and Differences," *The Linacre Quarterly* 59 (May 1992): 48–62, pages 50–51.

142 Andrea Z. Pereira et al., "The Difficult Decision Not to Prescribe Artificial Nutrition by Health Professionals and Family: Bioethical Aspects," *Frontiers in Nutrition* 9 (March 3, 2022): 781540, https://doi.org/10.3389/fnut.2022.781540, page 3.

143 Marianna Chaves, "Advance Directives: The Consecration of Autonomy and Dignity of the Human Being," *Medicine and Law* 32, no. 4 (2013): 515–524.

144 "2006 Act 169" (Pennsylvania General Assembly, 2006), www.legis.state.pa.us/cfdocs/Legis/LI/uconsCheck.cfm?txtType=HTM&yr=2006&sessInd=0&smthLwInd=0&act=169.

145 Sayuri Yokota et al., "Effects of Artificial Nutrition and Hydration on Survival in Patients with Head and Neck Cancer and Esophageal Cancer Admitted to Palliative Care Units," *Clinical Nutrition Open Science* 41 (February 2022): 33–43, https://doi.org/10.1016/j.nutos.2021.11.008.

146 Alexandria J. Bear, Elizabeth A. Bukowy, and Jayshil J. Patel, "Artificial Hydration at the End of Life," *Nutrition in Clinical Practice* 32, no. 5 (October 2017): 628–632, https://doi.org/10.1177/0884533617724741.

147 J. Blandford, "An Examination of the Revisionist Challenge to the Catholic Tradition on Providing Artificial Nutrition and Hydration to Patients in a Persistent Vegetative State," *Christian Bioethics* 17, no. 2 (August 1, 2011): 153–164, https://doi.org/10.1093/cb/cbr013.

148 J. Blandford, "An Examination of the Revisionist Challenge to the Catholic Tradition on Providing Artificial Nutrition and Hydration to Patients in a Persistent Vegetative State," *Christian Bioethics* 17, no. 2 (August 1, 2011): 153–164, https://doi.org/10.1093/cb/cbr013.

149 Archdiocese of Cincinnati, "Catholic Advance Healthcare Directive," https://resources.catholicaoc.org/wpfd_file/catholic-advanced-health-care-directive.

150 Ronald P. Hamel and James J. Walter, eds., *Artificial Nutrition and Hydration and the Permanently Unconscious Patient: The Catholic Debate* (Washington, DC: Georgetown University Press, 2007), page 204.

151 Michael A. Vaccari, "Artificial Respiration and AHN: Some Similarities and Differences," *The Linacre Quarterly* 59 (May 1992): 48–62, page 52.

152 David M. Zientek, "Artificial Nutrition and Hydration in Catholic Healthcare: Balancing Tradition, Recent Teaching, and Law," *HEC Forum* 25, no. 2 (June 2013): 145–159, https://doi.org/10.1007/s10730-013-9214-4.

153 Ronald P. Hamel and James J. Walter, eds., *Artificial Nutrition and Hydration and the Permanently Unconscious Patient: The Catholic Debate* (Washington, DC: Georgetown University Press, 2007), page 204.

154 Timothy E. Quill, Rebecca Dresser, and Dan W. Brock, "The Rule of Double Effect—A Critique of Its Role in End-of-Life Decision Making," *New England Journal of Medicine* 337, no. 24 (December 11, 1997): 1768–1771, https://doi.org/10.1056/NEJM199712113372413, page 1768–1769.

155 "Dr. William S. Husel Indicted for 25 Counts of Murder in Mount Carmel Hospital Patient Deaths. —Franklin County Prosecutor's Office," accessed August 26, 2022, https://prosecutor.franklincountyohio.gov/press-releases/1381.

156 Owen Dyer, "Ohio Doctor Is Charged with 25 Counts of Murder over Patients' Deaths," *BMJ*, June 11, 2019, l4170, https://doi.org/10.1136/bmj.l4170.

157 "Nurses Defend Ohio Doctor Accused of Murdering 25 Patients in Lawsuit against Hospital," accessed November 20, 2020, www.nbcnews.com/news/crime-courts/nurses-defend-ohio-doctor-accused-murdering-25-patients-lawsuit-against-n1102796.

158 "Nurses Defend Ohio Doctor Accused of Murdering 25 Patients in Lawsuit against Hospital," accessed November 20, 2020, www.nbcnews.com/news/crime-courts/nurses-defend-ohio-doctor-accused-murdering-25-patients-lawsuit-against-n1102796.

159 Margaret L. Campbell, Katherine K. Kero, and Thomas N. Templin, "Mild, Moderate, and Severe Intensity Cut-Points for the Respiratory Distress Observation Scale," *Heart & Lung—The Journal of Acute and Critical Care* 46, no. 1 (January 1, 2017): 14–17.

160 Qingyuan Zhuang et al., "Validity, Reliability, and Diagnostic Accuracy of the Respiratory Distress Observation Scale for Assessment of Dyspnea in Adult Palliative Care Patients," *Journal of Pain and Symptom Management* 57, no. 2 (February 2019): 304–310, https://doi.org/10.1016/j.jpainsymman.2018.10.506.

161 Mark A. Mazer, Chad M. Alligood, and Qiang Wu, "The Infusion of Opioids During Terminal Withdrawal of Mechanical Ventilation in the Medical Intensive Care Unit," *Journal of Pain and Symptom Management* 42, no. 1 (January 1, 2011): 44–51.

162 "Ohio Doctor Charged with 25 Murders Sues Hospital for Defamation," accessed November 20, 2020, www.nbcnews.com/news/us-news/ohio-doctor-charged-25-murders-sues-hospital-defamation-n1108291.

163 "Hearing Delayed on Motion to Dismiss Murder Charges against Ex-Mount Carmel Doctor" (Columbus, Ohio: 10 WBNS, October 20, 2020).

164 Steve Helling, "Why Did a Jury Acquit Dr. William Husel on 14 Murder Charges?," accessed August 26, 2022, https://people.com/crime/william-husel-doctor-accused-overdosing-patients-not-guilty.

165 Y. Tony Yang and Rebecca L. Haffajee, "Murder Liability for Prescribing Opioids: A Way Forward?," *Mayo Clinic Proceedings* 91, no. 10 (October 2016): 1331–1335, https://doi.org/10.1016/j.mayocp.2016.06.018.

166 Timothy E. Quill, Rebecca Dresser, and Dan W. Brock, "The Rule of Double Effect—A Critique of Its Role in End-of-Life Decision Making," *New England Journal of Medicine* 337, no. 24 (December 11, 1997): 1768–1771, https://doi.org/10.1056/NEJM199712113372413, page 1770–1771.

167 Robert Macauley, "The Role of the Principle of Double Effect in Ethics Education at US Medical Schools and Its Potential Impact on Pain Management at the End of Life," *Journal of Medical Ethics* 38, no. 3 (March 2012): 174–178, https://doi.org/10.1136/medethics-2011–100105, page 176.

168 Peter T. Hetzler et al., "A Report of Physicians' Beliefs about Physician-Assisted Suicide: A National Study," *Yale Journal of Biology and Medicine* 92, no. 4 (December 20, 2019), page 579.

169 Dana L. Abraham et al., "Association between Opioid Dose Escalation and Time to Death in a Comfort Measures Only Population," *American Journal of Health-System Pharmacy* 78, no. 3 (January 22, 2021): 203–209, https://doi.org/10.1093/ajhp/zxaa367, page 107.

170 Guy Schofield et al., "Palliative Opioid Use, Palliative Sedation and Euthanasia: Reaffirming the Distinction," *Journal of Medical Ethics* 46, no. 1 (January 2020): 48–50, https://doi.org/10.1136/medethics-2018–105256, page 49.

171 Robert Macauley, "The Role of the Principle of Double Effect in Ethics Education at US Medical Schools and Its Potential Impact on Pain Management at the End of Life," *Journal of Medical Ethics* 38, no. 3 (March 2012): 174–178, https://doi.org/10.1136/medethics-2011–100105, page 176.

172 Bernard Lo and Gordon Rubenfeld, "Palliative Sedation in Dying Patients: 'We Turn to It When Everything Else Hasn't Worked,'" *JAMA* 294, no. 14 (October 12, 2005), https://doi.org/10.1001/jama.294.14.1810, page 1812.

173 M. Maltoni et al., "Palliative Sedation Therapy Does Not Hasten Death: Results from a Prospective Multicenter Study," *Annals of Oncology* 20, no. 7 (July 1, 2009): 1163–1169, page 1168.

174 Jordan Potter, Steven Shields, and Renée Breen, "Palliative Sedation, Compassionate Extubation, and the Principle of Double Effect: An Ethical Analysis.," *American Journal of Hospice & Palliative Medicine* 38, no. 12 (December 2021): 1536–1540, https://doi.org/10.1177/1049909121998630, page 1536.

175 Jordan Potter, Steven Shields, and Renée Breen, "Palliative Sedation, Compassionate Extubation, and the Principle of Double Effect: An Ethical Analysis.," *American Journal of Hospice & Palliative Medicine* 38, no. 12 (December 2021): 1536–1540, https://doi.org/10.1177/1049909121998630, page 1538.

176 M. Maltoni et al., "Palliative Sedation Therapy Does Not Hasten Death: Results from a Prospective Multicenter Study," *Annals of Oncology* 20, no. 7 (July 1, 2009): 1163–1169, page 1166.

177 Hannah Faris et al., "Goods, Causes and Intentions: Problems with Applying the Doctrine of Double Effect to Palliative Sedation," *BMC Medical Ethics* 22, no. 1 (December 2021): 141, https://doi.org/10.1186/s12910-021-00709-0, page 5.
178 Gina Maria Noia, "The Principle of Double Effect within Catholic Moral Theology: A Response to Two Criticisms of the Principle in Relation to Palliative Sedation," *Journal of Moral Theology* 6, no. 2 (June 2017): 130–148, page 146.
179 Jordan Potter, Steven Shields, and Renée Breen, "Palliative Sedation, Compassionate Extubation, and the Principle of Double Effect: An Ethical Analysis.," *American Journal of Hospice & Palliative Medicine* 38, no. 12 (December 2021): 1536–1540, https://doi.org/10.1177/1049909121998630, page 1539.
180 Bernard Lo and Gordon Rubenfeld, "Palliative Sedation in Dying Patients: 'We Turn to It When Everything Else Hasn't Worked,'" *JAMA* 294, no. 14 (October 12, 2005), https://doi.org/10.1001/jama.294.14.1810, pages 1814–1815.

BIBLIOGRAPHY

Abraham, Dana L, Inmaculada Hernandez, Gina T. Ayers, and Jennifer A. Pruskowski. "Association between Opioid Dose Escalation and Time to Death in a Comfort Measures Only Population." *American Journal of Health-System Pharmacy* 78, no. 3 (January 22, 2021): 203–209. https://doi.org/10.1093/ajhp/zxaa367.

Afaya, Agani, Kennedy Diema Konlan, and Hyunok Kim Do. "Improving Patient Safety through Identifying Barriers to Reporting Medication Administration Errors among Nurses: An Integrative Review." *BMC Health Services Research* 21, no. 1 (December 1, 2021). https://doi.org/10.1186/s12913-021-07187-5.

Alexander, Irene. "Redefining Direct and Indirect Abortions through 'The Perspective of the Acting Person': A Misreading of *Veritatis Splendor*." *The Linacre Quarterly* 86, no. 1 (February 2019): 28–46. https://doi.org/10.1177/0024363919838852.

Arora, Sonal, et al. "Patient Safety Education 20 Years After the Institute of Medicine Report: Results From a Cross-Sectional National Survey." *Journal of Patient Safety* 17, no. 8 (December 2021): 1884–1888.

Baker, Paul A., Britta S. Ungern-Sternberg, and Thomas Engelhardt. "Primum Non Nocere ('first Do No Harm') with Oxygen Therapy." *Pediatric Anesthesia* 32, no. 2 (February 1, 2022): 101. https://doi.org/10.1111/pan.14367.

Baker, Sean, and Kimberly A. Lauffer. "DC-Based Religious and Secular Media Coverage of the District's Death with Dignity Act." *Journal of Media and Religion* 18, no. 3 (July 3, 2019): 75–84. https://doi.org/10.1080/15348423.2019.1678944.

Bassuni, Majid, and Ahmed-Hazem Helmy. "'Primum Non Nocere'—First Do No Harm—in the Time of SARS-CoV-2/COVID-19 Pandemic." *Egyptian Journal of Surgery* 39, no. 3 (July 2020): 513–514.

Bear, Alexandria J., Elizabeth A. Bukowy, and Jayshil J. Patel. "Artificial Hydration at the End of Life." *Nutrition in Clinical Practice* 32, no. 5 (October 2017): 628–632. https://doi.org/10.1177/0884533617724741.

Beauchamp, Tom L., and James F. Childress. *Principles of Biomedical Ethics*. Eighth edition. New York: Oxford University Press, 2019.

Ben-Jacob, Talia K., and Lars-Kristofer N. Peterson. "Drastic Changes in the Practice of End-of-Life Care during the COVID-19 Pandemic." *Journal of Critical Care* 67 (February 1, 2022): 195–197.

Berer, Marge. "Termination of Pregnancy as Emergency Obstetric Care: The Interpretation of Catholic Health Policy and the Consequences for Pregnant Women: *An Analysis of the Death of Savita Halappanavar in Ireland and Similar Cases*." *Reproductive Health Matters* 21, no. 41 (January 2013): 9–17. https://doi.org/10.1016/S0968-8080(13)41711-1.

Biswas, Nirbachita, Toheeb Mustapha, Jagdish Khubchandani, and James H. Price. "The Nature and Extent of COVID-19 Vaccination Hesitancy in Healthcare Workers." *Journal of Community Health* 46, no. 6 (December 2021): 1244–1251. https://doi.org/10.1007/s10900-021-00984-3.

Blandford, J. "An Examination of the Revisionist Challenge to the Catholic Tradition on Providing Artificial Nutrition and Hydration to Patients in a Persistent Vegetative State." *Christian Bioethics* 17, no. 2 (August 1, 2011): 153–164. https://doi.org/10.1093/cb/cbr013.

Bogatyńska-Kucharska, Anna. "The Doctrine of Double Effect: A Comparison of the Version of Thomas Aquinas and Contemporary Accounts as Formulated by Joseph Mangan and Joseph Boyle." *Forum Philosophicum* 25, no. 2 (December 4, 2020): 273–292. https://doi.org/10.35765/forphil.2020.2502.18.

Bufacchi, Vittorio. "Justice as Non-Maleficence." *Theoria* 67, no. 1 (March 1, 2020): 1. https://doi.org/10.3167/th.2020.6716201.

Campbell, Margaret L., Katherine K. Kero, and Thomas N. Templin. "Mild, Moderate, and Severe Intensity Cut-Points for the Respiratory Distress Observation Scale." *Heart & Lung—The Journal of Acute and Critical Care* 46, no. 1 (January 1, 2017): 14–17.

Cantor, Norman N. "'In the Matter of Karen Quinlan': A Comment." *BioScience* 26, no. 4 (April 1, 1976): 257–259. https://doi.org/10.2307/1297348.

Casey, Murray Joseph, and Todd A. Salzman. "Therapeutic, Prophylactic, Untoward, and Contraceptive Effects of Combined Oral Contraceptives: Catholic Teaching, Natural Law, and the Principle of Double Effect When Deciding to Prescribe and Use." *American Journal of Bioethics* 14, no. 7 (July 1, 2014): 20–34.

Cavanaugh, Pius. *The Life of the Angelic Doctor St. Thomas Aquinas*. No. 44 Barclay Street, NY: P.J. Kennedy and Sons, 1881.

Chaves, Marianna. "Advance Directives: The Consecration of Autonomy and Dignity of the Human Being." *Medicine and Law* 32, no. 4 (2013): 515–524.

Cherba, Maria, Boris H. J. M. Brummans, Michael P. Hier, Lauriane Giguère, Gabrielle Chartier, Hannah Jacobs, Véronique-Isabelle Forest, Alex Mlynarek, Khalil Sultanem, and Melissa Henry. "Framing Concerns about Body Image during Pre- and Post-Surgical Consultations for Head and Neck Cancer: A Qualitative Study of Patient–Physician Interactions." *Current Oncology* 29, no. 5 (May 5, 2022): 3341–3363. https://doi.org/10.3390/curroncol29050272.

Childress, James F. "Non-Heart-Beating Donors of Organs: Are the Distinctions Between Direct and Indirect Effects & Between Killing and Letting Die Relevant and Helpful?" *Kennedy Institute of Ethics Journal* 3, no. 2 (1993): 203–216. https://doi.org/10.1353/ken.0.0014.

Clancy, Michael. "Bishop Says Nun Excommunicated for Allowing Abortion." *National Catholic Reporter* 46, no. 16 (May 28, 2010): 1, 12.

Cohen-Almagor, Raphael. "First Do No Harm: Intentionally Shortening Lives of Patients without Their Explicit Request in Belgium." *Journal of Medical Ethics* 41, no. 8 (August 2015): 625–629. https://doi.org/10.1136/medethics-2014-102387.

Cole, Jennifer L. "Why the USA Should 'Drop the Pounds' to Improve Patient Safety in Adults." *Drugs & Therapy Perspectives* 36, no. 2 (February 1, 2020): 67–68. https://doi.org/10.1007/s40267-019-00703-y.

Coleman, Gerald D. "Direct and Indirect Abortion in the Roman Catholic Tradition: A Review of the Phoenix Case." *HEC Forum: HealthCare Ethics Committee Forum: An Interprofessional Journal on Healthcare Institutions' Ethical and Legal Issues* 25, no. 2 (June 1, 2013): 127–143. https://doi.org/10.1007/s10730-013-9211-7.

DePergola, Peter A. "Euthanasia, Assisted-Suicide, and Palliative Sedation: A Brief Clarification and Reinforcement of the Moral Logic." *Online Journal of Health Ethics* 14, no. 2 (November 1, 2018). https://doi.org/10.18785/ojhe.1402.04.

Dyer, Owen. "Ohio Doctor Is Charged with 25 Counts of Murder over Patients' Deaths." *BMJ*, June 11, 2019, l4170. https://doi.org/10.1136/bmj.l4170.

Emanuel, Ezekiel J., and David J. Skorton. "Mandating COVID-19 Vaccination for Health Care Workers." *Annals of Internal Medicine* 174, no. 9 (September 2021): 1308–1310. https://doi.org/10.7326/M21-3150.

Escobar, María Fernanda, María Paula Echavarría, María Andrea Zambrano, Isabella Ramos, and Juan Pedro Kusanovic. "Maternal Sepsis." *American Journal of Obstetrics & Gynecology MFM* 2, no. 3 (August 2020): 100149. https://doi.org/10.1016/j.ajogmf.2020.100149.

Faris, Hannah, Brian Dewar, Claire Dyason, David G. Dick, Ainsley Matthewson, Susan Lamb, and Michel C. F. Shamy. "Goods, Causes and Intentions: Problems with Applying the Doctrine of Double Effect to Palliative Sedation." *BMC Medical Ethics* 22, no. 1 (December 2021): 141. https://doi.org/10.1186/s12910-021-00709-0.

Fisher, Ian. "A Poet Crusades for the Right to Die His Way." *The New York Times*, December 20, 2006.

Flood, Maura A. "Treatment of the Vegetative Patient: The Legacies of Karen Quinlan, Nancy Cruzan and Terri Schiavo." *J. Health & Biomedical L. 1 (2005) / Journal of Health & Biomedical Law* 1, no. 2 (2005): 1–48.

Gearty, C. A. "Could Ireland Have Saved Savita?" *The Tablet* 266, no. 8974 (November 24, 2012): 12–13.

Gill, Michael B. "A Moral Defense of Oregon's Physician-Assisted Suicide Law." *Mortality* 10, no. 1 (February 2005): 53–67.

Gillon, Raanan. "The Principle of Double Effect and Medical Ethics." *BMJ* 292, no. 6514 (January 18, 1986): 193–194. https://doi.org/10.1136/bmj.292.6514.193.

Gillon, Raanan. "'Primum Non Nocere' and the Principle of Non-Maleficence." *British Medical Journal* 291, no. 6488 (July 13, 1985): 130–131.

Glasier, Anna. "Emergency Contraception: Clinical Outcomes." *Contraception* 87, no. 3 (March 2013): 309–13. https://doi.org/10.1016/j.contraception.2012.08.027.

Gordin, Eli A., Andrew Day, Lenka Stankova, Elizabeth Heitman, and John Sadler. "Care in the Time of Coronavirus: Ethical Considerations in Head and Neck Oncology." *Head & Neck* 42, no. 7 (July 2020): 1519–1525. https://doi.org/10.1002/hed.26272.

Hamel, Ronald P., and James J. Walter, eds. *Artificial Nutrition and Hydration and the Permanently Unconscious Patient: The Catholic Debate*. Washington, DC: Georgetown University Press, 2007.

Have, Mike van der, and Jeroen Maljaars. "Editorial: Opioids in Inflammatory Bowel Disease-Primum Non Nocere." *Alimentary Pharmacology & Therapeutics* 53, no. 7 (April 2021): 844–845. https://doi.org/10.1111/apt.16286.

Helling, Steve. "Why Did a Jury Acquit Dr. William Husel on 14 Murder Charges?" Accessed August 26, 2022. https://people.com/crime/william-husel-doctor-accused-overdosing-patients-not-guilty/.

Hernigou, Philippe. "Primum Non Nocere: Is It Really True with Corticosteroid Hip Injections?: Commentary on an Article by Kanu Okike, MD, MPH, et al.: 'Rapidly Destructive Hip Disease Following Intra-Articular Corticosteroid Injection of the Hip'." *Journal of Bone & Joint Surgery, American Volume* 103, no. 22 (November 17, 2021): e92.

Hetzler, Peter T., et al. "A Report of Physicians' Beliefs about Physician-Assisted Suicide: A National Study." *Yale Journal of Biology and Medicine* 92, no. 4 (December 20, 2019).

Horowitz, Alan C. "Medication Errors and Homicide: When Law and Medicine Collide." *Caring for the Ages* 23, no. 5 (June 2022): 1–3. https://doi.org/10.1016/j.carage.2022.04.033.

Horton, J. Bauer, Jeffrey E. Janis, and Rod J. Rohrich. "MOC-PS(SM) CME Article: Patient Safety in the Office-Based Setting:" *Plastic and Reconstructive Surgery* 122, no. Supplement (September 2008): 1–21. https://doi.org/10.1097/PRS.0b013e318183c118.

Jessup, Rebecca L., and Rachelle Buchbinder. "What If I Cannot Choose Wisely? Addressing Suboptimal Health Literacy in Our Patients to Reduce over-Diagnosis and Overtreatment: Health Literacy and Too Much Medicine." *Internal Medicine Journal* 48, no. 9 (September 2018): 1154–1157. https://doi.org/10.1111/imj.14025.

Jonsen, Albert R. *A Short History of Medical Ethics*. New York: Oxford University Press, 2000.

Keenan, James F. "The Function of the Principle of Double Effect." *Theological Studies* 54, no. 2 (June 1993): 294–315.

Kelly, David F. *Medical Care at the End of Life : A Catholic Perspective*. First edition. Georgetown University Press, 2006.

Kelly, David F., Gerard Magill, and H. ten Have. *Contemporary Catholic Health Care Ethics*. Second edition. Washington, DC: Georgetown University Press, 2013.

Kelman, Brett, and Hannah Norman. "Why Nurses Are Raging and Quitting After the RaDonda Vaught Verdict." *Biomedical Safety & Standards*, June 15, 2022, 81–83.

Kessler, Glenn. "The Claim That 98 Percent of Catholic Women Use Contraception: A Media Foul." *The Washington Post*, February 17, 2012.

Kim, Yujeong, and Eunmi Lee. "The Relationship between the Perception of Open Disclosure of Patient Safety Incidents, Perception of Patient Safety Culture, and Ethical Awareness in Nurses." *BMC Medical Ethics* 21, no. 1 (October 27, 2020). https://doi.org/10.1186/s12910-020-00546-7.

Kohn, Linda T., Janet Corrigan, and Molla S. Donaldson. *To Err Is Human: Building a Safer Health System*, 2000. http://site.ebrary.com/id/10038653.

Krishnan, Sheila, Erin M. Fricke, Marcos Cordoba, Laurie A. Chalifoux, and Reda E. Girgis. "Pulmonary Hypertension Complicating Pregnancy." *Current Pulmonology Reports* 10, no. 2 (June 1, 2021): 71–83. https://doi.org/10.1007/s13665-021-00275-1.

Kumar, Ajay, et al. "Euthanasia: A Debate—For and Against." *Journal of Postgraduate Medicine, Education and Research,* 55, no. 2 (June 2021): 91–96.

Laskowski-Jones, Linda. "Fatal Flaws." *Nursing*, June 2022, 6.

Latham, Stephen R. "U.S. Lawsuit Claims Federal Law Can Require Emergency Abortions." *Hastings Center Report* 52, no. 5 (September 2022): 4–5. https://doi.org/10.1002/hast.1414.

Lima Silva Nunes, Ranielle de, Ana Elisa Bauer de Camargo Silva, Juliana Carvalho de Lima, Dayse Edwiges Carvalho, Cristina Alves Bernardes, Tanielly Paula Sousa, Fernanda Raphael

Escobar Gimenes, and Ana Claudia Andrade Cordeiro Pires. "Factors Influencing the Patient Safety Climate in Intensive Care Units: Cross-Sectional Study." *BMC Nursing* 20, no. 1 (December 1, 2021). https://doi.org/10.1186/s12912-021-00643-x.

Lo, Bernard, and Gordon Rubenfeld. "Palliative Sedation in Dying Patients: 'We Turn to It When Everything Else Hasn't Worked.'" *JAMA* 294, no. 14 (October 12, 2005). https://doi.org/10.1001/jama.294.14.1810.

Macauley, Robert. "The Role of the Principle of Double Effect in Ethics Education at US Medical Schools and Its Potential Impact on Pain Management at the End of Life." *Journal of Medical Ethics* 38, no. 3 (March 2012): 174–178. https://doi.org/10.1136/medethics-2011-100105.

Magill, Gerard. "Threat of Imminent Death in Pregnancy: A Role for Double-Effect Reasoning." *Theological Studies* 72, no. 4 (December 2011): 848–878.

Maltoni, M., C. Pittureri, E. Scarpi, L. Piccinini, F. Martini, P. Turci, L. Montanari, O. Nanni, and D. Amadori. "Palliative Sedation Therapy Does Not Hasten Death: Results from a Prospective Multicenter Study." *Annals of Oncology* 20, no. 7 (July 1, 2009): 1163–1169.

Marimow, Ann E. "Supreme Court Sides with Doctors Convicted of Overprescribing Opioids." *The Washington Post*, June 28, 2022. Gale Academic OneFile.

Martin, Hannah B., and Daryl F. Sas. "Autonomy vs. Selflessness at the End of Life." *Ethics & Medicine: An International Journal of Bioethics* 31, no. 2 (June 22, 2015): 109.

Martin, Stephanie R., and Alexandra Edwards. "Pulmonary Hypertension and Pregnancy." *Obstetrics & Gynecology* 134, no. 5 (November 2019): 974–987.

Materstvedt, Lars Johan, and Morten Magelssen. "Medical Murder in Belgium and the Netherlands." *J Med Ethics* 42, no. 9 (September 2016).

Mazer, Mark A., Chad M. Alligood, and Qiang Wu. "The Infusion of Opioids During Terminal Withdrawal of Mechanical Ventilation in the Medical Intensive Care Unit." *Journal of Pain and Symptom Management* 42, no. 1 (January 1, 2011): 44–51.

McCradden, Melissa D, Shalmali Joshi, James A Anderson, Mjaye Mazwi, Anna Goldenberg, Randi Zlotnik Shaul, and Randi Zlotnik Shaul. "Patient Safety and Quality Improvement: Ethical Principles for a Regulatory Approach to Bias in Healthcare Machine Learning." *Journal of the American Medical Informatics Association* 27, no. 12 (December 2020): 2024–2027.

McDonnell, Orla, and Padraig Murphy. "Mediating Abortion Politics in Ireland: Media Framing of the Death of Savita Halappanavar." *Critical Discourse Studies* 16, no. 1 (January 2019): 1–20. https://doi.org/10.1080/17405904.2018.1521858.

Medina, Marco T., and Sir Salvador Moncada. "Hydroxychloroquine/Chloroquine as a Treatment Choice or Prophylaxis for Covid-19 at the Primary Care Level in Developing Countries: A Primum Non Nocere Dilemma." *Journal of the Neurological Sciences* 415 (August 15, 2020): N.PAG-N.PAG.

Merriam-Webster. *Merriam-Webster's Intermediate Dictionary*. Springfield, MA: Merriam-Webster, 2020.

Meyer, Harris. "Hospitals Fall Short of Patient-Safety Goals 20 Years after 'To Err Is Human.'" *Modern Healthcare*, November 11, 2019.

Montaldi, Daniel F. "A Defense of St Thomas and the Principle of Double Effect." *Journal of Religious Ethics* 14, no. 2 (1986): 296–332.

Moriates, Christopher, Krishan Soni, Andrew Lai, and Sumant Ranji. "The Value in the Evidence: Teaching Residents to 'Choose Wisely.'" *JAMA Internal Medicine* 173, no. 4 (February 25, 2013): 308. https://doi.org/10.1001/jamainternmed.2013.2286.

Noia, Gina Maria. "The Principle of Double Effect within Catholic Moral Theology: A Response to Two Criticisms of the Principle in Relation to Palliative Sedation." *Journal of Moral Theology* 6, no. 2 (June 2017): 130–148.

Olson, Olivia, Corinne Berry, and Nirbhay Kumar. "Addressing Parental Vaccine Hesitancy towards Childhood Vaccines in the United States: A Systematic Literature Review of Communication Interventions and Strategies." 2020. https://hsrc.himmelfarb.gwu.edu/sphhs_global_facpubs/543.

Pereira, Andrea Z., Selma Freire de Carvalho da Cunha, Henrique Grunspun, and Marco Aurelio Scarpinella Bueno. "The Difficult Decision Not to Prescribe Artificial Nutrition by Health Professionals and Family: Bioethical Aspects." *Frontiers in Nutrition* 9 (March 3, 2022): 781540. https://doi.org/10.3389/fnut.2022.781540.

Piccione, Joseph J. "An Exploration of the ERD, Fourth Edition Ethical and Religious Directives for Catholic Health Care Services." *The Journal of the Association of Professional Chaplains* 17, no. 1 (Summer 2001): 22–34.

Ponzo, Jenny. "Motherhood and Personhood: The Canonization of Gianna Beretta Molla and the Figurativization of Catholic Norms." *International Journal for the Semiotics of Law—Revue Internationale de Sémiotique Juridique*, February 5, 2021. https://doi.org/10.1007/s11196-020-09813-7.

Potter, Jordan G. (Jordan Gabriel). "The Principle of Double Effect in End-of-Life Care." *The National Catholic Bioethics Quarterly* 15, no. 3 (2015): 515–529.

Potter, Jordan, Steven Shields, and Renée Breen. "Palliative Sedation, Compassionate Extubation, and the Principle of Double Effect: An Ethical Analysis." *American Journal of Hospice & Palliative Medicine* 38, no. 12 (December 2021): 1536–1540. https://doi.org/10.1177/1049909121998630.

Prusak, Bernard G. "Double Effect, All over Again: The Case of Sister Margaret McBride." *Theoretical Medicine and Bioethics* 32, no. 4 (August 2011): 271–283. https://doi.org/10.1007/s11017-011-9183-z.

Quill, Timothy E., Rebecca Dresser, and Dan W. Brock. "The Rule of Double Effect—A Critique of Its Role in End-of-Life Decision Making." *New England Journal of Medicine* 337, no. 24 (December 11, 1997): 1768–1771. https://doi.org/10.1056/NEJM199712113372413.

Reed, P. A. "The Danger of Double Effect." *Christian Bioethics* 18, no. 3 (December 1, 2012): 287–300. https://doi.org/10.1093/cb/cbs021.

Roberts, Tom. "Ethicists Fault Bishop's Action in Phoenix Abortion Case." *National Catholic Reporter* 46, no. 17 (n.d.): 1, 12–13.

Rubin, Rita, et al. "How Caring for Patients Could Change in a Post-*Roe v Wade* US." *JAMA* 327, no. 21 (June 7, 2022): 2060–2062.

Schofield, Guy, Idris Baker, Rachel Bullock, Hannah Clare, Paul Clark, Derek Willis, Craig Gannon, and Rob George. "Palliative Opioid Use, Palliative Sedation and Euthanasia: Reaffirming the Distinction." *Journal of Medical Ethics* 46, no. 1 (January 2020): 48–50. https://doi.org/10.1136/medethics-2018-105256.

Shenoy, Amrita. "Patient Safety from the Perspective of Quality Management Frameworks: A Review." *Patient Safety in Surgery* 15, no. 1 (December 1, 2021). https://doi.org/10.1186/s13037-021-00286-6.

Shenoy, Amrita, Gopinath N. Shenoy, and Gayatri G. Shenoy. "The Impact of EMTALA on Medical Malpractice Framework Models: A Review." *Patient Safety in Surgery* 16, no. 1 (December 2022): 21. https://doi.org/10.1186/s13037-022-00325-w.

Skidmore, Samuel J., and Sharon E. Robinson Kurpius. "Euthanasia in an Aging America: An Ethical Challenge for Mental Health Counselors." *Journal of Mental Health Counseling* 43, no. 2 (April 1, 2021): 125–138. https://doi.org/10.17744/mehc.43.2.03.

Slosar, J. P. "Pregnancy Complications Can Bring on Complex Ethical Questions." *Catholic Health World* 26, no. 21 (2010).

Sofer, Dalia. "Is a Medical Mistake an Error or a Crime?" *AJN American Journal of Nursing* 119, no. 5 (May 2019): 12.

Sokol, Daniel. "Covid-19 Vaccination Should Be Mandatory for Healthcare Workers." *BMJ*, November 2, 2021, n2670. https://doi.org/10.1136/bmj.n2670.

Somasundaram, Praveena. "Explainer: What's next for Abortion Pills after the Fall of Roe." *The Washington Post*, July 9, 2022.

Sprengholz, Philipp, Lisa Felgendreff, Robert Böhm, and Cornelia Betsch. "Vaccination Policy Reactance: Predictors, Consequences, and Countermeasures." *Journal of Health Psychology* 27, no. 6 (May 2022): 1394–1407. https://doi.org/10.1177/13591053211044535.

Stangl, Rebecca. "Plan B and the Doctrine of Double Effect." *Hastings Center Report* 39, no. 4 (2009): 21–25. https://doi.org/10.1353/hcr.0.0162.

Stratta, Gregorio, Cinzia Monti, Piermario Salvini, Vittorio Vavassori, and Massimo Maria Grassi. "Multidisciplinary Management of Breast Cancer in a 103 Years Old Patient: The Ultimate 'Primum Non Nocere' Challenge." *Aging and Health Research* 1, no. 4 (December 1, 2021).

Sulmasy, Daniel P. "Death and Dignity in Catholic Christian Thought." *Medicine, Health Care and Philosophy* 20, no. 4 (December 2017): 537–543. https://doi.org/10.1007/s11019-016-9690-9.

Totenberg, Nina, and Sarah McCammon. "Supreme Court Overturns Roe v. Wade, Ending Right to Abortion Upheld for Decades." *NPR*, June 24, 2022, sec. Roe v. Wade and the future of reproductive rights in America. www.npr.org/2022/06/24/1102305878/supreme-court-abortion-roe-v-wade-decision-overturn.

Tuohey, John F. "A Fatal Conflict: Can Catholic Hospitals Refuse to Save Lives?" *Commonweal* 138 (January 28, 2011): 8.

United States Conference of Catholic Bishops. *Ethical and Religious Directives for Catholic Health Care Services*. Washington, DC: United States Conference of Catholic Bishops. Sixth Edition. June 2018.

Vaccari, Michael A. "Artificial Respiration and AHN: Some Similarities and Differences." *The Linacre Quarterly* 59 (May 1992): 48–62.

Viessman, Sara S. "New CME Requirements for Pennsylvania Physicians." *Lehigh Valley Medical Staff Progress Notes* 18, no. 11 (November 2004): 1.

Vincent, Charles. *Patient Safety*. Second edition. Chichester: Wiley-Blackwell, 2010.

Vives-Borràs, Miquel, and Alessandro Sionis. "Elderly Patients with Comorbidities and Acute Coronary Syndrome: Primum Non Nocere?" *REC: Interventional Cardiology (English Ed.)* 3, no. 1 (February 1, 2021): 3–4. https://doi.org/10.24875/RECICE.M20000167.

Webster, Craig S. "Existing Knowledge of Medication Error Must Be Better Translated Into Improved Patient Safety." *Frontiers in Medicine* 9 (2022): 870587. https://doi.org/10.3389/fmed.2022.870587.

Yang, Y. Tony, and Rebecca L. Haffajee. "Murder Liability for Prescribing Opioids: A Way Forward?" *Mayo Clinic Proceedings* 91, no. 10 (October 2016): 1331–1335. https://doi.org/10.1016/j.mayocp.2016.06.018.

Yokota, Sayuri, Koji Amano, Shunsuke Oyamada, Hiroto Ishiki, Isseki Maeda, Tomofumi Miura, Yutaka Hatano, et al. "Effects of Artificial Nutrition and Hydration on Survival in Patients with Head and Neck Cancer and Esophageal Cancer Admitted to Palliative Care Units." *Clinical Nutrition Open Science* 41 (February 2022): 33–43. https://doi.org/10.1016/j.nutos.2021.11.008.

Zhuang, Qingyuan, Grace Meijuan Yang, Shirlyn Hui-Shan Neo, and Yin Bun Cheung. "Validity, Reliability, and Diagnostic Accuracy of the Respiratory Distress Observation Scale for Assessment of Dyspnea in Adult Palliative Care Patients." *Journal of Pain and Symptom Management* 57, no. 2 (February 2019): 304–310. https://doi.org/10.1016/j.jpainsymman.2018.10.506.

Zientek, David M. "Artificial Nutrition and Hydration in Catholic Healthcare: Balancing Tradition, Recent Teaching, and Law." *HEC Forum* 25, no. 2 (June 2013): 145–159. https://doi.org/10.1007/s10730-013-9214-4.

Zilinski, Lisa. "Sister Margaret McBride." *Carnegie Mellon University Research Showcase*, January 2013.

Chapter 4
The Ethical Principle of Justice

INTRODUCTION

This chapter will look at the last ethical principle, justice. Along with autonomy, beneficence, and nonmaleficence, it is one of the basic tenets of healthcare ethics. More specifically, the focus will be on distributive justice and how it applies to healthcare. Social justice, criminal justice, political justice, and other types of justice will likely only receive brief comments, as this essay will focus on the distribution of healthcare as a finite commodity. For example, when the COVID-19 vaccine became available, there was a question regarding how to distribute it. Should healthcare workers receive it first? What about first responders, elderly patients, and the vulnerable? How about people in countries hardest hit by the virus?

First, there should be a discussion regarding whether or not the countries that make the vaccines should distribute them to other countries justly and if that benevolent distribution is sufficient. Although protecting one's population is good, stockpiling vital resources is wrong and can have global consequences. Public opinion regarding the distribution of the COVID-19 vaccine sees the world as one family, which is not only fair-minded but also most likely the best solution to the pandemic.[1] Nevertheless, justice also requires determining if these vaccines are privately owned by pharmaceutical companies or publicly owned and considered global public health goods. If the vaccines are publicly owned, the countries that produce them must give up the patents, allow poorer nations to manufacture them locally, and assist them with manufacturing them. Donating extra doses of COVID-19 vaccines to poorer nations is not enough; wealthy nations must provide these countries with methods to produce their own vaccines in the name of justice.[2] Therefore, distributive justice is not just donating vaccines to poorer countries; it also requires them to support other countries in developing their own vaccines. But why is that?

DOI: 10.4324/9781003654124-5

One reason is that the Roman Catholic Church has described social guidelines that mandate governments to form a society marked by peace, harmony, and justice toward all.[3] Called Catholic Social Teaching (CST), these moral principles regarding the universal sharing of the world's resources for the common good of society are the basis of the principle of distributive justice. Examining how COVID-19 vaccines were created revealed that pharmaceutical companies did not develop and finance their development alone. Instead, it was found that the collaboration of both private and publicly funded companies facilitated the rapid production of these vaccines. Therefore, this doctrine requires sharing ownership, suspending patents for the common good, and saving people's lives in less affluent countries. Vaccines are a global community factor and must be seen as a public health good. Following CST's principle that private ownership has both moral and social obligations, the US and other wealthy countries must insist that pharmaceutical companies give up their property rights for the common good and allow a vaccine distribution system that is moral and just.[4]

The next step is that once a nation has a vaccine supply, how do they fairly distribute it to the population? Germany and the US successfully developed and manufactured effective COVID-19 vaccines. Their respective people gave the highest consideration to concepts corresponding with utilitarian principles (that would promote the best outcomes), followed by egalitarian values (that which would be the fairest.) Overall, these results showed that the people from these countries prefer an equitable distribution of vaccines based on need.[5] However, even distinguishing between these two approaches can be problematic because it questions whether vaccines should be distributed to the most vulnerable or based on what would benefit society the most.

One tactic would be to give the vaccine first to those most vulnerable, those at the highest risk of dying from the virus. Because of this, high-risk groups were identified and given precedence over others. This group included elderly patients and those chronically ill.[6] However, after this cohort was managed, the distribution sequence became murky. Many argued that the well-being of the marginalized, lower rung of the social and economic ladder must be prioritized, especially during a crisis like this pandemic.[7] These authors were concerned about social justice's role in public health policymaking. Their conclusions emphasized the importance of the principles of distributive justice with pandemic-focused public health policymakers. They asked why social justice was not always applied to a pandemic vaccination program.[8] However, other approaches should be studied.

For example, some experts argued that prioritizing those at high risk of severe outcomes was a method that was likely to have negative consequences. This recommendation gave the initial limited vaccine supply to vulnerable populations, which vigorous isolation protocols could have served. It failed to promote the more important goal of saving the most people by containing the virus.[9] However, others argue that a predominately distributive justice approach could be problematic for vulnerable groups seeking immunization. An alternative method would include working with public health agencies that could, through dialogue, inclusiveness, and human interactions, affect the risk of death or serious complications during the pandemic and ensure all strategies are utilized in preventing illness and maintaining health.[10]

Things have changed regarding COVID-19 vaccines in the last two years of the pandemic, and now there are more vaccines than people who want them. Also, the vaccines do not appear to prevent disease or stop transmission because of newer coronavirus strains. However, they seem to inhibit severe illnesses and death.[11] However, the challenges with the original rollout of the vaccines serve as a timely introduction to understanding the ethical principle of distributive justice.

HISTORICAL BACKGROUND

The earliest writings about justice can be traced back to Plato (427–347 BCE) in *The Republic*. In what is called "dialogues," he discusses the two sides to justice.[12] First, justice is defined as a virtue of persons, depicted as the "harmonious ordering of the soul." Second, justice is the appropriate and harmonious ordering of political society, or "the first virtue of social institutions."[13] Therefore, he refers to justice as a personal virtue and a societal responsibility. In this paper, personal justice as a virtue will be explored, along with the topics of inequality and vulnerability. Also, on a societal or institutional level, justice regarding rationing and sustainability will be examined. Indeed, there is an intersection between the two, and the problem lies in resolving justice as a personal virtue with justice as a social responsibility.[14] Let us look at Plato's most famous student to define this subject further.

Aristotle (384–322 BCE) further describes justice's general nature in book V of the *Nicomachean Ethics*. He views justice as overcoming certain vices, such as cowardice or anger. Injustice is a defect of the character, and vices cannot only ruin a person, but their effects can also harm society. Therefore, justice concerns virtue precisely as it relates to others. Aristotle also introduces the term "distributive justice." He writes how the distribution of money and goods must follow a "geometric proportion" correlating to the "merits of the recipient."[15] Simply put, he sees justice as a personal and societal virtue that allows for the fair allocation of goods to those in need.

In Rome, a later disciple of Aristotle, Cicero (106–43 BCE),[16] described three domains of ethics: decorum, deontology, and public ethics. Decorum describes outward behaviors that show inner virtues, such as courage, respectfulness, and resoluteness. Deontology refers to morality associated with what one should do, expressed in rules and principles. Finally, Public Ethics looks beyond the person to the society where they live. As with the previous philosophers, Cicero states that the moral idea of justice involves the relationship between the individual and society.[17] Thomas Aquinas expressed this duality of moral responsibility over a thousand years later.

Thomas Aquinas (1224–1274 CE) sees justice as a personal virtue. He integrates multiple philosophical and theological sources to conclude that justice is "the perpetual and constant will to render to each one his right."[18] One author, Jean Porter, writes that Aquinas's theory of justice as a personal virtue differs from the current view of justice as a virtue of a group.[19] If justice is the virtue by which individuals relate to one another, then individuals acting in fundamentally unjust groups are behaving in an improper relationship with others and, therefore, unjust.[20] Thus, an individual cannot state that they are acting morally if their organization is not, nor can an organization divest itself of the actions of its members.

Aquinas then goes on to defend this position using the Bible. He warns that those in power who promote their own interests set an "evil example" to the group and that the maximum punishment shall be demanded. According to Micah 3:9–10: "Hear this you heads of the house of Jacob and rulers of the house of Israel, who abhor justice and pervert all equity, who build Zion with blood and Jerusalem with wrong."[21] So again, we see how individuals can subvert the group, and both can be seen as unjust. Finally, Aquinas defines how the Bible implores us to act justly.

Biblical justice not only encompasses but exceeds requirements to give others their due, including obligations to the poor, living as if we were a gift to others, and forming relationships that are not retaliatory. This directive defines the meaning of Biblical justice as the expression of all of those attributes by enlisting Jesus Christ's relationship with us at his death and resurrection. Of course, the modern concept of justice, by contrast, is secular and developed through reason, as opposed to Thomas's expression of the divine law, which is based on God's revelation to us.[22] Lastly, justice will be examined through the work of a contemporary American philosopher.

John Rawls (1921–2002)[23] has written extensively on justice. In his work *A Theory of Justice*, Rawls states, "Justice is the first virtue of social institutions, as truth is of systems of thought."[24] He sees justice as central to society and is crucial in structuring social institutions.[25] According to Rawls, a distributive justice theory should set standards for evaluating the distribution of goods within a society. Therefore, the distribution of economic benefits should be agreeable to all, regardless of their status or position. Specifically, no one should believe that "they or any of the others are taken advantage of, or forced to give in to claims which they do not regard as legitimate."[26] Keys to his philosophy, therefore, include fairness, cooperation, and the belief that even the disadvantaged have the means to live a good life. As with the other philosophers, he burdens society and the individuals that encompass it.

In this section, justice was investigated on a historical and philosophical basis. It seems clear that the authors view this moral principle as an individual and societal responsibility. However, the fair distribution of goods and services was looked at only broadly. In the next section, distributive justice will be explored in terms of how it relates more specifically to healthcare issues. In particular, there will be a discussion as to whether the abovementioned principles apply to healthcare concerns.

DISTRIBUTIVE JUSTICE DEFINED IN HEALTHCARE

The term distributive justice refers to the fair, equitable, and appropriate distribution of goods decided by defensible standards that promote the requirements of social cooperation. Its range includes policies that allow varied benefits and burdens, such as property, resources, taxation, privileges, and opportunities.[27]

First, there needs to be a brief discussion about equity versus equality. In the dictionary, *equitable* is defined as "dealing fairly and equally with all concerned," whereas *equal* is defined as "of the same measure, quantity, amount, or number as another."[28] That does not seem like much of a difference; however, the difference is enormous in reality. A closer look explains that *equity* involves distributing resources based on the recipients' needs, while *equality* means giving everyone the same resources.[29] So, should healthcare be equitable or equal? Perhaps the answer is both; some elements should be equitable, and others should be equal.

For instance, health equity refers to stopping institutional and discriminatory obstacles that lead to health inequities and inequality. The goal is to guarantee equal access to quality healthcare, even if this requires giving some people more resources than others.[30] For example, healthcare spending generally follows "the 80/20 rule," with 80% of all expenditures being incurred by only 20% of the population. This imbalance is because a small percentage of patients are troubled with severe chronic and complicated conditions that account for a disproportionate share of healthcare spending.[31] Spending as much healthcare for a healthy person as a sick person would not make sense.

Although costs should not be the same for all, some aspects of healthcare should not vary. Healthcare equality states everyone should have the same access to quality care and services.[32] A 2016 study revealed that some people felt that black and white people perceived pain differently. The authors reported that many white medical students and residents held beliefs about the genetic differences between races, which were untrue and unrealistic, and that these mistakes are associated with racial bias in pain perception. The fact that they believed that black people experienced less pain than their white counterparts could allow for undertreatment and other adverse outcomes.[33] Better education is needed to prevent this and other racial disparities.[34] So now that equity and equality have been defined, how do we assess distributive justice in healthcare?

In *Principles of Biomedical Ethics*, Beauchamp and Childress ask essential questions about healthcare access. For instance, should all play a role in access to healthcare resources? Many young, healthy people choose not to pay for health insurance, yet there are times when healthcare is needed. Most agree that the uninsured should be treated, even if they cannot pay. Nevertheless, questions arise regarding access to healthcare, specifically that people have the freedom to choose (or not choose) a health plan in a free-market economy.[35] Since these values indeed conflict, Beauchamp and Childress suggest that justice may have different objectives. A utilitarian approach would focus on advancing the common good. However, a libertarian approach would argue that healthcare is not a right and should be centered on a person's ability or willingness to pay for it. Finally, the communitarian and egalitarian approaches emphasize what is owed to a patient and the equal distribution of these resources.[36]

The authors conclude that no theory is superior, and each approach has pros and cons. They then propose what they refer to as the "fair opportunity rule," which is that no person should receive (or be denied) social benefits because of the person's "undeserved advantageous (or disadvantageous) properties." This rule is applied to mitigate the unfortunate effects of life's lotteries.[37] Therefore, Beauchamp and Childress conclude that everyone should be entitled to at least basic healthcare.

Other writers also look to find a balanced approach to justice. In their book *Contemporary Catholic Health Care Ethics*, the authors Kelly, Magill, and ten Have state three guidelines regarding distributive justice in healthcare. First, they recommend that our healthcare system have some form of national health insurance that guarantees everyone access to primary care regardless of the ability to pay. Second, this health insurance program should cover most medical treatments sensibly beneficial to the patient. Finally, there should be a provision to allow the affluent to get any treatment they want and to enable people to buy supplemental health insurance from private insurance companies to cover procedures the government program does not cover.[38] While this approach seems fair, defining a sensibly beneficial medical treatment from one that can only be purchased by the wealthy is problematic. However, such a program must also be fiscally sustainable or face failure.

So, a healthcare program based on justice needs to balance providing benefits to all in an economically responsible way since a program that fails benefits no one. The saying regarding doing "the greatest good for the greatest number" indicates the belief in increasing benefits, which indeed is a cause for discussion. One could maximize the number of people saved while simultaneously minimizing waste by giving the majority of medical resources to those most likely to stay alive. This "greatest good" principle would maximize benefits by considering patient differences in health status. Under this approach, distributive guidelines would increase life expectancy by giving preference based on age or health conditions.[39] This approach would ensure an equal opportunity for positive health outcomes and allow each patient's life to go as well as possible. However, doing this involves the difficult task of making comparisons and trade-offs between people, which balances the relevant considerations of individual needs and medical effectiveness.[40] Of course, not everyone will be happy with this approach. At some point, someone will have to say no to a medical treatment because it is too expensive and unlikely to help.

The other problem with justice is deciding what criteria should determine whether a patient should receive a requested treatment. This dilemma requires decisions about the treatment itself and the potential recipient. The treatment aspect should be safe, effective, and fiscally responsible. The other factor has to do with patient selection for controversial procedures. The age, medical condition, and ability to pay have already been mentioned, but should other criteria be investigated?

In a paper entitled "Patient Characteristics and the Allocation of Scarce Medical Resources," the authors explored patient characteristics that could decide potential treatment decisions. The study provided a questionnaire to participants that were asked to rank likely patients' eligibility to go on a kidney machine that could only accommodate a small percentage of patients. The results of the survey were intriguing and perhaps troubling. The variable that showed the most significant distinction was a history of mental illness; those with no history of mental illness were clearly favored over those with such a history. The second variable that separated patients was intelligence because it was believed that more intelligent people could contribute substantially to society. Finally, there was a small but significant preference for extroverts over introverts based on the assumption that extroverts were more optimistic, self-confident, easier to get along with, and more friendly than introverts.[41] Undoubtedly, it seems absurd that introverted, less intelligent patients with a history of mental illness should have fewer treatment options than extroverted, intelligent patients without such a history. Nevertheless, justice infers that not everyone can get everything demanded, and distribution decisions must be made. If not correctly made, these decisions can lead to healthcare inequities, especially with vulnerable populations. These ideas will be studied in the following sections.

PERSONAL JUSTICE

Justice has two sides: a personal virtue and a virtue of social institutions. Plato wrote about this in *The Republic*, and later Aquinas continued this idea. In this section, justice will be studied as a personal virtue. Professionals in all healthcare fields are obligated to take individual responsibility regarding fairness. In her book *Justice as a Virtue: A Thomistic Perspective*, Jean Porter states that Aquinas saw justice as a moral right with two elements: equality in interpersonal exchanges and strict obligations.[42] This segment will examine healthcare inequities and their root causes based on personal biases. The next part will study the elements that make specific populations vulnerable to these biases and offer solutions to overcome them.

Healthcare Inequities

The COVID-19 pandemic provides insight into healthcare disparities based on race and ethnicity. The Centers for Disease Control and Prevention (CDC) learned that the virus has unequal effects on communities of color. African Americans account for over a third of the cases, even though this group accounts for only 13% of the US population. The statistics for Hispanics are also similar nationwide. However, the CDC often does not include race and ethnicity in their COVID-19 reports. When Native Americans are counted, they are frequently included in the "other" category. Therefore, the health impact on communities of color is likely worse than is currently known.[43] COVID-19 has highlighted current disparities and risks for several groups, including the young, communities of color, and impoverished communities. If the CDC had provided this vital information, there would have been an opportunity to address the healthcare inequities that this pandemic has only exacerbated.[44] However, does this data show healthcare disparities or equities?

Healthcare disparities are roughly defined as population-specific differences in health outcomes, which may or may not be inequitable, meaning that the adverse outcomes may not necessarily be due to unequal care to these groups.[45] The National Institutes of Health (NIH) defines healthcare disparities as "differences in the incidence, prevalence, mortality, and burden of diseases and other adverse health conditions that exist among specific population groups in the United States." However, the lack of specific criteria for recognizing disparities and the relatively nonspecific descriptions of disparities used by federal agencies leave questions about what other factors might also be relevant.[46] In addition, because the amount of quality data is limited, one can conclude that in many cases, disparities in healthcare may not necessarily reflect healthcare inequities. Nevertheless, healthcare inequities exist, and there is good evidence to prove it.

As previously mentioned, some studies show that pain in black Americans is poorly diagnosed and treated compared to their white counterparts. In addition, wide-ranging studies have shown some reasons that could explain these fallacies, including status judgments, racial prejudice, and myths about the genetic differences between blacks and whites.[47] Most likely, this problem begins in medical school and could be remedied by good quality education.[48]

Besides race and ethnicity, there are other causes of healthcare disparities. For instance, the quality of care to obese patients appears to be affected by stigmatizing overweight people caused by the widespread weight bias (fat shaming) seen in our society. Such bias may result from an inadequate understanding of the reasons for obesity. Strategies including recognizing obesity as a chronic health disorder, improving education about the causes of obesity, and applying standard methods of evaluating the severity of obesity to guide treatment recommendations have been shown to reduce the weight bias and ultimate stigmatization of persons with obesity. Certainly, obese patients face risks secondary to their physical condition, and disparities will exist. First, however, inequities in treatment must be addressed.[49]

Another example of disparities and inequities can be seen in patients with developmental disabilities. Although the life span for individuals with developmental disabilities is similar to that of the general population, healthcare inequities have been reported. The prevalence of developmental disabilities among adults is rising due to improved care for infants and children.[50] However, people with developmental disabilities can be seen as a socially disadvantaged population that experiences healthcare inequities. This inequity is often due to the accessibility and quality of healthcare received. Healthcare inequities are worsened because this group is currently less likely to live in institutions because of the goal of placing them in the community. They need support from community agencies and providers to address unmet healthcare needs caused by decreased accessibility and limited financial resources.[51] As with other inequities in healthcare, better education is needed to remedy the situation.[52]

So, disparities can occur in healthcare without inequities because of challenges adherent to their unique circumstances, which will be discussed later in a section about vulnerable populations. However, healthcare inequities based on race, ethnicity, and other causes exist, which must be examined. One cause to address this is unconscious bias. By definition, this refers to societal stereotypes about specific cohorts of people outside their conscious awareness. It is felt that everyone holds unconscious beliefs about certain groups of people, and these biases originate from the inclination to categorize people.[53] However, it differs from prejudice, which is "an irrational attitude of hostility directed against an individual, a group, a race, or their supposed characteristics."[54] Bias is often imperceptible and hidden, yet once there is an understanding of unconscious bias, there can be an understanding of the significant harm it can promote. This bias can affect various issues, including contracting, meetings, teamwork, culture, performance evaluations, innovation, promotions, consensus-building, and healthcare delivery.[55] The simplest way to see unconscious bias is to look for its effects and outcomes, and this is where disparity and inequity come into play. Are the negative consequences seen due to a difference in the care provided, or are other factors at play?

Implicit bias can worsen health disparities, however, its extent among healthcare professionals is unknown.[56] The National Academy of Medicine describes team-based care as providing healthcare to individuals, families, and their communities, collaborating with at least two health providers to achieve shared goals and high-quality care. The five principles of team-based healthcare include "shared goals, clear roles, mutual trust, effective communication, and measurable processes and outcomes."[57] However, studies show that implicit bias may contribute to healthcare disparities by affecting medical providers' behavior, which causes differences in medical treatment because of race, ethnicity, gender, or other characteristics.[58]

Implicit biases are routinely triggered and unintentional. Providers often are unaware that they are responsible for this and will say that their medical decisions are exclusively science-based. Nevertheless, studies reveal that implicit biases are linked to unequal healthcare outcomes ranging from poorer quality encounters to a decreased frequency of receiving life-saving emergency medical treatments. Many authors argue that implicit biases persist because people lack personal awareness of them despite conscious virtuous attitudes or intentions.[59] One study looked at an educational intervention that reduced implicit race bias, which endures for at least two months. This data showed the conscious mind's power to overcome implicit bias intentionally. These findings provide hope for reducing race-based discrimination. Providing healthcare professionals with the proper training can stop the paradox of bias in a profession founded on the principle of justice.[60]

Implicit bias in healthcare is not just seen in the US; Canada, faced with similar challenges, has also sought solutions. The Royal College of Physicians and Surgeons defines a set of competencies Canadian physicians must possess to care for their patients effectively. One approach is the idea of health advocacy, described as promoting health equity for individuals and groups despite "race, ethnicity, religion, gender, sexual orientation, age, social class, economic status, or level of education."[61] For example, back in the US, it was found that COVID-19 disproportionately impacted communities of color and lower socioeconomic status. Therefore, some states revised how they distributed resources, including vaccines, to at-risk communities.[62]

Nevertheless, concentrating on equity rather than equality might be a better strategy to prevent the disparities seen in COVID-19. Noting that a significant problem with these communities is access to healthcare, the medical community must engage in outreach and anti-racism measures and listen to communities in need. The emphasis should be on implementing a distributive justice outline that treats all patients equitably, accounts for historical harm, and focuses on allocation and public health decision-making transparency.[63] Saying that more resources will be allocated to at-risk populations means little if that group does not know about this measure or cannot get to it. A more comprehensive program that includes community outreach, healthcare provider education, and better communication is needed to ensure that equity and justice goals are met.

This section examined the concepts of equity, equality, healthcare inequities, and healthcare disparities. In addition, implicit bias was also discussed. The reasons that make specific populations vulnerable will be studied in the next section. Understanding these groups is vital to help prevent healthcare inequities and honor the principle of distributive justice.

Vulnerability

To understand distributive justice more fully, we should look at those groups with the most to lose in an unfair system. In his book *Vulnerability: Challenging Bioethics*, Henk ten Have explains how this concept is relatively new in contemporary bioethics. He states that this concept first appeared as respect for persons as subjects for medical research." [64] However, this term is now applied to other groups, including older adults, people experiencing homelessness, and other countries.[65] This principle is often discussed regarding social determinants and their effect on healthcare outcomes. Social determinants of care include the circumstances in which one lives, learns, worships, and works and their impact on health risks and consequences. Unfortunately, the data shows that minority patients are disadvantaged and have higher risks of adverse outcomes.[66]

People who are vulnerable because of race and socioeconomic status are harmed by inaccessibility to justice, chronic health conditions, and lower life expectancy.[67] However, these healthcare disparities are not due solely to medical issues, as other health determinates are involved. Inner-city neighborhoods often have poor access to grocery stores, promoting poor food choices compared to better-supplied areas. This condition worsened in US urban areas during the racial protests honoring George Floyd in the summer of 2020. It is believed that 23.5 million people live in so-called "food deserts" and have difficulty finding culturally appropriate foods that meet their dietary needs. With limited options, many people living in these neighborhoods get their meals from fast-food restaurants, which contributes to higher rates of obesity, high blood pressure, and heart disease.[68] As nutrition is essential to health and recovery, these people are at greater risk for poor outcomes when they become ill.

Therefore, when looking at disparities, determinants of health such as economic and food stability, education, and community support are needed to assess the risks involved adequately.[69] Along with the social determinants of healthcare stated above, access to healthcare in poor neighborhoods remains a critical component. Several studies found that the percentage of African American residents living in the neighborhood was the leading factor in hospital closures between 1980 and 1987. Reducing hospital beds in African American communities further weakens their health by decreasing their access to healthcare. As hospitals leave these neighborhoods, the remaining hospitals are left to fill the gap, often stretching the hospitals' resources and ability to provide quality care. Consequently, the remaining hospitals are at risk of declining and delivering substandard care.[70]

Getting hospitals to stay in poor areas is challenging, and creative policies are needed. Specifically, state and federal regulators must examine institutional plans to close or relocate hospitals based on these plans' harm to these communities. This oversight would encourage hospitals to balance the benefits of closing and relocating these facilities to geographically better areas against the harmful effects on African American communities resulting from limited access to care.[71] However, this is not just a problem in urban areas, as these difficulties are also seen in rural areas.

What has been observed is that economic downturns can lead to people leaving the rural areas and moving to the city. The decrease in population implies lower patient volumes at hospitals, preventing hospitals from achieving profitability. Moreover, those left behind may be older, sicker, uninsured, or more reliant on Medicaid and Medicare, resulting in less favorable compensation for these hospitals, making them susceptible to closures.[72] Transportation is also a problem in rural areas compared with urban residents. Because these residents live in the country, they must often travel to the city to see a physician, especially specialists.[73] Ride-sharing services are beginning to increase in rural areas. In addition, because of the COVID-19 pandemic, the number of virtual visits has accelerated as more people choose to get their healthcare at home.[74]

INSTITUTIONAL JUSTICE

This section will discuss distributive justice in healthcare on an institutional level. As previously stated, Plato refers to justice as the appropriate and harmonious ordering of political society or "the first virtue of social institutions."[75] The reasons social institutions are responsible for justice can also be traced back to the Bible. In St. John's Gospel, Jesus tells Peter to "Feed my lambs, feed my sheep."[76] Therefore, organizations are duty-bound to make decisions that benefit the people they serve. However, they must find a way to remain fiscally sound. With this in mind, two topics will be explored: medical rationing and sustainability.

Organizational ethics gained recognition as part of the healthcare system during the disruptions in financing and organization in the 1990s. As a result, institutions struggled to be fiscally stable. However, organizational ethics in healthcare is distinct from simple business ethics. Just as healthcare professionals must follow a code of ethics, healthcare organizations, and systems must also meet ethical requirements to maintain their privileged position, including the right to provide and be paid for patient care.[77] Therefore, structural justice ethics often become part of the ethics committees at the institutional level. Organizational ethics committees can assist organizations in evaluating better, transforming, and ultimately satisfying their moral commitments to their patients and communities.[78]

When an organization commits to improving care in its community, it often involves elements such as team-based care and population health. These elements should be used to integrate health equity as a vital aspect of curricula, admissions, recruitment, and retention. In addition, community health indicators at local levels, such as the CDC's 500 Cities project, can help healthcare institutions understand their communities and patient populations.[79] Institutions need to be accountable to the communities they serve and those they teach. This accountability includes investing in programs for healthcare, research, funding, recruitment, and education of healthcare staff, including information about race and ethnicity and social determinants of healthcare. Organizations must also form trusting relationships and partnerships with their patients and communities.[80]

The challenge for institutions, however, is how to fund these programs. Often, this decision goes beyond equity, as the sickest patients are most likely the poorest. Promoting equality through the healthcare system could require a commitment to give the poor better access to care than the rich. That way, the well-being gap between rich and poor patients could be narrowed, and an equal society might be achieved. [81] Although this action is justified from a justice model, it is abysmal as a business action. To help close this financial gap, institutions often look at charity programs. Indeed, charity is a critical part of the ethic of Catholicism and other religions that sponsor hospitals; however, overreliance on it as a means of helping the poor is tough. A charity-dependent approach tends to minimize any discussion of society's responsibilities to social reform and the need to acknowledge the many structural injustices of our current economic system.[82]

Nevertheless, healthcare systems often face the burden of treating sick patients without the resources to pay for their care. Hospitals can only provide care for patients if they remain open and solvent; therefore, critical and often painful decisions must be made. The following two sections will look at rationing in healthcare and how distributive justice defines the ethical issues involved.

COVID-19 Rationing

The COVID-19 pandemic provided an excellent "classroom" as to how hospitals and healthcare systems use rationing in times of crisis and can provide insights regarding how rationing can be applied in future emergencies. For instance, in late February 2020, the United States warily observed how Italy handled dramatic shortages of ICU beds, medical staff, and ventilators because of COVID-19. The (CDC) predicted COVID-19 infections could cause between 2.4 million and 21 million Americans to be hospitalized and that no national criteria for rationing scarce medical resources existed. Based on the Italian experience, it was also predicted that between 10% and 25% of hospitalized patients would require ventilation.[83]

Therefore, there was grave concern that unexpected increases in hospital admissions during the first wave would flood the intensive care units (ICUs) in many countries, including the US. As a result, many countries employed emergency measures such as canceling non-COVID-related healthcare services, shifting hospital resources to COVID-related issues, and widespread public health restrictions, like masking and limiting public assemblies, to reduce transmission and hospital requirements.[84] Although these measures helped mitigate healthcare and ICU demands during the pandemic, there were some trade-offs. For example, non-COVID medical treatments were delayed, which could cause negative consequences for the patients involved. In addition, others argued that the extensive public health restrictions attacked one's civil liberties. Finally, how would the distribution of scarce resources such as ventilators and ICU beds be decided, and what were the ethics involved with these decisions?

Fortunately, the COVID pandemic did not lead to the severe rationing of healthcare that many predicted. However, I did come across one case that requires analysis. A 32-year-old male patient was admitted to the hospital with respiratory failure from COVID-19 pneumonia. He had multiple comorbidities, including diabetes and obesity, and had not been vaccinated. His condition worsened to the point that he required extracorporeal membrane oxygenation (ECMO), a machine that can provide oxygen to the person when their lungs have failed. ECMO is traditionally used until the lungs have recovered or as a bridge to a lung transplant. Unfortunately, his lungs did not improve, and he was not considered a candidate for transplantation.

Although he was comfortable on the ECMO, he faced a prolonged hospitalization in the Intensive Care Unit. The hospital faced an enormous cost for this type of protracted care; however, their main concern was the availability of ECMO for patients with a better chance of recovery. The clinical ethicists met with him and asked whether he would voluntarily agree to be withdrawn from the machine. The patient responded that he did not want to die and thought he had a good quality of life in the hospital. He was also worried by the possibility that the doctors would consider stopping his life support without his permission. The patient remained on ECMO until he died several weeks later from a blood clot that formed in the device's circuitry.[85]

Referring back to Beauchamp and Childress, the principles of distributive justice offer recommendations on how benefits and burdens can be distributed fairly, equitably, and suitably. They do this by presenting several different theories.[86] For example, Utilitarianism looks at criteria from multiple sources and prioritizes maximizing the public benefit. In contrast, Egalitarian theories of justice offer an alternative viewpoint by asserting that any benefits deemed valuable by members of a given group should be equally accessible to all. Therefore, an Egalitarian theory frequently focuses on the distribution of material benefits and insists that justice is based on considerations of need and equality. Consequently, allocating resources during a pandemic under an Egalitarian theory of justice would ensure that all scarce resources are equally distributed among all patients requiring them, regardless of the public benefit of this strategy.[87]

Other theories would emphasize different elements regarding the distribution of scarce resources. For example, should individuals who refuse to comply with public health guidelines be treated differently than those who do? This group could include COVID-19 deniers, those who refuse to wear masks, and those who decline to get vaccinated. According to the libertarianism school of thought, "all humans are naturally in a state of perfect freedom to order their actions and dispose of their possessions."[88] This declaration follows that those who would apply restrictions on their freedom are obligated to give good reasons for doing so.[89] Therefore, communitarians state that each person is obliged to their community and must support it. As the other three theories of distributive justice discussed, communitarianism is not an unbending belief system but an approach encompassing a variety of similar ideas. Nevertheless, communitarians are steadfast in their belief that community needs are more significant than personal goals and regard the group's desires as more important than individual freedom.[90] So, how can these theories be utilized for distributive justice during the pandemic?

A distributive justice structure can help facilitate decisions regarding distributing scarce resources. Under this framework, an appropriate comparative approach would look at how ill a patient is compared to others and how much they would benefit from treatment. In other words, the decision to treat a patient with effective but scarce resources should depend on whether the patient has the most significant need because of young age or poor health. It should also be based on the highest potential for survival or the effectiveness of treatment. Regrettably, this comparative approach is Utilitarian and overlooks the plight of the most ill because of their limited chance of survival even with these medical interventions. Indeed, this approach emphasizes the importance of efficiently stewarding resources, particularly in times of scarcity. Healthcare policies that adopt this distributive equity approach will show equal concern for all individuals, regardless of race, religion, economic class, or the designation stated by libertarian or communitarian theories. This approach recognizes that all individuals are worthy of satisfying their needs and bases treatment priority solely on medical issues and prognosis.[91] Still, even this approach has several problems.

The challenges caused by COVID-19 bring up bioethical dilemmas that have afflicted historically marginalized communities in the United States. How does one decide which patients are most needy AND can benefit from applying these limited resources, including ICU use and life support? Although these decisions should be nonbiased, the pandemic underscores the terrible impacts of longstanding health disparities on health outcomes since these differences can impact decisions to treat or not treat. In addition, the decision to use these resources is influenced by elements that affect people with disabilities from racial and ethnic minorities, including American Indian/Alaska Native communities.[92]

To illustrate this problem, we can examine how clinicians decide whether a patient is too ill to benefit from aggressive treatment. Emergency Department (ED) and ICU clinicians often utilize the Sequential Organ Failure Assessment (SOFA) tool. This tool looks at eight distinct parameters to calculate a value that predicts the likelihood of ICU mortality; the higher the score, the more likely a patient will not survive. This score is then used to assign patients to priority groups, with those not likely to survive often recommended for comfort measures only.[93] However, some would argue that the tool itself has elements that could be seen as biased.

The American College of Chest Physicians took issue with using SOFA in its current COVID-19 guide. They stated that "there is a growing body of evidence suggests such scoring systems are unlikely to predict critical care outcomes with sufficient accuracy … or be for a useful basis for triage decisions based upon the current protocol cut points."[94] The assessment also uses chronic illnesses as a condition that could harm minority populations. Finally, people with disabilities groups have expressed concerns, such as SOFA adding points to those with pre-existing speech disabilities that could impact treatment decisions for certain disabled groups.[95]

In conclusion, the distribution of limited resources during the pandemic should be fair, equitable, and based solely on helping those most ill and likely to benefit. However, current assessment tools like SOFA must be scrutinized to remove hidden biases affecting vulnerable populations. In addition, there needs to be a balance between utilitarian and egalitarian principles. An approach too heavily weighted on utilitarian principles would negatively affect vulnerable people by depriving them of beneficial treatments. Nevertheless, a process that is too heavily weighted on egalitarian principles could cause something called "ventilator affirmative action," which ultimately helps no one and deprives treatment to those it could benefit.

Non-COVID-19 Healthcare Rationing

While most people would not want to see anyone die from a curable disease because of a lack of healthcare, there appears to be very little agreement on how this should be accomplished. Instead, universal healthcare is often presented as a bulky economic burden that challenges what is good for society versus individuals' needs.[96] More often, the debate in the US is more about how medical care is paid for rather than whether it should be provided.[97] Nevertheless, it seems reasonable that a just society should provide universal access to a decent minimum healthcare package. Although it would be difficult to say what a basic package should contain, one could attempt to identify what must be made available to people for them to stay or become healthy. Unfortunately, this type of care is often presented as a basic need on the same level as providing food, water, and shelter.[98] Europe has not fully solved this problem either, as they struggle to provide basic healthcare to all. This fact is not just because some countries are wealthier than others but also because there is not enough basic care to provide for all.[99]

Beauchamp and Childress give three definitions of rationing. The first example they give is rationing because of a lack of resources.[100] This definition goes along with what is happening in some European countries where there is simply not enough basic healthcare to go around.[101] However, this type of rationing also includes shortages in healthcare because of a lack of funding. Rural areas in the US are deeply affected by this. Between January 2005 and July 2020, 171 rural hospitals closed nationwide.[102] The potential impact of local hospital closure on healthcare access in a rural community is critical to the community's health.

Nevertheless, certain inequities can exacerbate the problems associated with rural hospital closures. For example, reimbursement rates are higher if a Rural Health Clinic (RHC) is based in a small hospital. In addition, if the hospital closes, the incentive for expanding rural outpatient services often also goes away.[103]

The second type of rationing occurs when the government sets limits on certain goods and services, not market forces, as seen in the first. This type of rationing is seen in wartime when the government rations gasoline and food items. Still, it can also be seen if the government limits health insurance beyond some arbitrary amount. Finally, the third meaning of rationing refers to things with some degree of equitable distribution but allowing those who can afford them to purchase more.[104] This type of rationing can occur with certain types of treatment. For example, a cancer patient may get some treatment with their insurance and private funds but may be excluded from other treatments because of the high cost. The insurance company often makes these decisions based on various conditions, agreeing to pay for a treatment for some but not others. This type of rationing will be explored further.

The high cost of prescription medication poses challenges for distributive justice in many ways, but mainly by adding a barrier to treatment. This reality is valid for the 8.8% of Americans who lacked health insurance in 2017 and those whose insurance did not cover high-cost interventions. Often, clinicians have to petition insurance companies to get these treatments for their patients through a procedure called prior authorization. This time-consuming process may delay access to care, sometimes with adverse clinical consequences. A survey showed that 75% of doctors reported that these requirements could lead to patients abandoning treatment, and another 28% said that these requirements resulted in serious adverse events. Moreover, even if the insurance company chooses to cover the medication, many patients still incur high out-of-pocket costs that could limit their ability to afford treatment.[105]

In spinal muscular atrophy (SMA), motor cell degeneration in the spinal cord causes a progressive neuromuscular disorder. SMA has an incidence of 1 in 11,000 births and is the leading cause of inheritable infant mortality. Patients with SMA often develop proximal symmetric weakness and respiratory failure when it involves respiratory muscles. Despite its severity, many patients now survive into adulthood with advances in supportive treatment and new therapeutic interventions. It is estimated that adults comprise one-third of all patients with SMA.[106] One of these new therapeutic interventions is Nusinersen, which the US FDA approved in December 2016. The drug was later introduced in the European Union in 2017 and in China in 2019, and it has been credited for saving lives worldwide.[107]

Unfortunately, this medication is quite expensive. Nusinersen was initially priced at $750,000 for year one and $375,000 annually after that, not including costs required for administration since the medication must be given intrathecally (in the spinal canal). Because of its high price and complicated delivery, health systems face the challenge of prioritizing who should receive the drug first. For instance, should younger patients with less disability receive priority over older patients with more disability?[108] Should age be a valid reason for rationing, or should other variables be explored?

Some scholars say yes. American political philosopher Norman Daniels argues that age rationing is a practical way to deal with problems of resource scarcity under specific conditions. In the book *Just Health: Meeting Health Needs Fairly*, he contends that it is prudent to consider age and that it is a " morally permissible strategy to consider age when distributing resources although there is, of course, no prior moral obligation to pursue such a strategy."[109] Later, Daniels discusses an alternative to rationing by age: rationing by lottery.[110] Still, there are other ways clinicians have used to allocate limited resources fairly.

About 2.2 million adults were infected with hepatitis C virus (HCV) in the US from January 2017–to March 2020, and this rate is increasing, especially among young people with IV drug use. Without treatment, hepatitis C can lead to advanced liver disease, liver cancer, and death. However, effective therapeutic options are now available with new medications known as direct-acting antiviral (DAA) agents. It is now recommended that all patients with HCV infection, with few exceptions, receive this new treatment.[111] Unfortunately, in 2014, the price for this treatment exceeded $90,000, resulting in many insurance companies creating restrictions on access. Although the costs for hepatitis C treatments are better than in 2014, Medicaid still remains the least likely insurer to cover them. Nevertheless, this treatment is still expensive; however, if all eligible patients were treated, it would substantially lower future bad clinical outcomes and future costs, leading to considerable cost savings. Hepatitis C treatment eligibility restrictions have improved in some states, but others still have limited access to DAAs based on liver fibrosis qualifications, sobriety requirements, and medical specialist prescribing requirements.[112]

When DAAs first became available, various strategies were proposed to allow for fair distribution of this limited resource. Preferably, treatment-eligible patients with HCV would be provided with an educational session outlining the natural progression of HCV, stressing the importance of expediting treatment for the sickest patients and the safety of waiting for therapy in patients with early stages of the disease. Next, patients who have previously deferred therapy and new patients will be prioritized based on need, with patients with cirrhosis at one end of the spectrum and asymptomatic patients with mild fibrosis at the other. This system was felt to satisfy the principle of justice by prioritizing those with the highest medical needs.[113]

Cancer care is also costly, and there is great interest in improving treatment options and getting the best outcomes within a financially sustainable framework. Comparative effectiveness research (CER) has been suggested as a way to satisfy this dilemma.[114] The Institute of Medicine defines CER as "the generation and synthesis of evidence that compares the benefits and harms of alternative methods to prevent, diagnose, treat and monitor a clinical condition, or improve care delivery. The purpose of CER is to assist consumers, clinicians, purchasers, and policymakers to make informed decisions that will improve healthcare at both the individual and population levels."[115] Indeed, this appears to be a way to balance the high costs of treatment with a guide that establishes who would most benefit from the therapy clinically. Unfortunately, even if CER recommends a treatment, patients may be unable to pay for it if they lack insurance or if insurers refuse to pay. Nevertheless, CER attempts to balance physician discretion appropriately, patient autonomy, and system-level restrictions while considering where the benefit is marginal and limited by the financial cost.[116]

Finally, the least attractive way to allocate limited resources is by the "first come, first served" method. Still, unfortunately, that is how one valuable but limited resource is given: the intensive care unit (ICU). This allocation model has the potential for injustice; however, once a patient is admitted to an ICU, there is a presumption in favor of the continuation of treatment, even when the treatment may be futile. This situation may harm those waiting to get into the ICU, even if these patients were more likely to benefit from ICU treatment. Improper ICU bed utilization can lead to delays or denial for patients who could benefit from such care.[117] Although there is no absolute patient claim to continue care when it is futile, stopping it can be highly problematic.[118]

The US healthcare expenditure is currently almost 18% of the Gross National Product (GNP) and is expected to be 30% by 2030.[119] Critical care alone accounts for 20% of all healthcare costs and 1% of our GNP.[120] There are eight times as many beds per capita in the US than in other Western Nations, and elderly patients account for 60% of all ICU days.[121] People older than 65 years will double to 70 million in 2030. Because of these facts, the demand for ICU beds will increase substantially in the next decade. One way to mitigate these changes is to look at how many beds in the ICU are used for futile care. As stated above, these numbers are difficult to assess because of the lack of agreement on what constitutes medically futile care. In one study, the investigators felt that 11% of the ICU beds received futile care. The mortality rate for this group was 85%, with the survivors remaining in severely compromised health.[122]

Futile is an adjective meaning "incapable of producing any useful result; pointless."[123] Medical futility refers to treatments that are not likely to make the patient well. This definition seems simplistic, but it is often controversial in practice. As stated previously, this is now frequently called potentially inappropriate care. Physicians should be the guarantors of a treatment's therapeutic advantage. It should not be offered if a treatment does not have a benefit.[124] Nevertheless, even among physicians, there is no real consensus on futility. Some clinicians feel that an intervention is futile only if its chance for success is zero. In contrast, others will say an intervention is pointless even if the success rate is 13%.[125] When faced with rationing a scarce resource, the probability of success is a relevant criterion in deciding who should receive help.[126]

Can a hospital withhold resources when they feel the treatment is futile and that those resources could be used to help others? This case occurred at the hospital where I worked. An 85-year-old woman collapses after a sudden onset of abdominal pain. She has a history of multiple myeloma and stage IV kidney disease. She had refused dialysis in the past and was once under hospice care. In the ED, she was found to have a ruptured abdominal aortic aneurysm (AAA). Given the patient's age and comorbidities, her chance of survival was minimal and would likely include dialysis. The vascular surgeon has her in the OR and has already given her two massive transfusions. Each transfusion consists of six units of packed red blood cells plus fresh frozen plasma and platelets. When he requested a third, the blood bank refused, stating that the hospital is a Level 4 trauma center and that the request would cause a blood shortage that could jeopardize others. The surgeon angrily accused the blood bank of murder, but was the hospital correct in withholding the blood products under the principle of justice?

Scarce resources for specific treatments remain a reality in the US and other countries. How these resources are rationed is subject to the principle of distributive justice. Indeed, these resources should be allocated fairly, but "fairness" is often not easily determined. In this section, how resources are allocated is studied. The methods investigated include distribution models based on age, helping the sickest, helping those with the higher likelihood of benefit, and the "first come, first served" models. Unfortunately, none of these methods are entirely satisfying, and future studies will be needed to help resolve this continuing dilemma.

CONCLUSION

This chapter explores the ethical principle of justice from three different perspectives. First, it was looked at from a historical and somewhat philosophical background. Second, justice was examined regarding healthcare inequalities and vulnerable populations. Finally, the third section discussed justice regarding institutional decision-making regarding healthcare rationing and sustainability. This last section also looked at rationing that occurred during the COVID-19 pandemic.

Justice is sometimes challenging to understand as an ethical principle. How does one explain the fair distribution of healthcare goods and services? One argument would be that medical goods and services should be distributed to everyone equally. Others would say that some people should get a higher share because of need, and still, others would argue that some should get more because they are more likely to benefit. Should some people get more because they can and are willing to pay more? Should distribution decisions be based on benefits to the group or based on benefits to the individual? Using any of these arguments is likely to leave some groups feeling that they are being mistreated.

In a perfect world, everyone would receive everything they need or want without question. Trivial arguments like cost and availability would be seen as outrageous, outdated, and even laughable. All treatments would be available to all, and decisions about distribution would be, at worst, insignificant. However, healthcare has problems, and its very existence in the US is tenuous. On the one hand, treatment options continue to rise, and conditions once hopeless now have promising alternatives. The downside is that many of these miracle cures are expensive and unattainable to many Americans. In fact, the entire US healthcare system could collapse under its own weight. I have included a chapter that looks at the sustainability of US healthcare.

Surprisingly, many healthcare professionals pay little heed to costs. Nevertheless, the time is drawing near for tough decisions to be made. Understanding these dilemmas is essential for those who feel that healthcare continues to benefit all who need it in a way that will survive now and for future generations.

TAKE-HOME POINTS

- Justice is the first virtue of social institutions, as truth is of systems of thought. Justice is central to society and crucial in structuring social institutions.
- Justice is also a personal virtue and, as Aquinas describes, "the perpetual and constant will to render to each one his right."
- Health equity refers to stopping institutional and discriminatory obstacles that lead to health inequities and inequality. The goal is to guarantee equal access to quality healthcare, even if this requires giving some people more resources than others.
- Healthcare disparities are differences in the incidence, prevalence, mortality, and burden of diseases and other adverse health conditions that exist among specific population groups in the United States.
- Institutions need to be accountable to the communities they serve and those they teach. This accountability includes investing in programs for healthcare,

research, funding, recruitment, and education of healthcare staff, including information about race and ethnicity and social determinants of healthcare.

- The COVID-19 pandemic provides an excellent "classroom" as to how hospitals and healthcare systems use rationing in times of crisis and can provide insights regarding how rationing can be applied in future emergencies.
- The distribution of limited resources during the pandemic should be fair, equitable, and based solely on helping those most ill and likely to benefit. However, current assessment tools must be scrutinized to remove hidden biases affecting vulnerable populations.
- Beauchamp and Childress give three definitions of rationing: rationing because of a lack of resources, rationing because the government sets limits, such as in wartime, and rationing that allows some equitable distribution but also allows those who can afford them to purchase more.
- The worst way to allocate limited resources is by the "first come, first served" method, which often provides potentially inappropriate care to some while denying it to others that would most likely benefit.
- In a perfect world, everyone would receive everything they need or want without question. However, healthcare has a cost problem, and difficult decisions must be made for it to remain fair and sustainable.

NOTES

1 Matthias Klumpp, Ida G. Monfared, and Sebastian Vollmer, "Public Opinion on Global Distribution of COVID-19 Vaccines: Evidence from Two Nationally Representative Surveys in Germany and the United States," *Vaccine* 40, no. 16 (April 6, 2022): 2457–2461, page 2461.

2 Vivencio Ballano, "COVID-19 Vaccines, Public Health Goods and Catholic Social Teaching: Why Justice Must Prevail over Charity in the Global Vaccine Distribution," *HTS Theological Studies* 78, no. 4 (2022): 1–9, https://doi.org/10.4102/hts.v78i4.7065, page 3.

3 Vivencio Ballano, "COVID-19 Vaccines, Public Health Goods and Catholic Social Teaching: Why Justice Must Prevail over Charity in the Global Vaccine Distribution," *HTS Theological Studies* 78, no. 4 (2022): 1–9, https://doi.org/10.4102/hts.v78i4.7065, page 3.

4 Vivencio Ballano, "COVID-19 Vaccines, Public Health Goods and Catholic Social Teaching: Why Justice Must Prevail over Charity in the Global Vaccine Distribution," *HTS Theological Studies* 78, no. 4 (2022): 1–9, https://doi.org/10.4102/hts.v78i4.7065, page 9.

5 Matthias Klumpp, Ida G. Monfared, and Sebastian Vollmer, "Public Opinion on Global Distribution of COVID-19 Vaccines: Evidence from Two Nationally Representative Surveys in Germany and the United States," *Vaccine* 40, no. 16 (April 6, 2022): 2457–2461, page 2460.

6 Arne N. Akbar and Derek W. Gilroy, "Aging Immunity May Exacerbate COVID-19," *Science* 369, no. 6501 (July 17, 2020): 256–257, https://doi.org/10.1126/science.abb0762, page 256.

7 Ivan Efreaim A. Gozum and Jove Jim S. Aguas, *Philosophia: International Journal of Philosophy* 23, no. 1 (January 2022): 202–217, page 213.

8 Carmen Torrie et al., "Social Justice in Pandemic Immunization Policy: We're All in This Together," *Nursing Ethics* 28, no. 6 (September 2021): 924–934, page 925.

9 Rosamond Rhodes, "Justice in COVID-19 Vaccine Prioritisation: Rethinking the Approach," *Journal of Medical Ethics* 47, no. 9 (September 2021): 623–631, https://doi.org/10.1136/medethics-2020–107117, page 630.

10 Carmen Torrie et al., "Social Justice in Pandemic Immunization Policy: We're All in This Together," *Nursing Ethics* 28, no. 6 (September 2021): 924–934, page 931.

11 Nick Andrews et al., "Duration of Protection against Mild and Severe Disease by Covid-19 Vaccines," *New England Journal of Medicine* 386, no. 4 (January 27, 2022): 340–350, https://doi.org/10.1056/NEJMoa2115481, pages 340–350.

12 C. C. Meinwald, "Plato," 2022, www.britannica.com/biography/Plato.

13 Dominic Farrell, "Wanting the Common Good: Aquinas on General Justice," *Review of Metaphysics* 71, no. 3 (March 2018): 517–549, page 517.

14 Dominic Farrell, "Wanting the Common Good: Aquinas on General Justice," *Review of Metaphysics* 71, no. 3 (March 2018): 517–549, page 517.

15 Sean Coyle, "Corrective and Distributive Justice: From Aristotle to Modern Times," *Jurisprudence* 2, no. 2 (December 2011): 597–601, page 597.

16 John P. Balsdon, V. Dacre, and John Ferguson, "Cicero," 2022, www.britannica.com/biography/Cicero.

17 Albert R. Jonsen, *A Short History of Medical Ethics* (New York: Oxford University Press, 2000), page x.

18 "Whether Justice Is Fittingly Defined as Being the Perpetual and Constant Will to Render to Each One His Right?," accessed December 9, 2022, https://biblehub.com/library/aquinas/summa_theologica/whether_justice_is_fittingly_defined.htm.

19 Ryan Darr, "The Virtue of Justice and the Justice of Institutions: Aquinas on Money and Just Exchange," *Journal of the Society of Christian Ethics* 40, no. 1 (2020): 3–20, https://doi.org/10.5840/jsce202051925, page 4.

20 Ryan Darr, "The Virtue of Justice and the Justice of Institutions: Aquinas on Money and Just Exchange," *Journal of the Society of Christian Ethics* 40, no. 1 (2020): 3–20, https://doi.org/10.5840/jsce202051925, page 18.

21 Michael T. Dempsey, "Providence, Distributive Justice, and Divine Government in the Theology of Thomas Aquinas: Some Implications for Ecclesial Practice," *New Blackfriars* 90, no. 1027 (May 2009): 365–384, page 379.

22 Daniel Philpott, "Resurrecting Justice," *Journal of Moral Theology* 11, no. 1 (January 2022): 167–192, page 191.

23 B. Duignan, "John Rawls," 2022, www.britannica.com/biography/John-Rawls.

24 John Rawls, *A Theory of Justice* (Cambridge, MA : Belknap Press of Harvard University Press, 1971), page 387.

25 Ivan Efreaim A. Gozum and Jove Jim S. Aguas, *Philosophia: International Journal of Philosophy* 23, no. 1 (January 2022): 202–217, page 204.

26 Ronald Paul Hill, Robert M Peterson, and Kanwalroop Kathy Dhanda, "Global Consumption and Distributive Justice: A Rawlsian Perspective," *Human Rights Quarterly* 23, no. 1 (February 2001): 171–187, page 172.

27 Tom L. Beauchamp and James F. Childress, *Principles of Biomedical Ethics*, Eighth edition (New York: Oxford University Press, 2019), page 226.

28 Merriam-Webster, *Merriam-Webster's Intermediate Dictionary* (Springfield, MA: Merriam-Webster, 2020).

29 Ellen Gutoskey, "Equity vs. Equality: What's the Difference?," *Mental Floss*, June 11, 2020, www.mentalfloss.com/article/625404/equity-vs-equality-what-is-the-difference.

30 Jason Daniel-Ulloa and Zawn Villines, "Health Equity vs. Health Equality: Definitions, Examples, and More," December 15, 2021, www.medicalnewstoday.com/articles/health-equity-and-health-equality.

31 Thomas M. Robertson and Richard P. Lofgren, "Where Population Health Misses the Mark: Breaking the 80/20 Rule," *Academic Medicine* 90, no. 3 (March 2015): 277–278, https://doi.org/10.1097/ACM.0000000000000627, page 277.

32 Jason Daniel-Ulloa and Zawn Villines, "Health Equity vs. Health Equality: Definitions, Examples, and More," December 15, 2021, www.medicalnewstoday.com/articles/health-equity-and-health-equality.

33 Kelly M. Hoffman et al., "Racial Bias in Pain Assessment and Treatment Recommendations, and False Beliefs about Biological Differences between Blacks and Whites," *Proceedings of the National Academy of Sciences* 113, no. 16 (April 19, 2016): 4296–4301, https://doi.org/10.1073/pnas.1516047113, page 4300.

34 Jason Daniel-Ulloa and Zawn Villines, "Health Equity vs. Health Equality: Definitions, Examples, and More," December 15, 2021, www.medicalnewstoday.com/articles/health-equity-and-health-equality.

35 Tom L. Beauchamp and James F. Childress, *Principles of Biomedical Ethics*, Eighth edition (New York: Oxford University Press, 2019), page 266.

36 Tom L. Beauchamp and James F. Childress, *Principles of Biomedical Ethics*, Eighth edition (New York: Oxford University Press, 2019), pages 272–276.

37 Steven J. Baumrucker et al., "The Principle of Distributive Justice," *American Journal of Hospice & Palliative Medicine* 29, no. 2 (March 2012): 151–156, https://doi.org/10.1177/1049909111433307, pages 151–152.

38 David F. Kelly, Gerard Magill, and H. ten Have, *Contemporary Catholic Health Care Ethics*, 2nd ed (Washington, DC: Georgetown University Press, 2013), page 347.

39 Emma Culotta, "Understanding the Distributive Equity Framework for Allocating Scarce Medical Resources in Times of Crisis," *Texas Law Review* 100, no. 4 (March 2022): 803–837, page 808.

40 Emma Culotta, "Understanding the Distributive Equity Framework for Allocating Scarce Medical Resources in Times of Crisis," *Texas Law Review* 100, no. 4 (March 2022): 803–837, page 837.

41 A. Furnham, C. Thomas, and K. V. Petrides, "Patient Characteristics and the Allocation of Scarce Medical Resources," *Psychology, Health & Medicine* 7, no. 1 (February 2002): 99–106, page 105.

42 Jean Porter, *Justice as a Virtue: A Thomistic Perspective* (Grand Rapids, Michigan: William B. Eerdmans Publishing Company, 2016).

43 Lisa R. Fortuna et al., "Inequity and the Disproportionate Impact of COVID-19 on Communities of Color in the United States: The Need for a Trauma-Informed Social Justice Response," *Psychological Trauma: Theory, Research, Practice, and Policy* 12, no. 5 (July 2020): 443–445, https://doi.org/10.1037/tra0000889, page 443.

44 Lisa R. Fortuna et al., "Inequity and the Disproportionate Impact of COVID-19 on Communities of Color in the United States: The Need for a Trauma-Informed Social Justice Response," *Psychological Trauma: Theory, Research, Practice, and Policy* 12, no. 5 (July 2020): 443–445, https://doi.org/10.1037/tra0000889, page 445.

45 Melissa J. Bourne, Suzanne C. Smeltzer, and Michelle M. Kelly, "Healthcare Inequities among Adults with Developmental Disability: An Integrative Review with Implications for Nursing Education," *Nurse Education in Practice* 57 (November 1, 2021), page 1.

46 Paula A. Braveman et al., "Health Disparities and Health Equity: The Issue Is Justice," *American Journal of Public Health* 101, no. S1 (December 2011): S149–S155, https://doi.org/10.2105/AJPH.2010.300062, page 149.

47 Peter Mende-Siedlecki et al., "Perceptual Contributions to Racial Bias in Pain Recognition," *Journal of Experimental Psychology: General* 148, no. 5 (May 2019): 863–889, https://doi.org/10.1037/xge0000600, page 863.

48 Jason Daniel-Ulloa and Zawn Villines, "Health Equity vs. Health Equality: Definitions, Examples, and More," December 15, 2021, www.medicalnewstoday.com/articles/health-equity-and-health-equality.

49 Mary Forhan and Ximena Ramos Salas, "Inequities in Healthcare: A Review of Bias and Discrimination in Obesity Treatment," *Canadian Journal of Diabetes* 37, no. 3 (June 2013): 205–209, https://doi.org/10.1016/j.jcjd.2013.03.362, page 208.

50 Melissa J. Bourne, Suzanne C. Smeltzer, and Michelle M. Kelly, "Healthcare Inequities among Adults with Developmental Disability: An Integrative Review with Implications for Nursing Education," *Nurse Education in Practice* 57 (November 1, 2021), pages 1–2.

51 Melissa J. Bourne, Suzanne C. Smeltzer, and Michelle M. Kelly, "Healthcare Inequities among Adults with Developmental Disability: An Integrative Review with Implications for Nursing Education," *Nurse Education in Practice* 57 (November 1, 2021), pages 6–7.

52 Melissa J. Bourne, Suzanne C. Smeltzer, and Michelle M. Kelly, "Healthcare Inequities among Adults with Developmental Disability: An Integrative Review with Implications for Nursing Education," *Nurse Education in Practice* 57 (November 1, 2021), page 8.

53 Tracy Spears and Wally Schmader, "Unconscious Bias in Healthcare," *Physician Leadership Journal*, April 2021, page 22.

54 Merriam-Webster, *Merriam-Webster's Intermediate Dictionary* (Springfield, MA: Merriam-Webster, 2020).

55 Tracy Spears and Wally Schmader, "Unconscious Bias in Healthcare," *Physician Leadership Journal*, April 2021, page 22.

56 Brianna M. McQuade, Alan Schwartz, and Jennie B. Jarrett, "Acknowledging and Assessing Implicit Bias among Healthcare Professionals: A Randomized Controlled Trial," *Journal of Interprofessional Education & Practice* 24 (September 2021): 100452, https://doi.org/10.1016/j.xjep.2021.100452, page 1.

57 Brianna M. McQuade, Alan Schwartz, and Jennie B. Jarrett, "Acknowledging and Assessing Implicit Bias among Healthcare Professionals: A Randomized Controlled Trial," *Journal of Interprofessional Education & Practice* 24 (September 2021): 100452, https://doi.org/10.1016/j.xjep.2021.100452, page 4.

58 Elizabeth N. Chapman, Anna Kaatz, and Molly Carnes, "Physicians and Implicit Bias: How Doctors May Unwittingly Perpetuate Health Care Disparities," *Journal of General Internal Medicine* 28, no. 11 (November 2013): 1504–1510, https://doi.org/10.1007/s11606-013-2441-1, page 1504.

59 Patricia G. Devine et al., "Long-Term Reduction in Implicit Race Bias: A Prejudice Habit-Breaking Intervention," *Journal of Experimental Social Psychology* 48, no. 6 (November 2012): 1267–1278, https://doi.org/10.1016/j.jesp.2012.06.003, page 1267.

60 Patricia G. Devine et al., "Long-Term Reduction in Implicit Race Bias: A Prejudice Habit-Breaking Intervention," *Journal of Experimental Social Psychology* 48, no. 6 (November 2012): 1267–1278, https://doi.org/10.1016/j.jesp.2012.06.003, page 1277.

61 Victoria Nkunu and Kevin J. McLaughlin, "Why Do Some Physicians Choose to Tackle Inequities in Healthcare?," *International Journal for Equity in Health* 17, no. 1 (June 15, 2018), https://doi.org/10.1186/s12939-018-0790-4, page 5.

62 Derek Soled, "Distributive Justice as a Means of Combating Systemic Racism in Healthcare," *Voices in Bioethics* 7 (June 1, 2021), https://doi.org/10.52214/vib.v7i.8502, page 1.

63 Derek Soled, "Distributive Justice as a Means of Combating Systemic Racism in Healthcare," *Voices in Bioethics* 7 (June 1, 2021), https://doi.org/10.52214/vib.v7i.8502, page 4.

64 Henk ten Have, *Vulnerability: Challenging Bioethics* (New York: Routledge, 2016).

65 Henk ten Have, *Vulnerability: Challenging Bioethics* (New York: Routledge, 2016), page 4.

66 Anghela Z. Paredes et al., "Examining Healthcare Inequities Relative to United States Safety Net Hospitals," *The American Journal of Surgery* 220, no. 3 (September 1, 2020): 525–531, pages 529–530.

67 Yael Cannon, "Closing the Health Justice Gap: Access to Justice in Furtherance of Health Equity," *Columbia Human Rights Law Review* 53, no. 2 (Spring 2022), page 517.

68 Derrick Lane, "Looters Leave More Food Deserts In Black Communities," June 4, 2020, https://blackdoctor.org/looters-leave-more-food-deserts-in-black-communities.

69 Anghela Z. Paredes et al., "Examining Healthcare Inequities Relative to United States Safety Net Hospitals," *The American Journal of Surgery* 220, no. 3 (September 1, 2020): 525–531, pages 529–530.

70 Ruqaiijah Yearby, "Racial Disparities in Health Status and Access to Healthcare: The Continuation of Inequality in the United States Due to Structural Racism: Continuing Racial Health Disparities," *American Journal of Economics and Sociology* 77, no. 3–4 (May 2018): 1113–1152, https://doi.org/10.1111/ajes.12230, pages 1120–1121.

71 Ruqaiijah Yearby, "Racial Disparities in Health Status and Access to Healthcare: The Continuation of Inequality in the United States Due to Structural Racism: Continuing Racial Health Disparities," *American Journal of Economics and Sociology* 77, no. 3–4 (May 2018): 1113–1152, https://doi.org/10.1111/ajes.12230, page 1140.

72 Kritee Gujral and Anirban Basu, "Impact of Rural and Urban Hospital Closures on Inpatient Mortality" (Cambridge, MA: National Bureau of Economic Research, August 2019), https://doi.org/10.3386/w26182, page 1.

73 Mary K. Wolfe, Noreen C. McDonald, and G. Mark Holmes, "Transportation Barriers to Health Care in the United States: Findings From the National Health Interview Survey, 1997–2017," *American Journal of Public Health* 110, no. 6 (June 2020): 815–822, https://doi.org/10.2105/AJPH.2020.305579, page 816.

74 Hanadi Y. Hamadi et al., "Medicare and Telehealth: The Impact of COVID-19 Pandemic," *Journal of Evaluation in Clinical Practice* 28, no. 1 (February 2022): 43–48, https://doi.org/10.1111/jep.13634, pages 43–47.

75 Dominic Farrell, "Wanting the Common Good: Aquinas on General Justice," *Review of Metaphysics* 71, no. 3 (March 2018): 517–549, page 517.

76 Thomas A. Shannon, "Living the Vision: Health Care, Social Justice and Institutional Identity," *Christian Bioethics* 7, no. 1 (April 2001): 49–65, page 51.
77 Wendy DiChristina, "Structural Justice Ethics in Health Care," *Voices in Bioethics* 7 (June 2, 2021), https://doi.org/10.52214/vib.v7i.8404, page 1.
78 Wendy DiChristina, "Structural Justice Ethics in Health Care," *Voices in Bioethics* 7 (June 2, 2021), https://doi.org/10.52214/vib.v7i.8404, page 5.
79 Chyke A. Doubeni et al., "A Framework for Transforming Primary Care Health Care Professions Education and Training to Promote Health Equity," *Journal of Health Care for the Poor & Underserved* 31 (November 2, 2020): N.PAG-N.PAG, page 201.
80 Robert W Putsch and Linda Pololi, "Distributive Justice in American Healthcare: Institutions, Power, and the Equitable Care of Patients," *The American Journal of Managed Care* 10, no. Special (2004), https://doi.org/10.13016/QG6F-A6WO, page 51.
81 L. Chad Horne and Joseph Heath, "A Market Failures Approach to Justice in Health," *Politics, Philosophy & Economics* 21, no. 2 (May 2022): 165–189, https://doi.org/10.1177/1470594X221089670, page 174.
82 Thomas A. Shannon, "Living the Vision: Health Care, Social Justice and Institutional Identity," *Christian Bioethics* 7, no. 1 (April 2001): 49–65, page 62.
83 Emma Culotta, "Understanding the Distributive Equity Framework for Allocating Scarce Medical Resources in Times of Crisis," *Texas Law Review* 100, no. 4 (March 2022): 803–837, page 804.
84 Yves Saint James Aquino et al., "Ethical Guidance for Hard Decisions: A Critical Review of Early International COVID-19 ICU Triage Guidelines," *Health Care Analysis : HCA : Journal of Health Philosophy and Policy* 30, no. 2 (June 2022): 163–195, https://doi.org/10.1007/s10728-021-00442-0, page 164.
85 Joanna Smolenski, "Involuntary Withdrawal: A Bridge Too Far?," *Clinical Ethics Case Studies, Hastings Bioethics Forum*, 3, August 21, 2023.
86 Tom L. Beauchamp and James F. Childress, *Principles of Biomedical Ethics*, Eighth edition (New York: Oxford University Press, 2019), page 268.
87 Jeffrey Yuk-Chiu Yip, "Healthcare Resource Allocation in the COVID-19 Pandemic: Ethical Considerations from the Perspective of Distributive Justice within Public Health," *Public Health in Practice (Oxford, England)* 2 (November 2021): 100111, https://doi.org/10.1016/j.puhip.2021.100111, page 1.
88 John Locke, *Two Treatises of Government and A Letter Concerning Toleration: Locke* (New Haven, CT: Yale University Press, 2003), page 101.
89 Lukas J. Meier, "Systemising Triage: COVID-19 Guidelines and Their Underlying Theories of Distributive Justice," *Medicine, Health Care and Philosophy: A European Journal*, July 7, 2022, 1–12, https://doi.org/10.1007/s11019-022-10101-3, page 6.
90 Lukas J. Meier, "Systemising Triage: COVID-19 Guidelines and Their Underlying Theories of Distributive Justice," *Medicine, Health Care and Philosophy: A European Journal*, July 7, 2022, 1–12, https://doi.org/10.1007/s11019-022-10101-3, page 8.
91 Emma Culotta, "Understanding the Distributive Equity Framework for Allocating Scarce Medical Resources in Times of Crisis," *Texas Law Review* 100, no. 4 (March 2022): 803–837, page 837.
92 Maya Sabatello et al., "Disability, Ethics, and Health Care in the COVID-19 Pandemic," *American Journal of Public Health* 110, no. 10 (October 2020): 1523–1527, page 1526.

93 Harald Schmidt, Dorothy E. Roberts, and Nwamaka D Eneanya, "Rationing, Racism and Justice: Advancing the Debate around 'Colourblind' COVID-19 Ventilator Allocation," *Journal of Medical Ethics* 48, no. 2 (February 2022): 126–130, https://doi.org/10.1136/medethics-2020–106856, page 127.

94 R. C. Maves et al., "Triage of Scarce Critical Care Resources in COVID-19 an Implementation Guide for Regional Allocation: An Expert Panel Report of the Task Force for Mass Critical Care and the American College of Chest Physicians," *Chest* 158, no. 1 (2020): 212–225.

95 Harald Schmidt, Dorothy E. Roberts, and Nwamaka D Eneanya, "Rationing, Racism and Justice: Advancing the Debate around 'Colourblind' COVID-19 Ventilator Allocation," *Journal of Medical Ethics* 48, no. 2 (February 2022): 126–130, https://doi.org/10.1136/medethics-2020–106856, page 129.

96 Amie Leigh Zimmer, "Rethinking the Right to Health: Ableism and the Binary between Individual and Collective Rights," *Bioethics* 35, no. 8 (October 2021): 752–759, https://doi.org/10.1111/bioe.12922, page 759.

97 Scott L. Greer, Holly Jarman, and Peter D. Donnelly, "Lessons for the United States From Single-Payer Systems," *American Journal of Public Health* 109, no. 11 (November 2019): 1493–1496, https://doi.org/10.2105/AJPH.2019.305312, page 1493.

98 Allen Andrew A. Alvarez, "Threshold Considerations in Fair Allocation of Health Resources: Justice beyond Scarcity," *Bioethics* 21, no. 8 (October 2007): 426–438, https://doi.org/10.1111/j.1467–8519.2007.00580.x, page 11.

99 Stéphane Bauzon, "Classical Distributive Justice and the European Healthcare System: Rethinking the Foundations of European Health Care in an Age of Crises," *The Journal of Medicine and Philosophy* 40, no. 2 (April 2015): 190–200, https://doi.org/10.1093/jmp/jhu078, page 198.

100 Tom L. Beauchamp and James F. Childress, *Principles of Biomedical Ethics*, fifth edition (New York: Oxford University Press, 2001), page 253.

101 Stéphane Bauzon, "Classical Distributive Justice and the European Healthcare System: Rethinking the Foundations of European Health Care in an Age of Crises," *The Journal of Medicine and Philosophy* 40, no. 2 (April 2015): 190–200, https://doi.org/10.1093/jmp/jhu078.

102 Katherine E. M. Miller et al., "Access to Outpatient Services in Rural Communities Changes after Hospital Closure," *Health Services Research* 56, no. 5 (October 2021): 788–801, https://doi.org/10.1111/1475–6773.13694, page 789.

103 Katherine E. M. Miller et al., "Access to Outpatient Services in Rural Communities Changes after Hospital Closure," *Health Services Research* 56, no. 5 (October 2021): 788–801, https://doi.org/10.1111/1475–6773.13694, page 795.

104 Tom L. Beauchamp and James F. Childress, *Principles of Biomedical Ethics*, fifth edition (New York: Oxford University Press, 2001), page 253.

105 Amy Y. Tsou et al., "Ethical Perspectives on Costly Drugs and Health Care: AAN Position Statement," *Neurology* 97, no. 14 (October 5, 2021): 685–692, https://doi.org/10.1212/WNL.0000000000012571, page 686.

106 Nassim Rad, Haibi Cai, and Michael D. Weiss, "Management of Spinal Muscular Atrophy in the Adult Population," *Muscle & Nerve* 65, no. 5 (May 2022): 498–507, https://doi.org/10.1002/mus.27519.pages 498–499.

107 Jiaying Qiu et al., "History of Development of the Life-Saving Drug 'Nusinersen' in Spinal Muscular Atrophy," *Frontiers in Cellular Neuroscience* 16 (August 12, 2022): 942976, https://doi.org/10.3389/fncel.2022.942976, page 1.

108 Amy Y. Tsou et al., "Ethical Perspectives on Costly Drugs and Health Care: AAN Position Statement," *Neurology* 97, no. 14 (October 5, 2021): 685–692, https://doi.org/10.1212/WNL.0000000000012571, page 689.

109 S. Brauer, "Age Rationing and Prudential Lifespan Account in Norman Daniels' 'Just Health,'" *Journal of Medical Ethics* 35, no. 1 (January 1, 2009): 27–31, https://doi.org/10.1136/jme.2008.024398, page 2.

110 Norman Daniels, *Just Health: Meeting Health Needs Fairly*, ACLS Humanities E-Book. (Cambridge: Cambridge University Press, 2008), page 179–180.

111 William W. Thompson et al., "*Vital Signs:* Hepatitis C Treatment Among Insured Adults — United States, 2019–2020," *MMWR. Morbidity and Mortality Weekly Report* 71, no. 32 (August 12, 2022): 1011–1017, https://doi.org/10.15585/mmwr.mm7132e1, page 1011.

112 William W. Thompson et al., "*Vital Signs:* Hepatitis C Treatment Among Insured Adults — United States, 2019–2020," *MMWR. Morbidity and Mortality Weekly Report* 71, no. 32 (August 12, 2022): 1011–1017, https://doi.org/10.15585/mmwr.mm7132e1, page 1015.

113 Andrew Aronsohn and Donald Jensen, "Distributive Justice and the Arrival of Direct-Acting Antivirals: Who Should Be First in Line?," *Hepatology (Baltimore, Md.)* 53, no. 6 (June 2011): 1789–1791, https://doi.org/10.1002/hep.24374, page 1790.

114 Jeffrey Peppercorn et al., "Does Comparative Effectiveness Research Promote Rationing of Cancer Care?," *Lancet Oncology* 15, no. 3 (March 1, 2014): e132–e138, page e132.

115 Harold C. Sox, "Comparative Effectiveness Research: A Report From the Institute of Medicine," *Annals of Internal Medicine* 151, no. 3 (August 4, 2009): 203, https://doi.org/10.7326/0003-4819-151-3-200908040-00125, page 203.

116 Jeffrey Peppercorn et al., "Does Comparative Effectiveness Research Promote Rationing of Cancer Care?," *Lancet Oncology* 15, no. 3 (March 1, 2014): e132–e138, page e137.

117 Thanh N. Huynh et al., "The Opportunity Cost of Futile Treatment in the ICU," *Critical Care Medicine* 42, no. 9 (September 2014): 1977–1982, https://doi.org/10.1097/CCM.0000000000000402.

118 Lynette Cederquist, "The Role of Distributive Justice in 'Autonomy Versus Futility' Standoffs," *American Journal of Bioethics* 16, no. 7 (July 2016): 61–62, page 61.

119 Salimah H. Meghani and Pamela S. Hinds, "Policy Brief: The Institute of Medicine Report Dying in America: Improving Quality and Honoring Individual Preferences near the End of Life," *Nursing Outlook* 63, no. 1 (January 1, 2015): 51–59.

120 Thanh N. Huynh et al., "The Frequency and Cost of Treatment Perceived to Be Futile in Critical Care," *JAMA Internal Medicine* 173, no. 20 (November 11, 2013): 1887–1894, https://doi.org/10.1001/jamainternmed.2013.10261.

121 James L. Bernat, "Medical Futility: Definition, Determination, and Disputes in Critical Care," *Neurocritical Care* 2, no. 2 (2005): 198, https://doi.org/10.1385/ncc:2:2:198.

122 Thanh N. Huynh et al., "The Frequency and Cost of Treatment Perceived to Be Futile in Critical Care," *JAMA Internal Medicine* 173, no. 20 (November 11, 2013): 1887–1894, https://doi.org/10.1001/jamainternmed.2013.10261.

123 Merriam-Webster, Merriam-Webster's Intermediate Dictionary (Springfield, MA: Merriam-Webster, 2020).

124 David F. Kelly, Gerard Magill, and H. ten Have, *Contemporary Catholic Health Care Ethics*, second edition (Washington, DC: Georgetown University Press, 2013).

125 James L. Bernat, "Medical Futility: Definition, Determination, and Disputes in Critical Care," *Neurocritical Care* 2, no. 2 (2005): 198, https://doi.org/10.1385/ncc:2:2:198.

126 E. H. Elpern, B. Covert, and R. Kleinpell, "Moral Distress of Staff Nurses in a Medical Intensive Care Unit," *American Journal of Critical Care* 14, no. 6 (2005): 523–530.

BIBLIOGRAPHY

Akbar, Arne N., and Derek W. Gilroy. "Aging Immunity May Exacerbate COVID-19." *Science* 369, no. 6501 (July 17, 2020): 256–257. https://doi.org/10.1126/science.abb0762.

Alvarez, Allen Andrew A. "Threshold Considerations in Fair Allocation of Health Resources: Justice beyond Scarcity." *Bioethics* 21, no. 8 (October 2007): 426–438. https://doi.org/10.1111/j.1467-8519.2007.00580.x.

Andrews, Nick, Elise Tessier, Julia Stowe, Charlotte Gower, Freja Kirsebom, Ruth Simmons, Eileen Gallagher, et al. "Duration of Protection against Mild and Severe Disease by Covid-19 Vaccines." *New England Journal of Medicine* 386, no. 4 (January 27, 2022): 340–350. https://doi.org/10.1056/NEJMoa2115481.

Aquino, Yves Saint James, Wendy A. Rogers, Jackie Leach Scully, Farah Magrabi, and Stacy M. Carter. "Ethical Guidance for Hard Decisions: A Critical Review of Early International COVID-19 ICU Triage Guidelines." *Health Care Analysis* 30, no. 2 (June 2022): 163–295. https://doi.org/10.1007/s10728-021-00442-0.

Aronsohn, Andrew, and Donald Jensen. "Distributive Justice and the Arrival of Direct-Acting Antivirals: Who Should Be First in Line?" *Hepatology* 53, no. 6 (June 2011): 1789–1791. https://doi.org/10.1002/hep.24374.

Ballano, Vivencio. "COVID-19 Vaccines, Public Health Goods and Catholic Social Teaching: Why Justice Must Prevail over Charity in the Global Vaccine Distribution." *HTS Theological Studies* 78, no. 4 (2022): 1–9. https://doi.org/10.4102/hts.v78i4.7065.

Baumrucker, Steven J., Matt Stolick, Paige Mingle, Karrie A. Oertli, Gerald M. Morris, and Gregg VandeKieft. "The Principle of Distributive Justice." *American Journal of Hospice & Palliative Medicine* 29, no. 2 (March 2012): 151–156. https://doi.org/10.1177/1049909111433307.

Bauzon, Stéphane. "Classical Distributive Justice and the European Healthcare System: Rethinking the Foundations of European Health Care in an Age of Crises." *The Journal of Medicine and Philosophy* 40, no. 2 (April 2015): 190–200. https://doi.org/10.1093/jmp/jhu078.

Beauchamp, Tom L., and James F. Childress. *Principles of Biomedical Ethics*. Fifth edition. New York: Oxford University Press, 2001.

Beauchamp, Tom L., and James F. Childress. *Principles of Biomedical Ethics*. Eighth edition. New York: Oxford University Press, 2019.

Bernat, James L. "Medical Futility: Definition, Determination, and Disputes in Critical Care." *Neurocritical Care* 2, no. 2 (2005): 198. https://doi.org/10.1385/ncc:2:2:198.

Bourne, Melissa J., Suzanne C. Smeltzer, and Michelle M. Kelly. "Healthcare Inequities among Adults with Developmental Disability: An Integrative Review with Implications for Nursing Education." *Nurse Education in Practice* 57 (November 1, 2021).

Brauer, S. "Age Rationing and Prudential Lifespan Account in Norman Daniels' 'Just Health.'" *Journal of Medical Ethics* 35, no. 1 (January 1, 2009): 27–31. https://doi.org/10.1136/jme.2008.024398.

Braveman, Paula A., Shiriki Kumanyika, Jonathan Fielding, Thomas LaVeist, Luisa N. Borrell, Ron Manderscheid, and Adewale Troutman. "Health Disparities and Health Equity: The Issue Is Justice." *American Journal of Public Health* 101, no. S1 (December 2011): S149–S155. https://doi.org/10.2105/AJPH.2010.300062.

Cannon, Yael. "Closing the Health Justice Gap: Access to Justice in Furtherance of Health Equity." *Columbia Human Rights Law Review* 53, no. 2 (Spring 2022).

Cederquist, Lynette. "The Role of Distributive Justice in 'Autonomy Versus Futility' Standoffs." *American Journal of Bioethics* 16, no. 7 (July 2016): 61–62.

Chapman, Elizabeth N., Anna Kaatz, and Molly Carnes. "Physicians and Implicit Bias: How Doctors May Unwittingly Perpetuate Health Care Disparities." *Journal of General Internal Medicine* 28, no. 11 (November 2013): 1504–1510. https://doi.org/10.1007/s11606-013-2441-1.

Coyle, Sean. "Corrective and Distributive Justice: From Aristotle to Modern Times." *Jurisprudence* 2, no. 2 (December 2011): 597–601.

Culotta, Emma. "Understanding the Distributive Equity Framework for Allocating Scarce Medical Resources in Times of Crisis." *Texas Law Review* 100, no. 4 (March 2022): 803–837.

Daniels, Norman, 1942-. *Just Health: Meeting Health Needs Fairly*. ACLS Humanities E-Book. Cambridge: Cambridge University Press, 2008.

Daniel-Ulloa, Jason and Villines, Zawn. "Health Equity vs. Health Equality: Definitions, Examples, and More," December 15, 2021. www.medicalnewstoday.com/articles/health-equity-and-health-equality.

Darr, Ryan. "The Virtue of Justice and the Justice of Institutions: Aquinas on Money and Just Exchange." *Journal of the Society of Christian Ethics* 40, no. 1 (2020): 3–20. https://doi.org/10.5840/jsce202051925.

Dempsey, Michael T. "Providence, Distributive Justice, and Divine Government in the Theology of Thomas Aquinas: Some Implications for Ecclesial Practice." *New Blackfriars* 90, no. 1027 (May 2009): 365–384.

Devine, Patricia G., Patrick S. Forscher, Anthony J. Austin, and William T.L. Cox. "Long-Term Reduction in Implicit Race Bias: A Prejudice Habit-Breaking Intervention." *Journal of Experimental Social Psychology* 48, no. 6 (November 2012): 1267–1278. https://doi.org/10.1016/j.jesp.2012.06.003.

DiChristina, Wendy. "Structural Justice Ethics in Health Care." *Voices in Bioethics* 7 (June 2, 2021). https://doi.org/10.52214/vib.v7i.8404.

Doubeni, Chyke A., MD MPH, Tonya L Fancher, Paul Juarez, PhD, Christine Riedy, MA, et al. "A Framework for Transforming Primary Care Health Care Professions Education and Training to Promote Health Equity." *Journal of Health Care for the Poor & Underserved* 31 (November 2, 2020).

Farrell, Dominic. "Wanting the Common Good: Aquinas on General Justice." *Review of Metaphysics* 71, no. 3 (March 2018): 517–549.

Forhan, Mary, and Ximena Ramos Salas. "Inequities in Healthcare: A Review of Bias and Discrimination in Obesity Treatment." *Canadian Journal of Diabetes* 37, no. 3 (June 2013): 205–209. https://doi.org/10.1016/j.jcjd.2013.03.362.

Fortuna, Lisa R., Marina Tolou-Shams, Barbara Robles-Ramamurthy, and Michelle V. Porche. "Inequity and the Disproportionate Impact of COVID-19 on Communities of Color in the United States: The Need for a Trauma-Informed Social Justice Response." *Psychological Trauma: Theory, Research, Practice, and Policy* 12, no. 5 (July 2020): 443–445. https://doi.org/10.1037/tra0000889.

Furnham, A., C. Thomas, and K. V. Petrides. "Patient Characteristics and the Allocation of Scarce Medical Resources." *Psychology, Health & Medicine* 7, no. 1 (February 2002): 99–106.

Gozum, Ivan Efreaim A., and Jove Jim S. Aguas. *Philosophia: International Journal of Philosophy* 23, no. 1 (January 2022): 202–217.

Greer, Scott L., Holly Jarman, and Peter D. Donnelly. "Lessons for the United States From Single-Payer Systems." *American Journal of Public Health* 109, no. 11 (November 2019): 1493–1496. https://doi.org/10.2105/AJPH.2019.305312.

Gujral, Kritee, and Anirban Basu. "Impact of Rural and Urban Hospital Closures on Inpatient Mortality." Cambridge, MA: National Bureau of Economic Research, August 2019. https://doi.org/10.3386/w26182.

Gutoskey, Ellen. "Equity vs. Equality: What's the Difference? |." Mental Floss, June 11, 2020. www.mentalfloss.com/article/625404/equity-vs-equality-what-is-the-difference.

Hamadi, Hanadi Y., Mei Zhao, Donald Rob Haley, Ajani Dunn, Shyam Paryani, and Aaron Spaulding. "Medicare and Telehealth: The Impact of COVID -19 Pandemic." *Journal of Evaluation in Clinical Practice* 28, no. 1 (February 2022): 43–48. https://doi.org/10.1111/jep.13634.

Hill, Ronald Paul, Robert M Peterson, and Kanwalroop Kathy Dhanda. "Global Consumption and Distributive Justice: A Rawlsian Perspective." *Human Rights Quarterly* 23, no. 1 (February 2001): 171–187.

Hoffman, Kelly M., Sophie Trawalter, Jordan R. Axt, and M. Norman Oliver. "Racial Bias in Pain Assessment and Treatment Recommendations, and False Beliefs about Biological Differences between Blacks and Whites." *Proceedings of the National Academy of Sciences* 113, no. 16 (April 19, 2016): 4296–4301. https://doi.org/10.1073/pnas.1516047113.

Horne, L. Chad, and Joseph Heath. "A Market Failures Approach to Justice in Health." *Politics, Philosophy & Economics* 21, no. 2 (May 2022): 165–189. https://doi.org/10.1177/1470594X221089670.

Huynh, Thanh N., Eric C. Kleerup, Prince P. Raj, and Neil S. Wenger. "The Opportunity Cost of Futile Treatment in the ICU." *Critical Care Medicine* 42, no. 9 (September 2014): 1977–1982. https://doi.org/10.1097/CCM.0000000000000402.

Huynh, Thanh N., Kleerup Eric C., Wiley Joshua F., Savitsky Terrance D., Guse Diana, Garber Bryan J., and Wenger Neil S. "The Frequency and Cost of Treatment Perceived to Be Futile in Critical Care." *JAMA Internal Medicine* 173, no. 20 (November 11, 2013): 1887–1894. https://doi.org/10.1001/jamainternmed.2013.10261.

Jonsen, Albert R. *A Short History of Medical Ethics*. New York: Oxford University Press, 2000.

Kelly, David F., Gerard Magill, and H. ten Have. *Contemporary Catholic Health Care Ethics*. 2nd ed. Washington, DC: Georgetown University Press, 2013.

Klumpp, Matthias, Ida G. Monfared, and Sebastian Vollmer. "Public Opinion on Global Distribution of COVID-19 Vaccines: Evidence from Two Nationally Representative Surveys in Germany and the United States." *Vaccine* 40, no. 16 (April 6, 2022): 2457–2461.

Lane, Derrick. "Looters Leave More Food Deserts In Black Communities." June 4, 2020. https://blackdoctor.org/looters-leave-more-food-deserts-in-black-communities.

Locke, John. *Two Treatises of Government and A Letter Concerning Toleration: Locke*. New Haven, CT: Yale University Press, 2003.

Maves, R. C., et al. "Triage of Scarce Critical Care Resources in COVID-19 an Implementation Guide for Regional Allocation: An Expert Panel Report of the Task Force for Mass Critical Care and the American College of Chest Physicians." *Chest* 158, no. 1 (2020): 212–225.

McQuade, Brianna M., Alan Schwartz, and Jennie B. Jarrett. "Acknowledging and Assessing Implicit Bias among Healthcare Professionals: A Randomized Controlled Trial." *Journal of Interprofessional Education & Practice* 24 (September 2021): 100452. https://doi.org/10.1016/j.xjep.2021.100452.

Meghani, Salimah H., and Pamela S. Hinds. "Policy Brief: The Institute of Medicine Report Dying in America: Improving Quality and Honoring Individual Preferences near the End of Life." *Nursing Outlook* 63, no. 1 (January 1, 2015): 51–59.

Meier, Lukas J. "Systemising Triage: COVID-19 Guidelines and Their Underlying Theories of Distributive Justice." *Medicine, Health Care and Philosophy: A European Journal*, July 7, 2022, 1–12. https://doi.org/10.1007/s11019-022-10101-3.

Mende-Siedlecki, Peter, Jennie Qu-Lee, Robert Backer, and Jay J. Van Bavel. "Perceptual Contributions to Racial Bias in Pain Recognition." *Journal of Experimental Psychology: General* 148, no. 5 (May 2019): 863–889. https://doi.org/10.1037/xge0000600.

Merriam-Webster. *Merriam-Webster's Intermediate Dictionary*. Springfield, MA: Merriam-Webster, 2020.

Miller, Katherine E. M., Kyle L. Miller, Kathleen Knocke, George H. Pink, G. Mark Holmes, and Brystana G. Kaufman. "Access to Outpatient Services in Rural Communities Changes after Hospital Closure." *Health Services Research* 56, no. 5 (October 2021): 788–801. https://doi.org/10.1111/1475-6773.13694.

Nkunu, Victoria, and Kevin J. McLaughlin. "Why Do Some Physicians Choose to Tackle Inequities in Healthcare?" *International Journal for Equity in Health* 17, no. 1 (June 15, 2018). https://doi.org/10.1186/s12939-018-0790-4.

Paredes, Anghela Z., J. Madison Hyer, Adrian Diaz, Diamantis I. Tsilimigras, and Timothy M. Pawlik. "Examining Healthcare Inequities Relative to United States Safety Net Hospitals." *The American Journal of Surgery* 220, no. 3 (September 1, 2020): 525–531.

Peppercorn, Jeffrey, S Yousuf Zafar, Kevin Houck, Peter Ubel, and Neal J Meropol. "Does Comparative Effectiveness Research Promote Rationing of Cancer Care?" *Lancet Oncology* 15, no. 3 (March 1, 2014): e132–e138.

Philpott, Daniel. "Resurrecting Justice." *Journal of Moral Theology* 11, no. 1 (January 2022): 167–192.

Porter, Jean. *Justice as a Virtue: A Thomistic Perspective*. Grand Rapids, Michigan: William B. Eerdmans Publishing Company, 2016.

Putsch, Robert W, and Linda Pololi. "Distributive Justice in American Healthcare: Institutions, Power, and the Equitable Care of Patients." *The American Journal of Managed Care* 10, no. Special (2004). https://doi.org/10.13016/QG6F-A6WO.

Qiu, Jiaying, Liucheng Wu, Ruobing Qu, Tao Jiang, Jialin Bai, Lei Sheng, Pengchao Feng, and Junjie Sun. "History of Development of the Life-Saving Drug 'Nusinersen' in Spinal

Muscular Atrophy." *Frontiers in Cellular Neuroscience* 16 (August 12, 2022): 942976. https://doi.org/10.3389/fncel.2022.942976.

Rad, Nassim, Haibi Cai, and Michael D. Weiss. "Management of Spinal Muscular Atrophy in the Adult Population." *Muscle & Nerve* 65, no. 5 (May 2022): 498–507. https://doi.org/10.1002/mus.27519.

Rawls, John. *A Theory of Justice*. Cambridge, MA : Belknap Press of Harvard University Press, 1971.

Rhodes, Rosamond. "Justice in COVID-19 Vaccine Prioritisation: Rethinking the Approach." *Journal of Medical Ethics* 47, no. 9 (September 2021): 623–631. https://doi.org/10.1136/medethics-2020-107117.

Robertson, Thomas M., and Richard P. Lofgren. "Where Population Health Misses the Mark: Breaking the 80/20 Rule." *Academic Medicine* 90, no. 3 (March 2015): 277–278. https://doi.org/10.1097/ACM.0000000000000627.

Sabatello, Maya, Teresa Blankmeyer Burke, Katherine E. McDonald, and Paul S. Appelbaum. "Disability, Ethics, and Health Care in the COVID-19 Pandemic." *American Journal of Public Health* 110, no. 10 (October 2020): 1523–1527.

Schmidt, Harald, Dorothy E Roberts, and Nwamaka D Eneanya. "Rationing, Racism and Justice: Advancing the Debate around 'colourblind' COVID-19 Ventilator Allocation." *Journal of Medical Ethics* 48, no. 2 (February 2022): 126–130. https://doi.org/10.1136/medethics-2020-106856.

Shannon, Thomas A. "Living the Vision: Health Care, Social Justice and Institutional Identity." *Christian Bioethics* 7, no. 1 (April 2001): 49–65.

Smolenski, Joanna. "Involuntary Withdrawal: A Bridge Too Far?" *Clinical Ethics Case Studies, Hastings Bioethics Forum*, 3, August 21, 2023.

Soled, Derek. "Distributive Justice as a Means of Combating Systemic Racism in Healthcare." *Voices in Bioethics* 7 (June 1, 2021). https://doi.org/10.52214/vib.v7i.8502.

Sox, Harold C. "Comparative Effectiveness Research: A Report From the Institute of Medicine." *Annals of Internal Medicine* 151, no. 3 (August 4, 2009): 203. https://doi.org/10.7326/0003-4819-151-3-200908040-00125.

Spears, Tracy and Schmader, Wally. "Unconscious Bias in Healthcare." *Physician Leadership Journal*, April 2021.

Ten Have, H. *Vulnerability: Challenging Bioethics*. New York: Routledge, 2016.

Thompson, William W., Hasan Symum, Amy Sandul, DHSc, Neil Gupta, Priti Patel, Noele Nelson, Jonathan Mermin, and Carolyn Wester. "*Vital Signs:* Hepatitis C Treatment Among Insured Adults — United States, 2019–2020." *MMWR. Morbidity and Mortality Weekly Report* 71, no. 32 (August 12, 2022): 1011–1017. https://doi.org/10.15585/mmwr.mm7132e1.

Torrie, Carmen, Sharon Yanicki, Monique Sedgwick, and Lisa Howard. "Social Justice in Pandemic Immunization Policy: We're All in This Together." *Nursing Ethics* 28, no. 6 (September 2021): 924–934.

Tsou, Amy Y., William D. Graf, James A. Russell, and Leon G. Epstein. "Ethical Perspectives on Costly Drugs and Health Care: AAN Position Statement." *Neurology* 97, no. 14 (October 5, 2021): 685–692. https://doi.org/10.1212/WNL.0000000000012571.

Wolfe, Mary K., Noreen C. McDonald, and G. Mark Holmes. "Transportation Barriers to Health Care in the United States: Findings From the National Health Interview Survey, 1997–2017."

American Journal of Public Health 110, no. 6 (June 2020): 815–822. https://doi.org/10.2105/AJPH.2020.305579.

Yearby, Ruqaiijah. "Racial Disparities in Health Status and Access to Healthcare: The Continuation of Inequality in the United States Due to Structural Racism: Continuing Racial Health Disparities." *American Journal of Economics and Sociology* 77, no. 3–4 (May 2018): 1113–1152. https://doi.org/10.1111/ajes.12230.

Yuk-Chiu Yip, Jeffrey. "Healthcare Resource Allocation in the COVID-19 Pandemic: Ethical Considerations from the Perspective of Distributive Justice within Public Health." *Public Health in Practice (Oxford, England)* 2 (November 2021): 100111. https://doi.org/10.1016/j.puhip.2021.100111.

Zimmer, Amie Leigh. "Rethinking the Right to Health: Ableism and the Binary between Individual and Collective Rights." *Bioethics* 35, no. 8 (October 2021): 752–759. https://doi.org/10.1111/bioe.12922.

Chapter 5

Healthcare Ethics and Clinical Trials for Late-Stage Cancers

INTRODUCTION

Katherine is a vibrant 60-year-old patient of mine who recently found out that she has advanced cancer. Her oncologist told her that there were no chemotherapy or other treatments available for this diagnosis, but she would be eligible for a clinical trial. The study is being conducted by a university hospital about 60 miles away. It would involve her staying at a hotel near the hospital, paid for by the study, so that she can be closely monitored. Katherine was always a fighter and, at present, still feels strong and is excited about entering into a university study. She thinks that participating could help her and others with a similar diagnosis. However, her husband confides in you that he is secretly worried about his wife and feels that her decision will be burdensome and even dangerous to her; he asks you to talk her out of it.

This chapter will explore the ethical implications of patients with late-stage cancers and their choice of whether to participate in clinical trials for cancer research. Decades ago, as a young palliative care physician, I could not understand why any cancer patient would want to participate in a clinical trial. Once the cancer has progressed to an incurable stage, why not use that time to be comfortable and be with your family? I even questioned whether their choice was ethical. Was autonomy violated because the patient was under duress? Was beneficence violated because the treatment would most likely not benefit the patient? Was nonmaleficence violated because the trial could harm the patient? And finally, was justice violated because big pharma was the only one likely to benefit from the trial? As I spoke to more cancer patients and discussed their motives, I realized that I was acting paternalistic and ignoring their values. For some, participating in clinical trials was essential for them and how they define themselves with their new reality.

DOI: 10.4324/9781003654124-6

Cancer is a terrible disease and is the second leading cause of death in the United States. It was estimated that 608,570 Americans would die from cancer in 2021, corresponding to more than 1,600 daily deaths.[1] Most deaths are from lung, prostate, and colorectum cancers in men, and cancers of the lung, breast, and colorectum in women.[2] Furthermore, while cancer prognosis has significantly improved in the past decade, some cancers have limited treatment options. In addition, the prognosis is often poor and limited to weeks or months; infrequently, it can be measured in years.[3] When treatments are offered, they are frequently beset with severe side effects that can affect the quality of the limited amount of life available. Therefore, entering a clinical trial becomes a prospect when treatment options are scarce or even nil.[4]

The first section will start with a review of the clinical aspects of advanced cancer. It will include a discussion regarding the disease process, prognosis (real and perceived), prevalent symptoms, and available treatments. Indeed, knowledge of these illnesses is essential to decision-making. For example, some patients will opt for a plan emphasizing improving and maintaining a good quality of life, even if it means limiting their life expectancy. Other patients will look into aggressive therapies with the hope of prolonging life. Often, these choices are not binary, and many patients seek therapies to help them live longer with a manageable treatment burden. Mostly, these diseases are incurable and will ultimately cause the person's death. Oncologists often label treatments for incurable cancers as palliative with the goals of prolonging life or even lessening the symptom burden of the disease.[5] Patients sometimes choose to participate in a clinical trial when treatment options become limited. This section will look into the facts about clinical trials and the information given to patients. As a final discussion, the concept of compassionate use will be explored; participation criteria will also be discussed.[6]

The next section of this chapter will explore the ethical principles Beauchamp and Childress define, including autonomy, beneficence, nonmaleficence, and justice. The principles and benchmarks for ethical clinical research will also be included in the discussion in each section. These include "collaborative partnership, social value, scientific validity, fair participant selection, favorable risk-benefit ratio, informed consent, and respect for participants."[7]

The first part, which is dedicated to autonomy, for example, will look at the information given to the patient so that they can make genuinely informed consent to the protocol being offered. Indeed, patients are incredibly vulnerable at this time of their lives, and how the information is given to them regarding a trial is crucial. What are the patient's beliefs about the trial, and what motivates them to want to participate? Do the study designers and the oncologists use methods to persuade the patient or "nudge" them to participate ethically?[8]

The nonmaleficence portion of this chapter will look at the direct and indirect harm to the patient. Direct damage is self-explanatory and relates to the untoward effects of the cancer drug being tested.[9] The indirect effects, however, are more obscure. These could include staying near the testing site to participate in the trial. If disallowed by the drug trial protocol, it could also exclude specific palliative measures such as radiation treatments and corticosteroids. Next, in the beneficence section, this chapter will look at the benefits of joining a clinical trial for a cancer patient. Although it is difficult to predict any medical benefit in joining a clinical trial, patients continue to do so.[10] The benefit may be altruistic and the feeling that a person did something or participated in a program that could vastly benefit society. Other patients would note the intense feeling of their continual need to fight until the end.[11] Finally, in the justice segment of this chapter, the availability and even distribution of clinical trials will be investigated, along with how the benefits are distributed.[12]

BACKGROUND INFORMATION

This section will discuss the clinical aspects of late-stage cancers. Understanding the patient's journey is essential when talking about cancer research ethics. Therefore, this part will also explore clinical trials and the compassionate use of cancer therapies.

Medical Features of Late-Stage Cancers

An estimated 16.9 million individuals were living with cancer in the United States on January 1, 2019. Although the five-year relative cancer survival has improved over the past several decades for most cancer types, it remains a formidable disease.[13] Many factors are noted to influence survival in addition to cancer type, including age and stage at diagnosis, treatment, insurance status, comorbid health conditions, and financial resources. Cancer treatment has improved survival and can include localized therapies, such as surgery, radiation therapy, cryotherapy, and heat or chemical ablation. Treatment may also include systemic therapies such as chemotherapy, hormonal therapy, immune therapy, and targeted therapy, which can be used alone or in combination. Treatments that do not directly treat cancer, called palliative therapies, can be used to reduce side effects and address other patient and family quality of life concerns.[14]

Prognostication is problematic for more advanced cancers, although functional status has consistently been associated with survival. However, the length of survival may also depend on the underlying cancer. Patients with metastatic cancer with relatively good treatment options, such as prostate or breast cancer, may be considerably better off than those with pancreatic or biliary cancers, even those with poorer functional status. Nevertheless, some studies show improvement in the survival rate of these problematic cancers, although there is a lack of data on when these cancers affect people with significant comorbidities.[15]

Besides treatment of the underlying cancer, care goals may include alleviating suffering, enhancing the quality of life until death, and providing a comfortable death. Dealing with advanced cancer ultimately causes suffering to patients, their families, and the medical professionals caring for them.[16] Patients with incurable illnesses often deal with significant pain and other physical symptoms that can diminish their quality of life. Furthermore, many suffer from psychological distress and sometimes form an existential view that continued life is meaningless even if pain or other physical symptoms can be controlled. For the patient's families and loved ones, there is also emotional pain in this process, such as expected loss, watching the physical and emotional distress of the patient, and bearing the care responsibilities. Cancer patients may also be vulnerable because the physical distress from their illness can often impair their judgment and decision-making.[17]

Cancer patients often have uncertain prognoses, complex treatment regimens, and burdensome physical and non-physical symptoms. These factors can all lead to the assumption that this group is vulnerable. Therefore, when considering research options, they can be defined as a "subject at risk" because of the probability of harm that could be physical, psychological, or social.[18] Also, as with other patients with an extended illness, they can be unusually driven to take risks in return for the possibility of economic or physical benefits. They may be subject to undue influence from their physicians or family members, and they may be persuaded to agree to enroll in exploitative studies that do not distribute benefits and risks properly.[19] Many desperately seek a cure and are therefore motivated to take more chances. Thus, vulnerability may occur because of compromised consent due to insufficient comprehension or compromised risk assessment because of life conditions.[20] In addition, autonomy is compromised when people are desperate for treatments where there are none.[21] Therefore, since many cancer patients are clearly vulnerable, how can we justify their participation in clinical trials?

Clinical Trials Overview

Clinical trials are how new medications are tested for safety and efficacy, with four human phases. The aim of phase I trials is to find the highest dose of the study drug that patients tolerate when administered to human subjects for the first time. Often, these subjects are cancer patients with no other treatment options.[22] Phase II trials test whether the drug affects a specific diagnosis and what side effects it causes. Because multiple doses are tested in this phase, evaluating whether the drug will benefit these subjects is impossible. Apart from collecting additional safety information, Phase III trials determine whether the drug will provide any benefit. Finally, phase IV trials do further testing on an already approved drug.[23] As described above, patients are recruited to phase I and II trials even though the drug most likely will not help them as it is too early in the development phase.[24] These cases can be challenging; however, some safeguards were initiated.

The Belmont Report, published by the National Commission for the Protection of Human Subjects of Biomedical and Behavioral Research in 1978, documents moral principles as they apply to research with humans. Since then, it has given a clear and concise outline for examining ethical issues associated with medical studies.[25] First, the Belmont Report gives the principles for ethical research involving human subjects, such as respect for persons. This obligation requires informed consent from research subjects and additional protections for those who cannot consent. It also describes beneficence, which requires increasing research benefits while decreasing risks. Finally, it represents justice, which requires the fair allocation of benefits and burdens of medical research.[26]

The principle of respect for people requires that the choices an autonomous person makes cannot be ignored or in any way be made insignificant. In clinical cancer trials, this requirement cannot be overemphasized. This vital task demands that human subjects consent before investigators begin clinical trials. Therefore, this principle insists that the individual's informed consent be valid and examined regarding how information was disclosed, along with the understanding and voluntariness of the subject.[27] The selection of patients for cancer research should not exploit economically disadvantaged patients.[28] Cancer patients frequently face bankruptcy and could be placed in this category.[29] Another factor influencing a patient's willingness to participate in a clinical trial is trust in their physician. For instance, a cancer patient may be willing to try an experimental drug recommended by their trustworthy oncologist even though the chance of benefitting from the treatment is slim and could have harmful side effects.[30]

The trust that cancer patients put in their oncologists cannot be overlooked.[31] Some patients follow their physician's recommendation to participate because they want to be seen as a good patient who maintains a sense of optimism.[32] Trust occurs when the patient believes their physician will act ethically and professionally; there is a risk if that physician fails.[33] Also, the patient's confidence in investigators incorporates the full range of research conduct, including how the patients are enrolled and give informed consent. It also includes adopting research protocols that minimize risk, monitor safety, and report adverse events and unanticipated problems. Finally, it includes obeying the established regulations, guidelines, and policies already in place. Indeed, when human subjects distrust investigators, they are unlikely to participate in research studies, or if they do, they may not cooperate fully with the investigators.[34] Trust, therefore, is essential, and these responsibilities present an ethical challenge for researchers working with vulnerable cancer patients.

Compassionate Use

Sometimes, a patient can take advantage of an experimental medication outside clinical trials. This practice is often called "compassionate use." Expanding access to new medications creates hope for patients with immediately life-threatening diseases or conditions that allow treatments outside of clinical trials when no suitable alternative therapeutic options exist.[35] For example, the US Food and Drug Administration (FDA) website states that expanded access may be appropriate when the patient's life is in danger by their disease or condition, there is no other therapy to treat the disease, the patient is not a candidate to enter a clinical trial, the possibility to help the patient offsets the potential risks of treatment, and providing the new treatment will not affect any new trials of medications already in the pipeline for this indication. However, the FDA has not approved or found these medications safe and effective for their specific use. Furthermore, these drugs may or may not help treat the disease or condition and could cause severe, unexpected side effects.[36]

Compassionate use protocols, including those with a large population of patients, are often done after Phase III clinical trials. Technically, however, any investigational drug may be used compassionately at any phase in its development.[37] Therefore, compassionate use requests can occur from even the animal product testing phase up to the period nearing the end of clinical trials.[38] Often, questions are raised about the safety and efficacy of these experimental treatments. For example, a study of 1442 new drugs produced by fifty pharmaceutical firms found that the chance of these medications being approved was only 11.83%. Unfortunately, the percentage of failed drugs is significant, and many patients will take medicines that will later prove useless.[39]

One of the obstacles to compassionate use in the US is the Federal Drug Administration (FDA). However, even though the application process can be somewhat burdensome, the FDA ultimately approves 99% of compassionate use requests. The primary obstacle for patients is obtaining approval from the pharmaceutical company to get their new medication approved. The FDA will not act on these requests if they do not occur.[40]

Social media and computer search engines have profoundly increased the frequency of compassionate use requests. Specifically, this includes the growing trend of patients using social media to gain access to investigational drugs through various expanded access paths.[41] Once a possible new drug is found, patients may try to contact the researcher testing the agent or even try to contact a corporate executive to gain access. Sometimes, patients will even try to involve the local media in their pursuit or launch social media campaigns to draw attention, hoping that public pressure will convince private companies that own the new drug to allow it to be used.[42] Sadly, these are desperate people hoping that sympathy and compassion will provide them with a medication that could help them, no matter how slim the chance.

The choice for a cancer patient to go on compassionate use treatment is not easy. These patients already suffer from a disease with a poor prognosis and a high symptom burden. In addition, the medications that are utilized have an unproven safety and efficacy profile.[43] Therefore, the risk-benefit profile is even more uncertain than for patients in a clinical trial. However, patients can choose how they want to be treated, and medical professionals must comply with their choices. Or do they? The following sections of this paper will look at ethical principles that apply to patients with late-stage cancers.

ETHICAL ISSUES

Patients with late-stage cancers face many burdens, one of which may be the decision to participate in clinical trials. For them to participate in clinical trials is also problematic for the clinicians to run these trials. Therefore, as described by Beauchamp and Childress, a set of principles can be used as a baseline that explains general rules of common morality as they apply to medical decision-making. These principles can then function as guidelines for medical bioethics regarding clinical trials. These moral principles are: (1) respect for autonomy (can the cancer patient freely make decisions about their treatment?); (2) beneficence (what is the benefit of participating in a trial that may not help the patient?); (3) nonmaleficence (what is the harm in participating in a trial?); and (4) justice (are the benefits, risks, and participation in the trial evenly distributed?).[44]

Other sets of principles may also be used, and these are described in *The Oxford Textbook of Clinical Research Ethics*. These guidelines provide a comprehensive and organized way to define the ethical behavior needed for clinical trials, thereby minimizing (if not preventing) the possibility of ethical misconduct.[45] In addition, these general principles identify factors necessary to justify research as fundamentally ethical.

Autonomy

As Tom L. Beauchamp and James F. Childress stated in their book *Principles of Biomedical Ethics*, "The autonomous individual acts freely according to a self-chosen plan, analogous to how an independent government manages its territories and sets its policies. A person of diminished autonomy, by contrast, is in some respect controlled by others or incapable of deliberating or acting based on their desires and plans."[46] The writers further explain that convicts and mentally challenged individuals often have diminished autonomy. To have autonomy, an individual should have the freedom and the mental ability to make decisions on their behalf. They call these two conditions liberty, which is freedom from controlling influences, and agency, which is the capacity for purposeful action. So, ultimately, a sane person who is not a prisoner should be able to make decisions. However, this application gets complicated when dealing with the complexities involving patients with late-stage cancers.

One cannot make decisions about oneself without the correct information. Ideally, informed consent is a process of education based on communications between healthcare providers and a patient or their families that allows them to make the best possible decision regarding their care.[47] The need for accurate and thorough information is the foundation of one of the most discussed bioethical topics that are faced today. Even the name *informed consent* implies that one must be informed before consenting.[48] Autonomy requires the right to make self-governing choices and access to the instruments, such as sufficient information, that can help one make decisions.[49]

The information element refers to providing the best possible information and understanding the information disclosed. Additionally, the consent element refers to both a voluntary decision and an agreement to proceed. Legal, philosophical, medical, and psychological experts agree that the following elements are needed for informed consent: competence, disclosure, understanding, voluntariness, and consent.[50] Patients, therefore, can give informed consent to an intervention if, and perhaps only if, they have the capacity to act, receive thorough information, understand the information, act voluntarily, and consent to the treatment.[51]

In *The Oxford Textbook of Clinical Research Ethics*, informed consent is listed as one of the "principles and benchmarks for ethical clinical research." The authors state that "the purpose of informed consent is to show respect for the autonomy of individuals." To involve cancer patients in clinical trials without their consent is to treat them merely as a means to an end and deny them the opportunity to choose what goals they wish to pursue. When used correctly, informed consent allows patients to decide if and how they want to participate and respects them and their autonomy.[52]

Informed consent also involves the quality of the information that patients receive. One study showed that physicians judged patients' knowledge lower than the patients themselves did. One reason may have been that the physicians were more careful in grading a complete understanding of the information since that would be a high level to meet. However, physicians may also be aware of several details that they did not inform the patient about because of lack of time or to prevent what they thought to be information overload. As a result, the physician may have held back some details that they felt were not significant enough for the patient to know.

On the other hand, patients may not know what they do not know and, therefore, think they know more than they actually do.[53] Remarkably, however, neither the patients' nor their physicians' grading correlated with the patient's actual knowledge, as measured by a questionnaire in the study. These findings suggest that physicians must improve their ability to gauge patients' understanding of critical information to adjust how they give patients information individually.[54]

Valid informed consent requires that the consenting person consents voluntarily and without coercion.[55] So, how does that affect how physicians discuss clinical trials with their patients? One form of persuasion is referred to as a "nudge." Which is defined as "any aspect of the choice dialogue that predictably alters people's behavior without prohibiting any choices or significantly changing their economic incentives." Nudging is generally allowed and employed to promote items regarding public health in healthcare. Proponents of nudging argue that it can also encourage patients to give informed consent to their physicians' recommended treatments and improve patient compliance.[56]

Whereas public health nudging is intended to produce a direct health benefit for the public, the benefits for a cancer patient entering a clinical trial are unclear. Moreover, questions remain about how much public benefit there would need to be, what those public benefits are, and how likely these benefits would be to justify this type of nudging. Finally, while some of these techniques may be ethically acceptable, highly manipulative and deceptive techniques may be seen as unethical interference and be considered coercion.[57]

While coercion has no ethical place in informed consent, some routine actions by physicians need to be analyzed. For example, giving the patient only information supporting a particular decision is a type of coercion, as is attempting to decide the patient's preferred treatment choice and designing the information supporting this obvious patient choice.[58] While some may call these strategies nothing more than "friendly persuasion," they raise concerns about physicians applying improper persuasion techniques on an already susceptible subject and, therefore, can question the validity of the consent.[59]

Finally, some cancer patients regrettably find out their disease is incurable and are asked to participate in clinical trials with a palliative intent. The phrase "You have nothing to lose" is often used during these emotional discussions. One study looked at clinical trials with palliative or non-curative intent and identified a concern of both patients and professionals when "nothing to lose" was used. The authors provided insight into some of the issues that both parties share concerning what it means to "fight cancer" and the effect on their "trusting relationship." In addition, the study emphasized the obligation healthcare professionals have to ensure patients are fully informed regarding trial requirements and potential outcomes. Considering these patients' vulnerability, this task is more complicated and critical.[60]

Research policies relating to vulnerable subjects challenge inclusion and access on the one side and exclusion and protection on the other. Policies that prevent patients from entering clinical trials to protect them from harm or manipulation may actually cause harm to the group to which they belong. Without cancer research, the clinical gains that have occurred would not be possible. Not testing a population, even for altruistic reasons, could harm this group because it would lead to a lack of critical information. Essentially, this problem represents the moral tension between protecting vulnerable patients and promoting the common good, which often happens in medical research.[61] Therefore, the significance of framing vulnerability regarding flawed autonomy is twofold. First, recognizing vulnerability does not indicate that patients cannot participate in medical research or clinical trials. Cancer patients should be allowed to participate in clinical trials, even though their vulnerable circumstances are identified. Not allowing them to be included would go against their autonomy.

On the contrary, if a person lacks autonomy, their interests should be carefully assessed, and special protection should be given. The researcher must determine whether a patient can agree to participate in the clinical trial, even if multiple factors make them vulnerable. Allowing these individuals to participate demonstrates the fundamental ethical principle of respect for all people.[62] Careful decisions regarding allowing or not allowing certain classes of vulnerable people from research should be studied, considering how those choices will impact these individuals as well as other patients now and in the future. Failure to do so violates an individual's autonomy and may also prevent them from doing that one last profound act that gives their life meaning.

Beneficence

The term beneficence usually implies acts of mercy, kindness, and charity. Beneficence also typically includes acts of altruism, love, and humanity. It is generally understood that beneficent action consists of all actions intended to help a person. The principle of beneficence establishes a moral requirement to act for the benefit of others.[63] This section will explore why clinical trials for cancer patients fit into this category.

On the surface, the statement that clinical trials benefit the individual may be challenging to defend. Notwithstanding the rapid improvement of cancer treatment in recent years, including targeted therapy and immunotherapy, one assessment of the research literature found no evidence that treatment in clinical trials is any better than standard care.[64] These results, which align with older results by Peppercorn et al., demonstrated that many studies did not look at relevant confounders, were biased, and lacked transparency.[65] In other words, some studies tried to minimize any adverse outcomes and maximize the positive ones. The review also suggested that some participants believed there were collateral benefits, such as more office visits and studies. However, this did not establish an objective benefit of these trials over standard treatment. If these indirect effects (having more follow-ups, etc.) had had an overall positive value, this would have affected the results of the reviewed studies.[66]

Suppose there are no measurable positive effects for patients participating in trials. What are the reasons why they would do so? If it is altruism, patients should be encouraged to contribute to furthering knowledge to benefit future patients. However, when their burden is great, which is often the case in phase I trials, they may prefer to spend their remaining days on something more beneficial to their own quality of life—but that choice should be theirs.[67]

Nevertheless, many participants felt that staying positive was vital because they believed that expressing hope and having an optimistic attitude would ultimately improve their chances of having a therapeutic benefit. Some participants felt that there is a connection between hope and outcomes as established by science, even though the actual data are, at best, inconsistent. Studies stating that "hope helps" might be more likely to be reported in the media than in peer-reviewed studies. Nevertheless, these stories allow patients to believe that this is positively true. Furthermore, a widespread set of background cultural norms favors an optimistic attitude for patients, influencing their responses to inquiries about their expectations of therapeutic benefit upon enrolling in a clinical trial.[68] However, "hope is not a strategy," and more justification is needed to support beneficence in clinical trials.

Why do we do clinical research for cancer in the first place? Clinical research is not an end in itself; it has value because it provides knowledge that improves cancer treatment. Such breakthroughs ultimately define the benefits of research to society. However, the emphasis on the benefit to research participants has displaced the importance of assessing the research's benefit to society. Without social value, research exposes participants to harm with no other justification. However, transforming research results into treatment decisions that benefit society is complex, incremental, and often chaotic. More often than not, phase 1 studies are valuable because the data they generate inform additional research that could ultimately improve treatment goals for other patients, not those in the trials. In addition, priorities may change while a study is being conducted, and the cooperation of large groups is often needed to make changes based on research results.[69] So, even when there may be no measurable benefit to the individual patient, the research protocol can still be beneficial if it shows scientific validity.

The results produced by the trials need to be reliable and show valid data that others can interpret and use. If not, it will have no social value, and participants may be exposed to risks for no benefits. Therefore, research must be designed to provide valid and reliable data.[70] Ultimately, participation in clinical trials is consistent with the principle of beneficence, not because of its benefits to the individual cancer patient but because of its social value. National Cancer Institute director Norman E. Sharpless said optimistically in a speech:

> *I am happy to share the news, as you may have seen in last week's Annual Report to the Nation on the Status of Cancer, that we continue to see a steady decline in cancer mortality. In 1991, the cancer mortality rate was 215 deaths per 100,000 people in the US. In 2015, that number was down to 159. There is reason to believe that the number is even lower now and will continue to decline. This represents decreases in cancer death for men, women, and children and for all major ethnic groups. Almost every day, we learn of new discoveries, advances, and approaches that show promise. We have options. We have treatments. And sometimes, we do have a cure!*[71]

Nonmaleficence

According to Beauchamp and Childress, the principle of nonmaleficence establishes an obligation not to cause harm to others. In medical ethics, this principle is often linked with the phrase *primum non nocere* ("The first thing is to do no harm"; see Chapter 3).[72] The principle of nonmaleficence supports many more specific moral rules, such as do not kill, do not cause pain or suffering, do not incapacitate, do not cause offense, or deprive others of life's goods. Both the principle and its specifications in these moral rules are *prima facie*, not absolute.[73]

The *Oxford Textbook of Clinical Research* details how *favorable risk–benefit ratio* and *independent review* can be used to explain nonmaleficence during research further. The favorable risk–benefit ratio item asks, "Are the potential physical, psychological, social, and economic risks of the research for the individual participants delineated and their probability and magnitude quantified to the extent possible given the available data?" Conversely, "Are the potential physical, psychological, social, and economic benefits of the research for the individual participants delineated and their probability and magnitude quantified to the extent possible given the available data?"[74]

Similarly, the independent review item asks, "are the procedures for independent review established by law and regulation being properly followed?" This item also questions if the review process is "independent and competent." Is the review process "transparent," and are explanations given for the review committee's decisions? And finally, are multiple reviews minimized and resolved if they are not in agreement?[75]

The risks based on the clinical phase can be studied when dealing with clinical trials for cancer research. For example, are the possible benefits for patients justified by the dangers they may encounter when analyzing phase 2 and 3 research? If that is the case, then additional benefits of the research, such as social benefits to future patients and not the individual, need to be assessed. Therefore, fulfilling the value and validity requirements suggests that the accumulative advantages of the research outweigh its risks.[76] Nonmaleficence, thus, limits the risks to which research participants can be exposed for the sake of this goal.[77] However, what about phase 1 trials with minimal potential benefit to the patient?

As previously stated, phase I trials aim to find the trial drug's highest tolerated dose and safety, and the participants are most often cancer patients without other treatment options.[78] The principal objectives of phase I trials have usually been to characterize the safety of the drugs under investigation and find what dose to use in phase 2. Traditionally, determining this dose relies on the careful assessment of adverse events and utilizes what is called a "toxicity-driven endpoint," which is the maximum tolerated dose. Notably, this design was developed to investigate cytotoxic drugs, assuming that the toxic and effective doses were close, resulting in a narrow therapeutic index.[79] Often, this therapeutic index walks a fine line between being helpful or harmful to the patient.

To illustrate this, in one study, the participants had an average age of 64 years (range 30–89), and 50% (n = 121) of patients were male. Furthermore, the European Cooperative Oncology Group (ECOG) performance status of 44% of patients was either 0 (no symptoms) or 1 (minimal symptoms).[80] Even though these patients entered the Phase 1 trials with excellent performance status, the 90-day mortality rate was still 20%, emphasizing their poor prognosis even with an initial good functional status. Therefore, investigators must exercise caution while conducting early-phase trials by carefully discussing potential outcomes with patients and offering reasonable expectations based on clinical evidence.[81] In this study, there were some risks to the participants. Nine percent of the patients had mild, untoward effects from the treatment, 13% had moderate, and 2% had a severe impact. One patient died from a treatment-related death, accounting for 0.5% of the study group.[82]

Besides the adverse physical effects listed, other negative effects are more subtle. For example, when faced with incurable cancer with a poor prognosis, many would choose a more palliative approach over pursuing treatments with little chance of success. This approach would optimize the patient's quality of life and allow them to spend time with loved ones rather than chase therapies.[83] In an article that surveyed oncology nurses, One of the fundamental challenges was related to patients with progressive disease who were no longer responding to conventional treatments and enthusiastically agreed to participate in trailblazing drug trials, desperately hoping to receive some therapeutic benefit. Many nurses were concerned about what they saw as unrealistic hope and had concerns about the patient's health status being compromised by a push to get them in a research protocol. These nurses felt that patients often had unrealistic expectations and were, therefore, susceptible to participating in research with limited drug efficacy.[84]

However, other studies have shown that these patients are often very realistic about their limited chances of success and still choose to participate in phase 1 trials:

> *It does not appear that what most of our participants were doing when they reported high expectations of individual therapeutic benefit from participation in clinical trials was giving a confused report on their understanding trial*

> *statistics. If a patient can say, "I know that historically less than 5% of patients enrolled in phase I clinical trials have benefited," then the potential ethical problem is neither a failure of adequate disclosure by the investigators nor a failure of adequate comprehension by the patient. If this is true, then attempts to improve the informed consent process by new techniques of communication designed to improve comprehension may be missing the mark.*[85]

Nonmaleficence does not mean a patient will not get harmed in a clinical trial. However, ethical study designs measure the possible good to the individual participants and whether they outweigh the bad. If they do not, does the information gained from the study for society justify any harm to the individuals?[86] The principle of double effect (PDE) can also be used to defend clinical trials with cancer patients. As earlier stated, there is a risk to participants in these trials, including death.[87] The PDE explains that a single act can have two foreseen effects, one good and one bad (such as death), and is not always morally prohibited.[88] The potential clinical benefit of the trial is justification that the study is ethical. The final safeguard against nonmaleficence is an independent review as long as this assessment follows the law and is independent, competent, and transparent.[89]

Justice

As described by Beauchamp and Childress, the last principle of healthcare ethics is justice. Distributive Justice describes the "fair, equitable, and appropriate" allocation of resources. This principle involves policies fairly dispersing benefits and burdens, such as property, resources, taxation, privileges, and opportunities.[90] This section will look at how justice is applied to clinical cancer trials. It is important to note that research goals have shifted in recent years from deemphasizing risks to emphasizing the benefits of clinical trials. As a result, justice requires fair access to research. Both participation in research and access to research results has become as critical as protection from exploitation.[91]

Selecting participants for research trials should be done fairly and equally. Doing so will give the information generated the most excellent chance of producing valid and reliable data. Furthermore, by having a diverse study population, the information obtained from the study will yield results that reflect a diverse population. However, to get this value, groups that are vulnerable because of age, race, ethnicity, or economic deprivation must be allowed and encouraged to be part of these necessary scientific studies. Because of their vulnerability, safeguards must be in place for their protection, but excluding them just because they are vulnerable should be opposed.[92]

Developing drugs to benefit cancer patients has become a complex, multi-organization-based venture; it is also big business. Getting patients into cancer trials is also challenging because of the unique features, vulnerabilities, and needs of the people involved. However, because of the complexity of drug development and its cost, it is tempting to exclude certain people defined racially, pathologically, economically, or geographically to allow the study to proceed with fewer obstacles.[93] Therefore, study designs must find a way to include these people and somehow remain fiscally sound.

From the standpoint of cancer patients, deciding whether to participate in a clinical trial is right for them depends on a complex set of factors. Therefore, the research team must reach out to vulnerable populations that are often not well-educated about these scientific studies. In fact, this population is often misled about the potential risks or benefits of joining a cancer drug trial. Therefore, the absolute risk and benefit of joining are critical components of clinical trials that must be assessed. However, discussing these items can sometimes mislead patients, mainly when the available information is exaggerated to be overly pessimistic (they are just using you as a guinea pig) or excessively optimistic (you will be miraculously cured). Therefore, the messaging for clinical trials should not be aimed at directly getting more patients to sign up for experimental research. Instead, future research should aim to develop, apply, and refine audience-based messaging to reduce the inequities that cause certain groups to be underrepresented.[94]

A Maryland-based study looked at this in patients with cancer in their community. The National Cancer Institute (NCI) sponsored treatment trials between 1999 and 2002 and found that certain groups participated more than others. These groups included pediatric and adolescent age groups, white patients, female patients (for sex-specific tumors), patients with private health insurance, and patients living in the Baltimore-Washington region. Additionally, between 1999 and 2002, there was an estimated decline (8.9% per year) in the percentage of black patients participating in cancer treatment trials.[95] Therefore, the decrease in enrollment of African American patients needs to be assessed. Some reasons noted in the study included distrust, lack of available trials, limited information, age, and exclusionary criteria for comorbidity.[96]

For example, not having insurance coverage and trial reimbursement is an actual and perceived barrier to joining a drug study. Generally, most Maryland patients with cancer in the treatment trials had some insurance coverage; however, the study found that Medicaid covered a lower proportion of the patients than expected.[97] This information appears to show a bias against those economically disadvantaged and on Medicaid. Furthermore, these findings could explain why black clinical trial enrollment has declined. Therefore, there is a need to improve targeted educational and outreach efforts to communities to under-served communities. Likewise, community-based health professionals should provide information about trial availability and promote trial participation, recruitment, and retention. Finally, educational efforts should inform both minorities and community physicians about the clinical trials offered and encourage trust, health literacy, and community understanding of the importance of participating in clinical research not just for the individual but also for their community.[98]

How this education is done also needs to be examined. The most commonly used jargon for clinical trials can be unduly pessimistic, such as treatment by "trial and error" or being a subject in a medical experiment. Similarly, expressions like, patients are guinea pigs, and these are last resort treatments are used. People from these underserved communities also expressed clear, unfavorable responses to words that equate randomization with a dice roll or the use of other gambling metaphors. Dumbing-down approaches can also be troubling, suggesting that the potential value of culturally grounded vernacular used for teaching about clinical trials needs to be studied. Therefore, there are many ethical implications involved with recruiting cancer patients that this Maryland study brought to light.[99]

In the long run, how patients in vulnerable and underrepresented populations are recruited is consistent with the term collaborative partnership described in *The Oxford Textbook of Clinical Research Ethics*.[100] A messaging problem affects the recruitment of minorities and other vulnerable populations. This issue can affect the validity of the clinical trial and deprive this population of the research benefits. Therefore, the study designers should ask how to get the community involved in planning and participating in the research. These individuals should then be able to share the results but also use the results to improve health. Finally, will the community's values, circumstances, culture, and social practices be respected, and will the benefits of the study be shared with the community?[101] By attending to these essential items, researchers can design studies that fulfill the principle of justice for the communities that they serve.

CONCLUSION

In this chapter, the ethical aspects of cancer research were explored. Cancer is a devastating diagnosis that causes physical and non-physical pain to its victims. This condition makes this population vulnerable, compromising clinical research ethics.[102] However, clinical research is needed because cancer research will not progress without it. The first part of the chapter explored the background characteristics of cancer patients, research trials, and the compassionate use of experimental medications.

The second part of this chapter looked deeper into the ethical dilemmas involved, utilizing the principles established by Beauchamp and Childress: autonomy, nonmaleficence, maleficence, and justice.[103] These principles were also discussed in the context of the eight research guidelines described in *The Oxford Textbook of Clinical Research Ethics*.[104] The autonomy section addressed the concept of the cancer patient's vulnerability. Even though these patients face many challenges, physically, mentally, emotionally, and even economically, the fact remains that these people do have the ability to choose to be in clinical trials. Therefore, although precautions are needed, preventing this group from participating in clinical trials would violate their autonomy.

In the following sections, beneficence and nonmaleficence were studied. Under the beneficence section, the question was asked: can patients ethically be placed in clinical trials (such as phase 1 trials) where there is no chance for the trial to benefit the individual participant?[105] The answer to this, of course, is that the social value of the research makes this research principled. Under nonmaleficence, there was a discussion about how this principle may differ when medical treatment is compared to research. There is always some risk when patients enter into clinical research trials. Significant untoward effects and even death have occurred even with appropriate safeguards. However, the PDE can be applied since the research goal is to help people and not harm them.

In the final section, distributive justice (or justice) was explored. Once this aspect was examined regarding the exploitation of vulnerable patients, the ethical concern was more regarding protection. However, as research protocols have become less dangerous, the emphasis now involves allowing vulnerable populations to benefit from research. Therefore, better recruitment practices that do not discriminate against socially and economically disadvantaged groups must be implemented under the justice principle.[106] These practices will also allow this group to receive the benefits from the study fairly.

Suggestions for Further Research

Recognizing that these patients are at the end of their lives needs to be more carefully considered in clinical trials. Although the exploration and vigorous recording of possible medical outcomes is critical for informed decision-making, quality of life (QOL) is rarely mentioned as a factor or a therapeutic goal. Sadly, this factor is more important for the patients than the investigators. In addition, the language used regarding prognosis is frequently over-optimistic and unrelated to patients with comorbidities and decreased functional status.[107]

Previous studies have shown a patient's failure to understand the reason for phase 1 trials, alternatives to treatment trials, and realistic benefit and risk expectations. In addition, individuals must be made aware that they have the right to withdraw from or not enter a trial. It also has been found that despite a patient's terminal illness and an average survival of just several months, oncologists rarely discuss prognosis during phase 1 trials. For example, a national poll of 600 respondents found that physicians see clinical trials as a treatment of last resort, even if they are available in early treatment phases where there is almost no possibility for any clinical improvement.[108]

One study examined the effect of quality palliative care treatment for patients with solid tumors participating in phase 1 clinical trials. Incorporating palliative care with these patients can improve their QOL by addressing physical symptoms and emotional distress. Also, these patients can receive additional education about topics rarely discussed in clinical trials, such as QOL domains, which include physical, social, psychological, and spiritual well-being. Based on these educational sessions, referrals can be made to social work, nutritional services, and chaplains to help improve the patient's QOL.[109] Future studies of patients with late-stage cancers need to add palliative care referrals to their study protocols and remember that they are dealing not just with late-stage cancers but, instead, *patients* with late-stage cancers. This common oversight needs to be resolved.

TAKE-HOME POINTS

- Cancer treatment has improved survival and can include localized therapies, such as surgery, radiation therapy, cryotherapy, and heat or chemical ablation. Treatment may also include systemic therapies such as chemotherapy, hormonal therapy, immune therapy, and targeted therapy, which can be used alone or in combination.
- Phase I trials find the highest dose of the study drug that patients tolerate. Often, these subjects are cancer patients with no other treatment options.
- Phase II trials test whether the drug affects a specific diagnosis and what side effects it causes. Because multiple doses are tested in this phase, evaluating whether the drug will benefit these subjects is not possible.
- Phase III trials determine whether the drug will benefit cancer patients.
- Phase IV trials do further testing on an already approved drug.

- Compassionate use allows expanded access to experimental medication, which may be appropriate when the patient's life is in danger by their disease or condition, there is no other therapy to treat the disease, the patient is not a candidate to enter a clinical trial, the possibility to help the patient offsets the potential risks of treatment, and providing the new treatment will not affect any new trials of medications already in the pipeline for this indication.
- These moral principles for clinical trials include: (1) respect for autonomy (can the cancer patient freely make decisions about their treatment?); (2) beneficence (what is the benefit of participating in a trial that may not help the patient?); (3) nonmaleficence (what is the harm in participating in a trial?); and (4) justice (are the benefits, risks, and participation in the trial evenly distributed?).
- Recognizing that these patients are at the end of their lives needs to be more carefully considered in clinical trials. Although the exploration and vigorous recording of possible medical outcomes is critical for informed decision-making, quality of life (QOL) is rarely mentioned as a factor or a therapeutic goal and should be included.

NOTES

1 Rebecca L. Siegel et al., "Cancer Statistics, 2021," *CA: A Cancer Journal for Clinicians* 71, no. 1 (January 2021): 7–33, https://doi.org/10.3322/caac.21654, page 7.
2 Rebecca L. Siegel et al., "Cancer Statistics, 2021," *CA: A Cancer Journal for Clinicians* 71, no. 1 (January 2021): 7–33, https://doi.org/10.3322/caac.21654, page 9.
3 Emily J. Martin and Eric Widera, "Prognostication in Serious Illness," *Medical Clinics of North America* 104, no. 3 (May 2020): 391–403, https://doi.org/10.1016/j.mcna.2019.12.002.
4 Zandra Engelbak Nielsen and Connie Bøttcher Berthelsen, "Cancer Patients' Perceptions of Factors Influencing Their Decisions on Participation in Clinical Drug Trials: A Qualitative Meta-Synthesis," *Journal of Clinical Nursing* 28, no. 13–14 (July 2019): 2443–2461, https://doi.org/10.1111/jocn.14785, page 2444.
5 Rebecca L. Siegel et al., "Cancer Statistics, 2021," *CA: A Cancer Journal for Clinicians* 71, no. 1 (January 2021): 7–33, https://doi.org/10.3322/caac.21654, page 12.
6 Jan Borysowski, Hans-Jorg Ehni, and Andrzej Gorski, "Ethics Review in Compassionate Use," *BMC Medicine* 15, no. 1 (July 24, 2017), https://doi.org/10.1186/s12916-017-0910–9, page 2.
7 Ezekiel J. Emanuel, *The Oxford Textbook of Clinical Research Ethics* (Oxford: Oxford University Press, 2008), page 126.
8 Maxwell J. Mehlman, Eric Kodish, and Jessica Berg, "Ethical Issues in the Use of Nudges to Obtain Informed Consent for Biomedical Research," *Ethics & Human Research* 40, no. 3 (June 2018): 1–5.
9 Siddharth Menon et al., "Recruitment, Outcomes, and Toxicity Trends in Phase I Oncology Trials: Six-year Experience in a Large Institution," *Cancer Reports*, July 10, 2021, https://doi.org/10.1002/cnr2.1465, pages 1–8.
10 Zandra Engelbak Nielsen et al., "Are Cancer Patients Better Off If They Participate in Clinical Trials? A Mixed Methods Study," *BMC Cancer* 20, no. 1 (May 8, 2020): 1–17.

11 Daniel P. Sulmasy et al., "The Culture of Faith and Hope: Patients' Justifications for Their High Estimations of Expected Therapeutic Benefit When Enrolling in Early Phase Oncology Trials," *Cancer* 116, no. 15 (April 29, 2010): 3702–3711, https://doi.org/10.1002/cncr.25201, page 3710.
12 Claudia R. Baquet, Gary L. Ellison, and Shiraz I. Mishra, "Analysis of Maryland Cancer Patient Participation in National Cancer Institute-Supported Cancer Treatment Clinical Trials," *Journal of Health Care for the Poor and Underserved* 20, no. 2A (2009): 120–134, https://doi.org/10.1353/hpu.0.0162, pages 120–134.
13 "Cancer Treatment & Survivorship Facts & Figures 2019–2021" (American Cancer Society, 2019).
14 Rebecca L. Siegel et al., "Cancer Statistics, 2021," *CA: A Cancer Journal for Clinicians* 71, no. 1 (January 2021): 7–33, https://doi.org/10.3322/caac.21654, page 4.
15 Rebecca L. Siegel et al., "Cancer Statistics, 2021," *CA: A Cancer Journal for Clinicians* 71, no. 1 (January 2021): 7–33, https://doi.org/10.3322/caac.21654, page 4.
16 Nathan I. Cherny et al., eds., *Oxford Textbook of Palliative Medicine*, Fifth edition (Oxford: Oxford University Press, 2015), page 35.
17 David B. Resnik, *The Ethics of Research with Human Subjects: Protecting People, Advancing Science, Promoting Trust*, vol. 74, International Library of Ethics, Law, and the New Medicine (Cham: Springer International Publishing, 2018), https://doi.org/10.1007/978-3-319–68756-8, page 218.
18 Henk ten Have, *Vulnerability: Challenging Bioethics* (New York: Routledge, 2016), page 40.
19 David B. Resnik, *The Ethics of Research with Human Subjects: Protecting People, Advancing Science, Promoting Trust*, vol. 74, International Library of Ethics, Law, and the New Medicine (Cham: Springer International Publishing, 2018), https://doi.org/10.1007/978-3-319–68756-8, page 218.
20 Henk ten Have, *Vulnerability: Challenging Bioethics* (New York: Routledge, 2016), page 41.
21 Henk ten Have, *Vulnerability: Challenging Bioethics* (New York: Routledge, 2016), page 42.
22 Cancer Research UK, "About Cancer: Phases of Clinical Trials," 2015, www.cancerresearchuk.org/about-cancer/find-a-clinical-trial/what-clinical-trials-are/phases-of-clinical-trials#phase1.
23 US Food and Drug Administration, "The Drug Development Process, Step 3: Clinical Research," 2018, www.scribd.com/document/629430798/Step-3-FDA-Clinical-Research-Drugs.
24 Zandra Engelbak Nielsen and Connie Bøttcher Berthelsen, "Cancer Patients' Perceptions of Factors Influencing Their Decisions on Participation in Clinical Drug Trials: A Qualitative Meta-Synthesis," *Journal of Clinical Nursing* 28, no. 13–14 (July 2019): 2443–2461, https://doi.org/10.1111/jocn.14785, page 2444.
25 Ezekiel J. Emanuel, *The Oxford Textbook of Clinical Research Ethics* (Oxford: Oxford University Press, 2008), page 149.
26 Ezekiel J. Emanuel, *The Oxford Textbook of Clinical Research Ethics* (Oxford: Oxford University Press, 2008), page 27.
27 Ezekiel J. Emanuel, *The Oxford Textbook of Clinical Research Ethics* (Oxford: Oxford University Press, 2008), page 153.
28 Ezekiel J. Emanuel, *The Oxford Textbook of Clinical Research Ethics* (Oxford: Oxford University Press, 2008), page 377.
29 Matthew P. Banegas et al., "For Working-Age Cancer Survivors, Medical Debt And Bankruptcy Create Financial Hardships," *Health Affairs* 35, no. 1 (January 2016): 54–61, https://doi.org/10.1377/hlthaff.2015.0830.
30 David B. Resnik, *The Ethics of Research with Human Subjects: Protecting People, Advancing Science, Promoting Trust*, vol. 74, International Library of Ethics, Law, and the New Medicine (Cham: Springer International Publishing, 2018), https://doi.org/10.1007/978-3-319–68756-8, page 218.

31 Jennifer A. H. Bell et al, "Perceptions of and Decision Making about Clinical Trials in Adolescent and Young Adults with Cancer: A Qualitative Analysis," *BMC Cancer* 18, no. 629 (June 4, 2018): 2–18, page 2451.
32 Daniel P. Sulmasy et al., "The Culture of Faith and Hope: Patients' Justifications for Their High Estimations of Expected Therapeutic Benefit When Enrolling in Early Phase Oncology Trials," *Cancer* 116, no. 15 (April 29, 2010): 3702–3711, https://doi.org/10.1002/cncr.25201, page 3710.
33 David B. Resnik, *The Ethics of Research with Human Subjects: Protecting People, Advancing Science, Promoting Trust*, vol. 74, International Library of Ethics, Law, and the New Medicine (Cham: Springer International Publishing, 2018), https://doi.org/10.1007/978-3-319–68756-8, page 88.
34 David B. Resnik, *The Ethics of Research with Human Subjects: Protecting People, Advancing Science, Promoting Trust*, vol. 74, International Library of Ethics, Law, and the New Medicine (Cham: Springer International Publishing, 2018), https://doi.org/10.1007/978-3-319–68756-8, page 90.
35 "US Food and Drug Administration. Expanded Access (Compassionate Use)." (https://wwww.fda.gov/news-events/public-health-focus, 2017).
36 "US Food and Drug Administration. Expanded Access (Compassionate Use)."
37 Borysowski, Ehni, and Gorski, "Ethics Review in Compassionate Use." pages 1–7.
38 Arthur L. Caplan and Amrit Ray, "The Ethical Challenges of Compassionate Use," *JAMA* 315, no. 10 (March 8, 2016): 979, https://doi.org/10.1001/jama.2016.0416.
39 Borysowski, Ehni, and Gorski, "Ethics Review in Compassionate Use." pages 1–7.
40 Caplan and Ray, "The Ethical Challenges of Compassionate Use."
41 Tim K. Mackey and Virginia J. Schoenfeld, "Going 'Social' to Access Experimental and Potentially Life-Saving Treatment: An Assessment of the Policy and Online Patient Advocacy Environment for Expanded Access," *BMC Medicine* 14, no. 1 (December 2016): 17, s12916-016-0568-8, https://doi.org/10.1186/s12916-016-0568-8, pages 2–10.
42 Caplan and Ray, "The Ethical Challenges of Compassionate Use."
43 Borysowski, Ehni, and Gorski, "Ethics Review in Compassionate Use." page 6.
44 Tom L. Beauchamp and James F. Childress, *Principles of Biomedical Ethics*, fifth edition (New York: Oxford University Press, 2001), page 12.
45 Ezekiel J. Emanuel, *The Oxford Textbook of Clinical Research Ethics* (Oxford: Oxford University Press, 2008), page 126.
46 Tom L. Beauchamp and James F. Childress, *Principles of Biomedical Ethics*, eighth edition (New York: Oxford University Press, 2019), page 99.
47 H Vikas et al., "How Informed Is the Informed Consent?," *Journal of Family Medicine and Primary Care* 10, no. 6 (2021): 2299, https://doi.org/10.4103/jfmpc.jfmpc_2393_20.
48 Maura Priest, "Autonomy-Centered Healthcare," *HEC Forum : An Interdisciplinary Journal on Hospitals' Ethical and Legal Issues* 30, no. 3 (September 2018): 297–318, https://doi.org/10.1007/s10730-018-9355–6, page 300.
49 Maura Priest, "Autonomy-Centered Healthcare," *HEC Forum : An Interdisciplinary Journal on Hospitals' Ethical and Legal Issues* 30, no. 3 (September 2018): 297–318, https://doi.org/10.1007/s10730-018-9355–6, page 301.
50 E. K. White "A Reason for Hope? A Legal and Ethical Implementation of the HIV Organ Policy Equity Act," www.researchgate.net/publication/306212883_A_reason_for_hope_A_legal_and_ethical_implementation_of_the_HIV_organ_policy_equity_act.
51 Tom L. Beauchamp and James F. Childress, *Principles of Biomedical Ethics*, eighth edition (New York: Oxford University Press, 2019), page 122.
52 Ezekiel J. Emanuel, "What Makes Clinical Research Ethical?," *JAMA* 283, no. 20 (May 24, 2000): 2701, https://doi.org/10.1001/jama.283.20.2701, page 130.
53 Pia Dellson et al., "Patients' and Physicians' Disagreement on Patients' Understanding of Clinical Cancer Trial Information: A Pairwise Pilot Study of Mirroring Subjective Assessments Compared with Objective Measurements," *Trials* 20, no. 1 (May 29, 2019), https://doi.org/10.1186/s13063-019-3416-2, page 8.

54 Pia Dellson et al., "Patients' and Physicians' Disagreement on Patients' Understanding of Clinical Cancer Trial Information: A Pairwise Pilot Study of Mirroring Subjective Assessments Compared with Objective Measurements," *Trials* 20, no. 1 (May 29, 2019), https://doi.org/10.1186/s13063-019-3416-2, page 9.
55 Ezekiel J. Emanuel, *The Oxford Textbook of Clinical Research Ethics* (Oxford: Oxford University Press, 2008), page 131.
56 Maxwell J. Mehlman, Eric Kodish, and Jessica Berg, "Ethical Issues in the Use of Nudges to Obtain Informed Consent for Biomedical Research," *Ethics & Human Research* 40, no. 3 (May–June 2018), pages 1–6.
57 Maxwell J. Mehlman, Eric Kodish, and Jessica Berg, "Ethical Issues in the Use of Nudges to Obtain Informed Consent for Biomedical Research," *Ethics & Human Research* 40, no. 3 (May–June 2018), pages 1–6.
58 R. F. Brown et al., "Developing Ethical Strategies to Assist Oncologists in Seeking Informed Consent to Cancer Clinical Trials," *Social Science & Medicine* 58, no. 2 (January 2004): 379–390, https://doi.org/10.1016/S0277–9536(03)00204-1, pages 379–390.
59 R. F. Brown et al., "Developing Ethical Strategies to Assist Oncologists in Seeking Informed Consent to Cancer Clinical Trials," *Social Science & Medicine* 58, no. 2 (January 2004): 379–390, https://doi.org/10.1016/S0277–9536(03)00204-1.
60 Mary Murphy et al., "Nothing to Lose: A Grounded Theory Study of Patients' and Healthcare Professionals' Perspectives of Being Involved in the Consent Process for Oncology Trials with Non-Curative Intent," *BMC Palliative Care* 19, no. 1 (October 30, 2020), page 8.
61 David B. Resnik, *The Ethics of Research with Human Subjects: Protecting People, Advancing Science, Promoting Trust*, vol. 74, International Library of Ethics, Law, and the New Medicine (Cham: Springer International Publishing, 2018), https://doi.org/10.1007/978-3-319–68756-8, page 233.
62 Henk ten Have, *Vulnerability: Challenging Bioethics* (New York: Routledge, 2016), page 66.
63 Tom L. Beauchamp and James F. Childress, *Principles of Biomedical Ethics*, fifth edition (New York: Oxford University Press, 2001), page 166.
64 Zandra Engelbak Nielsen and Connie Bøttcher Berthelsen, "Cancer Patients' Perceptions of Factors Influencing Their Decisions on Participation in Clinical Drug Trials: A Qualitative Meta-Synthesis," *Journal of Clinical Nursing* 28, no. 13–14 (July 2019): 2443–2461, https://doi.org/10.1111/jocn.14785, page 15.
65 Jeffrey M. Peppercorn et al., "Comparison of Outcomes in Cancer Patients Treated within and Outside Clinical Trials: Conceptual Framework and Structured Review," *The Lancet* 363, no. 9405 (January 2004): 263–270, https://doi.org/10.1016/S0140–6736(03)15383-4, page 269.
66 Zandra Engelbak Nielsen and Connie Bøttcher Berthelsen, "Cancer Patients' Perceptions of Factors Influencing Their Decisions on Participation in Clinical Drug Trials: A Qualitative Meta-Synthesis," *Journal of Clinical Nursing* 28, no. 13–14 (July 2019): 2443–2461, https://doi.org/10.1111/jocn.14785, page 15.
67 Zandra Engelbak Nielsen and Connie Bøttcher Berthelsen, "Cancer Patients' Perceptions of Factors Influencing Their Decisions on Participation in Clinical Drug Trials: A Qualitative Meta-Synthesis," *Journal of Clinical Nursing* 28, no. 13–14 (July 2019): 2443–2461, https://doi.org/10.1111/jocn.14785, page 15.
68 Daniel P. Sulmasy et al., "The Culture of Faith and Hope: Patients' Justifications for Their High Estimations of Expected Therapeutic Benefit When Enrolling in Early Phase Oncology Trials," *Cancer* 116, no. 15 (April 29, 2010): 3702–3711, https://doi.org/10.1002/cncr.25201, page 9.
69 Ezekiel J. Emanuel, *The Oxford Textbook of Clinical Research Ethics* (Oxford: Oxford University Press, 2008), page 127.
70 Ezekiel J. Emanuel, *The Oxford Textbook of Clinical Research Ethics* (Oxford: Oxford University Press, 2008), page 128.
71 Norman E. Sharpless, "The Power and Promise of Cancer Research," *Vital Speeches of the Day* 84, no. 9 (September 2018): 253–256.

72 Tom L. Beauchamp and James F. Childress, *Principles of Biomedical Ethics*, fifth edition (New York: Oxford University Press, 2001), page 113.
73 Tom L. Beauchamp and James F. Childress, *Principles of Biomedical Ethics*, fifth edition (New York: Oxford University Press, 2001), page 117.
74 Ezekiel J. Emanuel, *The Oxford Textbook of Clinical Research Ethics* (Oxford: Oxford University Press, 2008), page 126.
75 Ezekiel J. Emanuel, *The Oxford Textbook of Clinical Research Ethics* (Oxford: Oxford University Press, 2008), page 126.
76 Ezekiel J. Emanuel, "What Makes Clinical Research Ethical?," *JAMA* 283, no. 20 (May 24, 2000): 2701, https://doi.org/10.1001/jama.283.20.2701, page 2705.
77 Ezekiel J. Emanuel, *The Oxford Textbook of Clinical Research Ethics* (Oxford: Oxford University Press, 2008), page 266.
78 Cancer Research UK, "About Cancer: Phases of Clinical Trials," 2015, www.cancerresearchuk.org/about-cancer/find-a-clinical-trial/what-clinical-trials-are/phases-of-clinical-trials#phase1.
79 Siddharth Menon et al., "Recruitment, Outcomes, and Toxicity Trends in Phase I Oncology Trials: Six-year Experience in a Large Institution," *Cancer Reports*, July 10, 2021, https://doi.org/10.1002/cnr2.1465, pages 1–9.
80 Siddharth Menon et al., "Recruitment, Outcomes, and Toxicity Trends in Phase I Oncology Trials: Six-year Experience in a Large Institution," *Cancer Reports*, July 10, 2021, https://doi.org/10.1002/cnr2.1465, pages 1–9.
81 Siddharth Menon et al., "Recruitment, Outcomes, and Toxicity Trends in Phase I Oncology Trials: Six-year Experience in a Large Institution," *Cancer Reports*, July 10, 2021, https://doi.org/10.1002/cnr2.1465, pages 1–9.
82 Siddharth Menon et al., "Recruitment, Outcomes, and Toxicity Trends in Phase I Oncology Trials: Six-year Experience in a Large Institution," *Cancer Reports*, July 10, 2021, https://doi.org/10.1002/cnr2.1465, pages 1–9.
83 Ann M. Berger, John L. Shuster, and Jamie H. Von Roenn, *Principles and Practice of Palliative Care and Supportive Oncology* (Philadelphia, PA: Lippincott, Williams & Wilkins), page 593.
84 Tove E. Godskesen et al., "When Nursing Care and Clinical Trials Coincide: A Qualitative Study of the Views of Nordic Oncology and Hematology Nurses on Ethical Work Challenges," *Journal of Empirical Research on Human Research Ethics* 13, no. 5 (December 2018): 475–485, https://doi.org/10.1177/1556264618783555, page 8.
85 Daniel P. Sulmasy et al., "The Culture of Faith and Hope: Patients' Justifications for Their High Estimations of Expected Therapeutic Benefit When Enrolling in Early Phase Oncology Trials," *Cancer* 116, no. 15 (April 29, 2010): 3702–3711, https://doi.org/10.1002/cncr.25201, page 11.
86 Ezekiel J. Emanuel, *The Oxford Textbook of Clinical Research Ethics* (Oxford: Oxford University Press, 2008), 126.
87 Siddharth Menon et al., "Recruitment, Outcomes, and Toxicity Trends in Phase I Oncology Trials: Six-year Experience in a Large Institution," *Cancer Reports*, July 10, 2021, https://doi.org/10.1002/cnr2.1465, pages 1–9.
88 Tom L. Beauchamp and James F. Childress, *Principles of Biomedical Ethics*, fifth edition (New York: Oxford University Press, 2001), page 129.
89 Ezekiel J. Emanuel, *The Oxford Textbook of Clinical Research Ethics* (Oxford: Oxford University Press, 2008), page 126.
90 Tom L. Beauchamp and James F. Childress, *Principles of Biomedical Ethics*, fifth edition (New York: Oxford University Press, 2001), page 226.
91 Tom L. Beauchamp and James F. Childress, *Principles of Biomedical Ethics*, fifth edition (New York: Oxford University Press, 2001), page 227.

92 Ezekiel J. Emanuel, *The Oxford Textbook of Clinical Research Ethics* (Oxford: Oxford University Press, 2008), page 126.

93 Gordon Jayson and John Harris, "How Participants in Cancer Trials Are Chosen: Ethics and Conflicting Interests," *Nature Reviews Cancer* 6 (April 2006): 330–336, page 335.

94 Janice L. Krieger, "Last Resort or Roll of the Die? Exploring the Role of Metaphors in Cancer Clinical Trials Education Among Medically Underserved Populations," *Journal of Health Communication* 19, no. 10 (October 2014): 1161–1177, page 1174.

95 Claudia R. Baquet, Gary L. Ellison, and Shiraz I. Mishra, "Analysis of Maryland Cancer Patient Participation in National Cancer Institute-Supported Cancer Treatment Clinical Trials," *Journal of Health Care for the Poor and Underserved* 20, no. 2A (2009): 120–134, https://doi.org/10.1353/hpu.0.0162, page 120.

96 Claudia R. Baquet, Gary L. Ellison, and Shiraz I. Mishra, "Analysis of Maryland Cancer Patient Participation in National Cancer Institute-Supported Cancer Treatment Clinical Trials," *Journal of Health Care for the Poor and Underserved* 20, no. 2A (2009): 120–134, https://doi.org/10.1353/hpu.0.0162, page 131.

97 Claudia R. Baquet, Gary L. Ellison, and Shiraz I. Mishra, "Analysis of Maryland Cancer Patient Participation in National Cancer Institute-Supported Cancer Treatment Clinical Trials," *Journal of Health Care for the Poor and Underserved* 20, no. 2A (2009): 120–134, https://doi.org/10.1353/hpu.0.0162, page 131.

98 Claudia R. Baquet, Gary L. Ellison, and Shiraz I. Mishra, "Analysis of Maryland Cancer Patient Participation in National Cancer Institute-Supported Cancer Treatment Clinical Trials," *Journal of Health Care for the Poor and Underserved* 20, no. 2A (2009): 120–134, https://doi.org/10.1353/hpu.0.0162, page 132.

99 Janice L. Krieger, "Last Resort or Roll of the Die? Exploring the Role of Metaphors in Cancer Clinical Trials Education Among Medically Underserved Populations," *Journal of Health Communication* 19, no. 10 (October 2014): 1161–1177, page 1161.

100 Ezekiel J. Emanuel, *The Oxford Textbook of Clinical Research Ethics* (Oxford: Oxford University Press, 2008).

101 Ezekiel J. Emanuel, *The Oxford Textbook of Clinical Research Ethics* (Oxford: Oxford University Press, 2008), page 126.

102 Tove E. Godskesen et al., "The Culture of Hope and Ethical Challenges in Clinical Trials: A Qualitative Study of Oncologists and Haematologists' Views," *Clinical Ethics* 15, no. 1 (March 2020): 29–38, https://doi.org/10.1177/1477750919897379.

103 Tom L. Beauchamp and James F. Childress, *Principles of Biomedical Ethics*, fifth edition (New York: Oxford University Press, 2001), page 226.

104 Ezekiel J. Emanuel, *The Oxford Textbook of Clinical Research Ethics* (Oxford: Oxford University Press, 2008), page 126.

105 Zandra Engelbak Nielsen et al., "Are Cancer Patients Better Off If They Participate in Clinical Trials? A Mixed Methods Study," *BMC Cancer* 20, no. 1 (May 8, 2020): 1–17.

106 Janice L. Krieger, "Last Resort or Roll of the Die? Exploring the Role of Metaphors in Cancer Clinical Trials Education Among Medically Underserved Populations," *Journal of Health Communication* 19, no. 10 (October 2014): 1161–1177.

107 Jan Gaertner et al., "The Role of End-of-Life Issues in the Design and Reporting of Cancer Clinical Trials: A Structured Literature Review," *PLoS ONE* 10, no. 9 (September 1, 2015), https://doi.org/10.1371/journal.pone.0136640.

108 Betty R. Ferrell et al., "Palliative Care and Phase 1 Trials: Intervention to Improve Quality of Life and Provide Education," *Clinical Journal of Oncology Nursing* 21, no. 4 (August 2017): 473–479, page 474.

109 Betty R. Ferrell et al., "Palliative Care and Phase 1 Trials: Intervention to Improve Quality of Life and Provide Education," *Clinical Journal of Oncology Nursing* 21, no. 4 (August 2017): 473–479, page 478.

BIBLIOGRAPHY

Banegas, Matthew P., Gery P. Guy Jr., Janet S. de Moor, Donatus U. Ekwueme, Katherine S. Virgo, Erin E. Kent, Stephanie Nutt, Zhiyuan Zheng, Ruth Rechis, and K. Robin Yabroff. "For Working-Age Cancer Survivors, Medical Debt And Bankruptcy Create Financial Hardships." *Health Affairs* 35, no. 1 (January 2016): 54–61. https://doi.org/10.1377/hlthaff.2015.0830.

Baquet, Claudia R., Gary L. Ellison, and Shiraz I. Mishra. "Analysis of Maryland Cancer Patient Participation in National Cancer Institute-Supported Cancer Treatment Clinical Trials." *Journal of Health Care for the Poor and Underserved* 20, no. 2A (2009): 120–134. https://doi.org/10.1353/hpu.0.0162.

Beauchamp, Tom L., and James F. Childress. *Principles of Biomedical Ethics*. Fifth edition. New York: Oxford University Press, 2001.

Beauchamp, Tom L., and James F. Childress. *Principles of Biomedical Ethics*. Eighth edition. New York: Oxford University Press, 2019.

Berger, Ann M., John L. Shuster, and Jamie H. Von Roenn. *Principles and Practice of Palliative Care and Supportive Oncology*. Philadelphia, PA: Lippincott, Williams & Wilkins.

Borysowski, Jan, Hans-Jorg Ehni, and Andrzej Gorski. "Ethics Review in Compassionate Use." *BMC Medicine* 15, no. 1 (July 24, 2017). https://doi.org/10.1186/s12916-017-0910-9.

Brown, R. F, P. N. Butow, D. G. Butt, A. R. Moore, and M. H. N. Tattersall. "Developing Ethical Strategies to Assist Oncologists in Seeking Informed Consent to Cancer Clinical Trials." *Social Science & Medicine* 58, no. 2 (January 2004): 379–390. https://doi.org/10.1016/S0277-9536(03)00204-1.

Caplan, Arthur L., and Amrit Ray. "The Ethical Challenges of Compassionate Use." *JAMA* 315, no. 10 (March 8, 2016): 979. https://doi.org/10.1001/jama.2016.0416.

Cherny, Nathan I., Marie Fallon, Stein Kaasa, Russell K. Portenoy, and David Currow, eds. *Oxford Textbook of Palliative Medicine*. Fifth edition. Oxford: Oxford University Press, 2015.

Dellson, Pia, Christina Carlsson, Mef Nilbert, and Helena Jernstrom. "Patients' and Physicians' Disagreement on Patients' Understanding of Clinical Cancer Trial Information: A Pairwise Pilot Study of Mirroring Subjective Assessments Compared with Objective Measurements." *Trials* 20, no. 1 (May 29, 2019). https://doi.org/10.1186/s13063-019-3416-2.

Emanuel, Ezekiel J. *The Oxford Textbook of Clinical Research Ethics. [Electronic Resource]*. Oxford University Press, 2008.

Emanuel, Ezekiel J. "What Makes Clinical Research Ethical?" *JAMA* 283, no. 20 (May 24, 2000): 2701. https://doi.org/10.1001/jama.283.20.2701.

Engelbak Nielsen, Zandra, Stefan Eriksson, Laurine Bente Schram Harsløf, Suzanne Petri, Gert Helgesson, Margrete Mangset, and Tove E. Godskesen. "Are Cancer Patients Better off If They Participate in Clinical Trials? A Mixed Methods Study." *BMC Cancer* 20, no. 1 (May 8, 2020): 1–17.

Ferrell, Betty R., Vincent Chung, Marianna Koczywas, Anna Cathy Williams, Denise Gallagher, Patricia Fischer, and Thomas J. Smith. "Palliative Care and Phase 1 Trials: Intervention to Improve Quality of Life and Provide Education." *Clinical Journal of Oncology Nursing* 21, no. 4 (August 2017): 473–479.

Gaertner, Jan, Vera Weingärtner, Stefan Lange, Elke Hausner, Ansgar Gerhardus, Steffen T. Simon, Raymond Voltz, Gerhild Becker, and Norbert Schmacke. "The Role of End-of-Life

Issues in the Design and Reporting of Cancer Clinical Trials: A Structured Literature Review." *PLoS ONE* 10, no. 9 (September 1, 2015). https://doi.org/10.1371/journal.pone.0136640.

Godskesen, Tove E., Suzanne Petri, Stefan Eriksson, Arja Halkoaho, Margrete Mangset, and Zandra E. Nielsen. "The Culture of Hope and Ethical Challenges in Clinical Trials: A Qualitative Study of Oncologists and Haematologists' Views." *Clinical Ethics* 15, no. 1 (March 2020): 29–38. https://doi.org/10.1177/1477750919897379.

Godskesen, Tove E., Suzanne Petri, Stefan Eriksson, Arja Halkoaho, Margrete Mangset, Merja Pirinen, and Zandra Engelbak Nielsen. "When Nursing Care and Clinical Trials Coincide: A Qualitative Study of the Views of Nordic Oncology and Hematology Nurses on Ethical Work Challenges." *Journal of Empirical Research on Human Research Ethics* 13, no. 5 (December 2018): 475–485. https://doi.org/10.1177/1556264618783555.

Jayson, Gordon, and John Harris. "How Participants in Cancer Trials Are Chosen: Ethics and Conflicting Interests." *Nature Reviews Cancer* 6 (April 2006): 330–336.

Jennifer A.H. Bell et al. "Perceptions of and Decision Making about Clinical Trials in Adolescent and Young Adults with Cancer: A Qualitative Analysis." *BMC Cancer* 18, no. 629 (June 4, 2018): 2–18.

Krieger, Janice L. "Last Resort or Roll of the Die? Exploring the Role of Metaphors in Cancer Clinical Trials Education Among Medically Underserved Populations." *Journal of Health Communication* 19, no. 10 (October 2014): 1161–1177.

Mackey, Tim K., and Virginia J. Schoenfeld. "Going 'Social' to Access Experimental and Potentially Life-Saving Treatment: An Assessment of the Policy and Online Patient Advocacy Environment for Expanded Access." *BMC Medicine* 14, no. 1 (December 2016): 17, s12916-016-0568-8. https://doi.org/10.1186/s12916-016-0568-8.

Martin, Emily J., and Eric Widera. "Prognostication in Serious Illness." *Medical Clinics of North America* 104, no. 3 (May 2020): 391–403. https://doi.org/10.1016/j.mcna.2019.12.002.

Maxwell J. Mehlman, Eric Kodish, and Jessica Berg. "Ethical Issues in the Use of Nudges to Obtain Informed Consent for Biomedical Research." *Ethics & Human Research* 40, no. 3 (June 2018): 1–5.

Menon, Siddharth, Amy Davies, Sophia Frentzas, Cheryl-Ann Hawkins, Eva Segelov, Daphne Day, and Ben Markman. "Recruitment, Outcomes, and Toxicity Trends in Phase I Oncology Trials: Six-year Experience in a Large Institution." *Cancer Reports*, July 10, 2021. https://doi.org/10.1002/cnr2.1465.

Murphy, Mary, Eilís McCaughan, Matthew A Carson, Monica Donovan, Richard H Wilson, and Donna Fitzsimons. "Nothing to Lose: A Grounded Theory Study of Patients' and Healthcare Professionals' Perspectives of Being Involved in the Consent Process for Oncology Trials with Non-Curative Intent." *BMC Palliative Care* 19, no. 1 (October 30, 2020).

Nielsen, Zandra Engelbak, and Connie Bøttcher Berthelsen. "Cancer Patients' Perceptions of Factors Influencing Their Decisions on Participation in Clinical Drug Trials: A Qualitative Meta-Synthesis." *Journal of Clinical Nursing* 28, no. 13–14 (July 2019): 2443–2461. https://doi.org/10.1111/jocn.14785.

Peppercorn, Jeffrey M., Jane C. Weeks, E. Francis Cook, and Steven Joffe. "Comparison of Outcomes in Cancer Patients Treated within and Outside Clinical Trials: Conceptual Framework and Structured Review." *The Lancet* 363, no. 9405 (January 2004): 263–270. https://doi.org/10.1016/S0140-6736(03)15383-4.

Priest, Maura. "Autonomy-Centered Healthcare." *HEC Forum : An Interdisciplinary Journal on Hospitals' Ethical and Legal Issues* 30, no. 3 (September 2018): 297–318. https://doi.org/10.1007/s10730-018-9355-6.

Resnik, David B. *The Ethics of Research with Human Subjects: Protecting People, Advancing Science, Promoting Trust*. Vol. 74. International Library of Ethics, Law, and the New Medicine. Cham: Springer International Publishing, 2018. https://doi.org/10.1007/978-3-319-68756-8.

Sharpless, Norman E. "The Power and Promise of Cancer Research." *Vital Speeches of the Day* 84, no. 9 (September 2018): 253–256.

Siegel, Rebecca L., Kimberly D. Miller, Hannah E. Fuchs, and Ahmedin Jemal. "Cancer Statistics, 2021." *CA: A Cancer Journal for Clinicians* 71, no. 1 (January 2021): 7–33. https://doi.org/10.3322/caac.21654.

Sulmasy, Daniel P., Alan B. Astrow, M. Kai He, Damon M. Seils, Neal J. Meropol, Ellyn Micco, and Kevin P. Weinfurt. "The Culture of Faith and Hope: Patients' Justifications for Their High Estimations of Expected Therapeutic Benefit When Enrolling in Early Phase Oncology Trials." *Cancer* 116, no. 15 (April 29, 2010): 3702–3711. https://doi.org/10.1002/cncr.25201.

Ten Have, H. *Vulnerability: Challenging Bioethics*. London; New York: Routledge, Taylor & Francis Group, 2016.

Vikas, H, Ananth Kini, Nishant Sharma, Naveen R. Gowda, and Anant Gupta. "How Informed Is the Informed Consent?" *Journal of Family Medicine and Primary Care* 10, no. 6 (2021): 2299. https://doi.org/10.4103/jfmpc.jfmpc_2393_20.

Chapter 6

The Bioethical Dilemma of Medical Futility in the ICU

INTRODUCTION

This is the second clinical chapter that discusses an issue that encompasses multiple ethical principles. Although the intensive care units (ICUs) may only have a small fraction of the beds in an average American hospital, they are responsible for a significant amount of the hospital's budget. However, the burdens are more than financial. It is also where most of the hospital deaths occur.[1] In addition, the emotional toll of prolonged ICU stays is daunting and affects the patients, families, and the unit's staff.

Some studies have suggested a high percentage of care in the ICU that is futile or medically ineffective. Yet, there is no clear definition of what is considered futile care.[2] This additional burden adds to the severity of this problem. This chapter will explore the issue of futile care in the ICU. It will also look into the possible causes of why this may be occurring. A better understanding of this problem is essential for finding future solutions.

WHAT IS MEDICAL FUTILITY IN THE ICU, AND WHAT IS THE HARM?

Most people wish to die at home, yet almost a third of patients will die in the hospital.[3] Nothing is more tragic than a patient dying after a prolonged ICU stay. The patient may be kept alive using "organ support technology" or machines during that time. These machines could include mechanical ventilation, dialysis, and left ventricular assist devices (LADs). If this technology helps the patient return to a healthy condition, it is a triumph for medical technology. However, the patient often languishes in this state for a prolonged time. The patient may be medically sedated, unconscious, or in severe delirium for much of this time. The chance of recovery is nil, yet there is hesitancy to stop the current treatment. At some

DOI: 10.4324/9781003654124-7

point, all treatment options will end, and someone (maybe out of exhaustion) will say, "There is nothing more to do." This "person" could be one of the physicians, a family member, a nurse, a chaplain, or a myriad of individuals involved in the patient's care. Rarely is it the patient. When death does occur, there may be some relief, but there is also a considerable burden.

Definition of Medical Futility

Futile is an adjective meaning "incapable of producing any useful result; pointless."[4] Medical futility refers to actions that are unlikely to make the patient well. This definition seems simplistic, but it is often controversial in practice. Physicians should be the guarantors of whether a treatment has a therapeutic advantage. If a treatment does not benefit, it should not be offered.

Nevertheless, even among physicians, there is no real consensus on what futility means. Some clinicians feel that an intervention is futile only if its chance for success is zero. In contrast, others will say an intervention is pointless even if the success rate is 13%.[5] There is also controversy about whether the treatment has a high success and whether it is beneficial. For example, dialysis always does something to a patient. It can correct electrolyte imbalances and remove fluid very effectively. Ventilators can keep a patient alive whose lungs have failed. Antibiotics are very effective in killing bacteria. The list goes on and on, and every specialist has their own "tool" they can offer. The question is not whether these "tools" will do something but whether the patient will improve. Even if the treatment is successful, it is medically futile if it does not make the patient well.[6] Just because a patient has a physiologic response to a treatment, does it make that treatment medically appropriate? Painting the RMS Titanic's staterooms would brighten the rooms and make them pretty but would otherwise have no effect once it hits the iceberg!

Because of this controversy, many have proposed replacing futile with more precise terminology such as *inappropriate* or *potentially inappropriate*[7] (this was previously discussed in Chapter 2). Patients and their families may find this terminology more comfortable to understand. It also seems that many researchers and writers have accepted this term because it is less judgmental and opens up further discussion. However, in this discussion, I use the term futile to emphasize treatments that no one expects to have any change in the outcome. Also, the usefulness of this word substitution alone is questionable and most likely tends to oversimplify the dilemma. Furthermore, communication with patients and families will be even more difficult if clinicians spend too much time debating terminology and its meaning. Futile or potentially inappropriate? I will let the reader decide which is correct under the given context and circumstances.

Cost of the Problem: Economically and Emotionally

The United States' expenditure for healthcare is currently almost 18% of our Gross National Product (GNP) and is expected to be 30% by 2030.[8] Critical care alone accounts for 20% of all healthcare costs and 1% of our GNP.[9] We have eight times as many beds per capita than other Western Nations, and elderly patients account for 60% of all ICU days.[10] People who are older than 65 years will double to 70 million in 2030. Because of these facts, the demand for ICU beds will increase substantially in the next decade. One way to mitigate these changes is to look at how many beds in the ICU are used for futile care. As stated above, these numbers are difficult to assess because of the lack of agreement on what constitutes medically futile care. In one study, the investigators felt that 11% of the ICU beds received futile care. The mortality rate for this group was 85%, with the survivors remaining in severely compromised health.[11] There is also an opportunity loss when ICU beds are used for futile treatment.[12] Patients who could benefit from therapy in the ICU are delayed from admission because of a bed shortage. This dilemma affects patients in the Emergency Department, patients being transferred from the floor, and patients requesting a transfer from another institution. The mortality and morbidity from this delay are unclear but could be significant.

The emotional cost of futile care in the ICU is significant and includes patients, their families, and the entire ICU staff. This tension is made worse by long lengths of stay preceding the patient's death. High rates of stress occur in families of patients admitted to the ICU.[13] Post traumatic stress disorder (PTSD) symptoms were prevalent in 47.8% when family members were required to make end-of-life decisions.[14] Stress is also seen in the ICU staff when families demand that everything be done because they are waiting for a miracle.[15] ICU nurses provide significant care for their patients. They define futile care as "useless, ineffective caregiving with wastage of resources and torment of both patients and nurses having nursing and medical aspects." Burnout, moral distress, and ethical conflicts are among the consequences they face.[16] Finally, ICU physicians (intensivists) face difficulties attending to patients receiving potentially futile care.[17] These conflicts include disagreements regarding whether the care provided is genuinely futile and communications with the family.[18]

Ethical Implications

Multiple bioethical problems occur when patients are perceived to be receiving futile care in the ICU. Autonomy is the patient's or their surrogates' right to make healthcare decisions. Many times, this is the cause of ethical conflicts concerning ICU care. Even though this right is widely respected, it does imply that patients or their families can demand medically ineffective treatments.[19] Difficulties can also arise when the treatments given conflict with the patient's previous wishes. Very few critically ill patients can make their own decisions, causing the ICU to rely on surrogate decision-makers.[20] It is often difficult to tell if their proxies correctly represent the patient's self-interest.

Beneficence is also of concern when providing medically inappropriate care. Some physicians feel that all treatments to keep someone alive are necessary, even if the benefits are questionable.[21] However, providing treatments that are not nonbeneficial to a dying patient is not good practice. Finally, distributive justice is an ethical concern concerning futile care in the ICU. These beds are a limited resource that needs appropriate use. Improper ICU bed utilization can lead to delays or denial for patients who could benefit from such care.[22] Also, by definition, futile care is expensive and adds to the burden of our rapidly expanding healthcare budget. When potentially medically inappropriate care is suspected, these ethical principles must be part of the dialog.

Causes

We have previously discussed the stress involved with critically ill patients and the need for end-of-life decision-making for physicians, nurses, and family members.[23] Ideally, physicians and the ICU team will have family meetings to discuss the case in depth with those involved with current and future decisions. The goal is to share clinical information and walk the family through the maze of variables that are likely to occur. In addition, the family must share information about the patient with the team regarding what they would want if they could speak for themselves. Unfortunately, heuristics sometimes get involved, negatively affecting the decision-making process on multiple levels.[24]

Patient and Family Issues

Dealing with end-of-life decisions is extremely difficult. Families are encouraged to have discussions with loved ones before a crisis occurs. Advance care planning is essential to this process. This process includes choosing a healthcare proxy to make healthcare decisions for patients when they can no longer make them themselves. A living will is often added to specify choices when the person is terminally ill or permanently unconscious. The quality of the conversation with loved ones regarding future healthcare can significantly enhance the family member's decision-making ability.[25] Most patients feel that discussing end-of-life decisions with their family is essential, but only one-third of patients will complete an advance directive or have these crucial conversations.[26]

Family members often lack the essential information to make end-of-life decisions. These discussions are complicated, and it is usually easier to avoid them. Having a family member in an ICU can be devastating. Families then have the difficult task of dealing with a loved one's severe illness and then being asked to make difficult choices.[27] Frequently, relatives are emotionally unprepared to make these decisions and will choose aggressive care, hoping to buy time. Unfortunately, this tactic only delays the need to make difficult decisions. The ICU team is occasionally complicit with this plan to avoid a struggle and will extend aggressive care, wasting time, effort, and resources.[28]

Heuristic decision-making may also play a role in the family. Relatives may use these decision-making techniques as a fallback because of their severe stress. An *anchoring* heuristic can occur based on a character trait. If the patient was stubborn, the family may conclude that they should continue aggressive treatment. For example, Dad was always a fighter. A *bandwagon* heuristic can occur if a single family member can enlist others. Even if some family members feel the treatment is futile, they may go along with the crowd. Finally, there may be a *neglect of the probability* heuristic. Suppose the decision-maker was told there is only a 1% chance of survival. In that case, they might decide to continue aggressive care because there is still a chance.[29] A careful discussion with the family may help understand why a decision was made and whether it remains valid under further debate and scrutiny.

Physician Issues

Physicians ultimately play a substantial role in the utilization of ICU beds. Their decisions affect the care of the patients currently in the ICU and patients who will require ICU admission in the immediate future. Therefore, stewardship regarding access to and discharge from the ICU is essential. Intensivists appear to do a better job with this dilemma than other types of physicians.[30] In "closed units" (only intensivists can admit and manage patients) or open units with a mandatory intensivist consultation, mortality rates and lengths of stay are improved. Intensivists are motivated to provide the best possible care and to use limited resources responsibly.

When families request medically ineffective care, physicians feel distressed for multiple reasons.[31] Clinicians will state that they do not want to make patients suffer. However, most patients can be sedated to near unconsciousness to prevent this from occurring. They will also note that they would not want this type of care if they were the patient. Finally, they are concerned about the economic costs and use of medical resources. Other reasons for distress can arise from the physician's disappointment that the family does not trust their clinical assessment and feels that they are being forced to do something unethical or even repugnant. Communication with the family is vital when there is discordance regarding ICU treatment. However, most families will ultimately agree with the ICU staff,[32] which suggests that there are reasons with the physicians themselves regarding futile care.

Physicians are poor prognosticators even with an incredible amount of data at their fingertips. Most are over-optimistic and can be off by a factor of five or more.[33] In ICU medicine, multiple metrics can be performed to predict outcomes with varying degrees of accuracy. Some require clinical determinants, whereas others appear to be more subjective. One study found it very accurate if the physicians, nurses, residents, and advanced clinical practitioners (nurse practitioners and physician assistants) agreed on a single day that the patient was likely to die before discharge.

Nevertheless, there may also be a degree of heuristic decision-making involved. These could include an *anchoring* heuristic, "I once had a patient that was like and did well," or a *bandwagon* where one team member pushes to keep going, especially if that person is the Intensivist. Physicians list other reasons for continuing futile care. These include the feeling that physicians are trained to treat, often are inexperienced with death and dying, do not want to give up hope, feel death is the enemy, worry about legal consequences, are poor communicators, are compelled to do everything possible, may have an emotional attachment to patients, goes against their personality, may have had personal experiences with dying family members, or believe that their religion demands it.[34] These reasons are problematic in many ways. Emotional reasons are almost always involved when families insist on medically ineffective care. The treatment may not be helpful as it will not return the patient to a state of wellness, but at least it is wanted. However, it is neither useful nor wanted when physicians insist on futile care.

COMMUNICATION

The first section of this chapter discussed the scope of futile care in the ICU and its associated financial and economic burden.[35] It also referenced the causes of the problem with physicians, patients, and their families.[36] This section will look at some of the root causes of the dilemma. Next, the discussion will examine physicians' and healthcare workers' communication problems with these discussions and possible solutions. Finally, defining hope, realistic goals, and the compassionate use of technology will be reviewed.

As a palliative care physician who practiced in a hospital that was also a regional trauma center, I once received a stat consult on a Monday morning regarding a man who had spent the weekend in the Trauma ICU, even though he was brain dead. The family had refused to take him off the ventilator. The staff was concerned that he was taking up a bed they may need later because it was summertime (when most traffic accidents occur). The beds were already full from the weekend. Other consults required my immediate attention, so a palliative care certified nurse went to the ICU to gather more information. I saw her later that morning, and she stated that she had taken care of the problem and that the consult was "canceled." (I do not think it was a legitimate consult in the first place since the patient had already died!) I asked my colleague, a very experienced RN, how she resolved the problem so quickly. She replied that she merely explained to the family that brain-dead meant he was dead and would not wake up.[37] Hearing this, they promptly allowed the team to take him off the ventilator.

This story illustrates how difficult these discussions can be. If someone had merely sat down with the family over the weekend and thoroughly explained the situation, this problem could have been solved quickly.[38] This family did not have unrealistic expectations; they just were not given the correct information to decide. Although much technical data was shared with the poor man's relatives, it was not the information needed.

Defining Realistic Hope

Nobody can predict outcomes in the ICU with 100% accuracy, which means that physicians, patients, and surrogates often have to make decisions based on inadequate, pedantic, and sometimes misleading information. For intensivists, two skills are needed: foreseeing and foretelling. Foreseeing can be defined as assessing the probability that someone will benefit from aggressive and sophisticated treatment in the short run (i.e., ICU mortality) and in the long run (i.e., post-discharge mortality). Foretelling is the ability to communicate that information to facilitate decision-making.[39] Futile care occurs when these two tasks are either delayed or ignored altogether. [40] Therefore, clinicians' challenges are twofold: having the clinical knowledge to make accurate assessments and the communication skills needed to present this highly technical data effectively and sympathetically, which allows for realistic hope.

If it were known that a patient had either a zero percent chance or a one hundred percent chance of recovery, this would be a simple discussion. Resources would be withheld for the former, and the person would be kept comfortable and allowed to die; for the latter, all would be done on that person's behalf, knowing without a doubt that this approach would be successful. However, these conditions rarely occur in real life, and most patients will fall somewhere between being greater than zero and less than one hundred.[41] Dealing with the "in-between" requires hope. To be considered "realistic hope," three components should be present: the desire for something to happen (my loved one will get better), the chance or probability of that happening, and a pathway for that to occur.

For the desire component, the question can be asked, "What are you hoping for?" If the patient was well before whatever acute incident put them in the ICU, the goal might be to get them back to being well again. If the person was sickly before this event, the hope might be that they return to some ability to function less than baseline. If the patient was significantly debilitated at baseline, then the goals need to be realistically explored. Hoping that this last individual becomes well is most likely unrealistic. The second aspect is the probability of success. However, that may not be clear, and the chance for success may not be equal among different cases. A young, healthy patient who becomes desperately ill may have only a slight chance of recovery. Yet, there would be an enormous push to get that person to recover.[42]

In contrast, an individual who is not quite as ill but has a low baseline functionally may have a less likely recovery chance. Finally, is there a pathway for the patient to recover? Many critically ill patients in the ICU have multiple problems, and recovery would mean that most, if not all, of these problems must be resolved. If one vital organ system has failed, and there is no way for it to be managed or recovered, then it should be stated that there is no pathway to recovery.[43] Taking care of all the other problems is futile as there is no discernible path to have the patient become well.

Intensivists do have tools to help them predict ICU outcomes. The APACHE (Acute Physiology and Chronic Health) score is widely used in the ICU. This evaluation examines the patient's illness, age, and related comorbidities. This study and others provide a framework to characterize a patient's illness's severity and are frequently updated to improve accuracy. However, they are not perfect and are only meant to act as a guide.[44]

Other research programs have looked to identify patients admitted to the ICU who are at high risk for a poor prognosis proactively. One study looked at patients that had the following complications: ICU admission after ten or more days in the hospital, patients greater than eighty years old with two life-threatening comorbidities (congestive heart failure, chronic obstructive pulmonary disease, or end-stage renal disease), active stage IV malignancy, a resuscitated cardiac arrest, or an intracranial hemorrhage requiring mechanical ventilation.[45] A similar study looked at patients with global cerebral ischemia after CPR and patients with multi-system organ failure.[46] And finally, a third study looked at patients with terminal dementia.[47] The results of all three of these studies were the same; if one can identify specific conditions associated with a poor prognosis early, one can decrease the ICU length of stay with no effect on the mortality rate. In this subset of patients, switching from aggressive care to comfort measures only reduced the length of stay in the ICU, in some cases, by over 50%; it did not affect overall mortality.

This approach is proactive because decisions were made early rather than the standard practice of waiting and seeing what happens. This practice is successful because specific patients will not benefit from increased time in the ICU and the foretelling; that is, how this information was communicated to their families.

Setting Appropriate Goals

The foretelling component of communication skills in the ICU is perhaps more complicated than foreseeing. Dealing with distraught families is a demanding yet vital component of quality ICU care. Families struggle to make decisions following their loved ones' wishes, but this information is often unavailable. Most patients have not completed an advance directive to designate an appropriate healthcare proxy and list their end-of-life preferences. This problem is acutely real if the onset of the severe illness is sudden. Even if advance directives are present, the information may be unclear.[48] Often, these documents are completed without the patient's requisite conversations with family. Family members are, therefore, faced with the responsibility of making difficult decisions under duress.[49]

To counter this, physicians need to have skills in empathic communication, effective sharing of prognosis, and a decision-making approach based on families' communication styles and preferences.[50] It is essential for healthcare professionals that these are competencies to be learned and not talents that people have when they are born.[51] These skills not only help curb futile ICU care but can also improve family satisfaction and bereavement outcomes.

Previously, it has been discussed that physicians have some tools to help determine patient prognosis the foreseeing. However, physicians often withhold this information, thinking it would prevent families from maintaining hope. Physicians may also fail to admit that the prognosis is poor and take on a passive, wait-and-see attitude.[52] However, as a rule, most surrogates want prognostic information, even if it is lacking or uncertain.[53] Families need time to cognitively understand an ICU patient's complex issues and process them emotionally. Delaying this information is not compassionate or helpful.[54]

How decisions are made is also essential. Most surrogates favor a shared decision-making process. This procedure involves sharing clinical data, asking for the family's decision-making input, and giving recommendations. There is distress at either end of the spectrum. Some physicians take an informative role, giving families data and requiring them to make difficult decisions without the physician's contribution. Other clinicians will provide very little information and make the patient's decisions with little surrogate input, the directive, or the paternalistic approach. The preferred way is to be facilitative, where the physician guides the decision-making, or collaborative, where recommendations are given.[55] These last two positions may be difficult for some physicians as it involves allowing surrogates (who are not intensivists or, most often, not even doctors!) to participate in the decision-making process.

In his book *Vital Conversations*, Dennis Rosen makes this poignant observation:

> *People in the early years of their medical careers have invested an incredible amount of time and energy and pain in their training, and they have been taught that what they've learned in medical school is the only legitimate way to approach health problems. I think that is why some young physicians go through the roof when … patients reject what we have to offer them because it intimates that what Western medicine has to offer is not much.*[56]

Ethically, the concept of patient autonomy dictates a shared decision-making approach. Earlier crucial conversations with families may help to prevent futile ICU care.

Finally, a few more points should be made regarding surrogate decision-makers. Most patients are too ill to make decisions in the ICU; therefore, the team must rely on family members.[57] As stated before, this is very distressing for families, and the validity of these decisions can be questioned.[58] The two approaches used for this are the "best interest" model, which asks what is best for your loved one, and the "substituted judgment" model, which asks what your loved one would tell us to do in this situation if they could. Unfortunately, both these flawed models may not make the decision-making process any easier. A proposed third way is the "substituted interest and best judgment" model that asks, tell us about your loved one.[59] By using this third approach, decisions can be made based on the patient's values. This process is more empathetic and allows the family to discuss what is essential to the patient. It also enables the intensivists to formulate and offer recommendations based on these values.

COMPASSIONATE USE OF TECHNOLOGY

This section will discuss two relatively new technologies concerning futile care. These two procedures are extracorporeal membrane oxygenation, or ECMO, and left ventricular device, or LVAD. Although lifesaving and beneficial to many, both these procedures can lead to markedly prolonged and often futile treatment in the ICU. This technology can also raise ethical questions regarding autonomy and beneficence.

ECMO is used in severe cardiopulmonary failure cases and involves mechanically oxygenating the blood when the lungs can no longer do so, even with full ventilator support. Rarely semi-elective (the patient chooses to have it), this procedure is often utilized in an emergency to save a life. Because of this, the patient usually cannot participate in the decision-making process. Positive outcomes occur if the lungs can improve from their acute injury or a lung transplant can be performed. Ethical issues arise when neither of these possible positive outcomes can occur. The role of surrogates demanding this procedure for their loved ones is controversial, especially when the perceived prognosis is poor.[60] Many physicians will cite beneficence as the reason to proceed with the course, as there is a chance that the patient could come off the ventilator and associated sedation to the point where they can help with decision-making. Autonomy could be utilized further with the patient and not the surrogates on whether to continue. However, because of the high cost of this procedure, institutions need to address affordability and sustainability.[61] This conundrum would involve the bioethical problem of distributive justice.

The FDA approved LVADs and similar devices in 1984 as a bridge to transplantation. These machines were meant to keep a cardiac patient alive until a suitable heart donor was found and lifesaving cardiac transplantation could be performed.[62] More recently, LVADs have been used for "destination therapy," meaning that the patient is not a candidate for a heart transplant. The patients can decide to choose this procedure electively to treat their heart failure. Having an LVAD can improve quality of life, decrease hospitalizations, and prolong life expectancy. However, complications can lead to a prolonged and futile ICU admission called "destination zero." A decision can often be made proactively with the patient or their surrogates to deactivate the LVAD under specific circumstances when certain conditions occur, such as sepsis, bleeding, or severe neurologic complications.[63] This type of discussion is so important that in 2009, the Centers for Medicaid and Medicare

Services directed the involvement of palliative care when patients are considered for LVADs as destination therapy because of the difficulties of maintaining EOL care in this patient subset. Having these conversations is essential in preventing future futile care and removes the patient's surrogate burden.

INSTITUTIONAL MATTERS

This section will look into concerns regarding reimbursement and legal issues. These are bureaucratic and look at ICU care in broad terms. As previously stated, the United States spends enormous amounts of money on healthcare.[64] In the United States, even though the number of hospital beds has decreased over the past decade, the number of ICU beds has increased.[65] Therefore, interventions that target reducing costs in the ICU by decreasing futile care are of great interest.

Reimbursement Concerns

Understanding and evaluating diminishing futile care interventions' impact on ICU costs is essential for hospitals and healthcare systems operating on a tight budget. Although few would argue the value of decreasing futile ICU care ethically,[66] hospitals must ask how these well-meaning interventions will affect their bottom line. This information is vital as healthcare systems decide how to utilize their resources. As demand for ICU beds grows, is it better to spend money to build more beds or look at programs that decrease futile ICU care, freeing up more existing beds?

Length of stay (LOS) in the ICU is one of the most common goals for evaluating methods to decrease futile care.[67] This data is significant for patients, families, clinicians, and healthcare systems, as its effects are substantial. Extended ICU stays are expensive to hospitals, insurance companies, and society and, more notably, are correlated with symptoms of pain, stress, and anxiety for patients and families.[68]

Strategies to decrease LOS can have a substantial financial impact. This fact is significant because the cost of prolonged ICU services may be higher than the compensation but also because prolonged LOS has been associated with other outcomes, including higher rates of hospital-related complications and infections, delirium, and pressure ulcers. In addition to these adverse patient outcomes, they can negatively affect the value-based payments (VBP) reimbursement model, which can also be costly to hospitals. Therefore, reducing the LOS in the ICU could increase overall profits for the hospital and perhaps even providers in programs offered by the Affordable Care Act (ACA). These strategies could include more active roles in ethics, palliative care, and ICU-based hospice environments.[69]

Many studies about hospital and ICU costs use total costs as their endpoint. However, demonstrating reductions in total costs can be misleading since an intervention will not affect all costs equally. While the terminology may differ, three cost categories are generally noted: indirect, direct fixed, and direct variable costs. Indirect costs represent expenses the hospital encounters regardless of patient volume; examples include building maintenance and administrative salaries shared by all hospital sections. Direct fixed costs represent the hospital's costs for having an ICU but are unrelated to patient volume; examples can include staff expenses and equipment such as mechanical ventilators. Finally, direct variable costs can change based on patient volume, types of patients, and treatment decisions; examples include lab work, supplies, and drugs.[70]

It is estimated that direct variable costs are roughly 20% of total ICU costs, with the rest being direct fixed and indirect costs. Therefore, from the hospital's standpoint, open beds have complex economic consequences under the current volume-based fee-for-service (FFS) reimbursement because hospitals must continue to pay direct fixed and indirect costs regardless of whether they are empty. Ultimately, there could be a decrease in direct fixed and indirect costs if the hospital can avoid the expense of adding new ICU beds. However, in the FFS setting, there may be little financial benefit in reducing ICU utilization, even when the care is futile.[71]

However, FFS payment models are under fire, and future payment models, such as those proposed by the ACA, will most likely affect this paradigm. The increase in health insurance coverage, emphasis on quality and cost-effectiveness, and change of reimbursement, including reimbursement models that link pay and performance along with those centered on episodic care, will permanently alter care delivery in hospital ICUs across the country for years to come.[72]

Population demographics can also affect cost analysis for institutions. It has been shown that significantly greater costs are seen with African Americans and Hispanics compared to non-Hispanic Whites. This result is consistent with other studies, and further research is needed to determine whether this is due to patient preferences, disparities in access to medical services, differences in preventative care and provider continuity, or other factors.

It was also found that there was no association between costs and having an advance directive or a discussion of end-of-life care preferences. However, the data does not provide sufficient detail to evaluate the possibility that some patients, despite their illness, could retain the capacity to choose intensive treatment, which would cancel out the use of the living will. Nevertheless, for the subset of patients with a living will, 92% stated a comfort-focused care preference. As documented in living wills, these data suggest that patient preferences correlate poorly with the treatment delivered.[73] As noted in this chapter, ICU communication must be improved.[74]

Finally, strategies to improve LOS can add to the value of an organization because these programs enhance the quality of care provided, reduce the cost of treating patients with life-limiting illnesses, and help the organization meet credentialing requirements such as pain management standards from the Joint Commission.[75] In conclusion, decreasing futile care in the ICU can financially benefit a healthcare system. Diligence is needed to monitor these benefits as healthcare reimbursement and delivery systems emerge and evolve.

Legal Issues

Twenty percent of Americans die during or shortly after an ICU stay, and often, decisions to forgo life-sustaining therapies (DFLSTs) are involved.[76] These choices include do-not-resuscitate orders, withholding or withdrawing mechanical ventilation, or other specific interventions. These decisions also include redirecting care's principal goals from curative to comfort. Studies have shown that most patients dying in the ICU do so after a DFLST.[77] Because deaths are involved, there is concern about whether physicians could be prosecuted, not just sued, as a result. Doctors have stated that they (or their colleagues) gave ineffective treatment because they worried about legal consequences for refusing patient or family demands. This concern was related to patient and family factors and the doctors' level of risk tolerance.[78]

The reality is that between 1990 and 1997, seven doctors were charged with murdering terminally ill patients, although there were only ten indictments in the previous 55 years.[79] A survey of palliative medicine physicians showed that 4% had been formally investigated for hastening a patient's death when that was not their intention. Thirteen involved using opiates for symptom relief, and six for prescribing various medications for comfort associated with removing mechanical ventilation. A colleague initiated the charges against the physicians in one-third of these cases.[80] For example, a palliative care colleague stated that a cardiologist refused to sign the death certificate of a patient actively dying with end-stage heart disease because she gave the patient morphine for her dyspnea; he told her that if he completed the document, he would put "euthanasia" as the cause of death.[81] Although these accusations exist, is there any legal validity?

In the early 1950s, physicians developed cardiopulmonary resuscitation (CPR) techniques and created intensive care units (ICUs) where patients needing ventilation support and cardiac monitoring could be better treated. While these efforts helped some patients to recover and leave the hospital, many others ended up on ventilators indefinitely, creating a new dilemma. At the time, the prevailing understanding in medical ethics was that physicians were obligated to continue this treatment as long as respiration and circulation could be supported. Furthermore, since stopping these treatments would cause death, physicians believed that "pulling the plug" could lead to a charge of criminal homicide.[82]

While some physicians accepted that patients could decline treatment, many still insisted that once treatment had been started, it could not be stopped if doing so would result in a patient's death. One of the early contributions of medical ethicists to the topic was insisting that withholding and withdrawing life-sustaining treatment were morally equal.[83] They argued that the prevailing contrary position that these two acts were not equal could discourage physicians from starting a trial of therapy (which could save some lives) out of concern that they would be locked into continuing the treatment even if it did not achieve the aim that justified trying it in the first place.[84]

Whether ventilator support should be continued even if there was little chance of recovery gained public attention in the summer of 1975 when a dispute over the care of an unconscious 21-year-old woman, Karen Ann Quinlan, appeared on the front page of newspapers nationwide. That April, she had attended a party where she took Valium and alcohol. Her friends took her home, where later she became unconscious and was rushed to the hospital.

Unfortunately, she remained unconscious and was eventually diagnosed with a persistent vegetative state (PVS). Her parents were Catholic, and after consulting with their parish priest four months later, they informed the physicians that they regarded the ventilator as an "extraordinary means" of keeping her alive and wanted it removed.[85] Her physicians, however, were unwilling to do this because they had been informed by the Morris County (NJ) prosecutors that if the patient died (as they expected she would) after the ventilator was removed, they would be prosecuted for criminal homicide. The Quinlans' tragedy became public when they petitioned the court to allow the removal of their daughter's life support. The decision came about a year later when, on March 31, 1976, the New Jersey Supreme Court granted their request, holding that the constitutionally protected "right to privacy," which had been previously only recognized in the context of contraception and abortion, was broad enough to include their request to remove

Karen's life support and allow her to die.[86] However, the New Jersey court imposed a critical condition before the Quinlans' instructions could be honored: that the physicians' diagnosis must be confirmed by a hospital "ethics committee." Hospitals nationwide responded by appointing such committees, which typically consisted of physicians, nurses, a lawyer, a chaplain, and some laypersons drawn from the community. This group was charged with ensuring that decisions to forgo treatment are ethically grounded and follow proper procedures and with helping to resolve disagreements between (or within) the treatment team and the patient's next of kin.[87]

Subsequently, in 1984, two physicians were charged with homicide following the removal of life support. Two doctors accused in the Los Angeles Judicial District filed a writ of prohibition with murder and conspiracy to commit murder.[88] In a preliminary hearing, the magistrate dismissed the complaint. However, on the motion of the people, the Superior Court ordered the magistrate to reinstate the complaint. The patient, Clarence Herbert, underwent surgery to close an ileostomy, and while in the recovery room, he suffered a cardio-respiratory arrest. He was revived by a team of physicians and nurses and placed on life support equipment. Three days later, a team of physicians, including the two charged with homicide, determined that Herbert was in a "deep comatose state from which he was not likely to recover." After the doctors informed the family of the poor prognosis, the family met and wrote a request to remove Herbert from the life-sustaining machines. Accordingly, the two physicians ordered removing the ventilator and other life-sustaining equipment. Two days later, after consultation with the family, the physicians ordered the removal of intravenous tubing, which provided hydration and nourishment.[89] The California Court of Appeals dismissed the complaint against the physicians, holding that removing the life-supporting equipment and intravenous feeding lines, "though intentional and with the knowledge that the patient would die, was not an unlawful failure to perform a legal duty."[90]

The Quinlan and Herbert cases were similar in that surrogates acted on behalf of incapacitated patients. Similar cases sometimes arise after months or even years of treatment when a permanently unconscious patient's family finally gives up hope and asks the physicians to remove life support. For the family (and perhaps the physicians), the problem was not that the patient was near death but rather that the patient, as a person, had "died" long before. The family no longer believed that the continuation of treatment was respecting the patient's wishes or interests.[91] Incompetent persons have the same rights as competent persons concerning the decision to decline potential life-sustaining procedures. Still, there needs to be some discussion regarding who has the authority to make such decisions.

One view is that since the family must live with the decision, the law should provide only general guidelines allowing the family to make the decision. A second view places responsibility upon the physicians alone. A third view involves a shared decision made by the family and physicians. In the Quinlan case, the New Jersey court suggested that a third party, the hospital ethics committee, should participate in the decision to withdraw medical treatment. Utilizing the Quinlan approach, life support equipment could be withdrawn without the threat of civil or criminal liability upon the concurrence of all three parties involved. Regardless of who the courts decide who the lawful decision-maker is when the treatment offers no reasonable hope of recovery from the patient's vegetative state, the treatment is characterized as medically ineffective and, therefore, extraordinary care. Thus, its removal imposes no criminal liability on the physician to continue treatment.[92]

Besides legal concerns regarding the DFLSTs, there have been court cases regarding the patient's comfort after removing life support. Some studies show no correlation between the amount of sedation/analgesia and survival duration after the wean. When medications such as opioids and benzodiazepines are carefully titrated to the patient's comfort, the patient's life will most likely not be shortened.[93] However, although necessary for the patient's comfort, what if these medications do shorten their life?

Physicians often rely on Thomas Aquinas' principle of double effect, which states that it may be permissible to bring about as a foreseeable side effect a harmful event (the patient's death) that would be impermissible to cause intentionally, significantly when the potential benefit (the patient's comfort) outweighs the side effect's harm. It assumes that shortening the dying process to ameliorate terminal suffering is entirely justifiable.[94] PDE will be discussed more thoroughly in the chapter on nonmaleficence. However, clinicians may neither fully appreciate nor accept that the double effect seems to many to be a philosophical "double-talk."

Probably thousands of physicians and millions of Americans believe that citing this or any principle to justify shortening someone's life is improper. Such individuals often instead maintain philosophies that are either *vitalist*, believing that human existence needs to be kept as long as possible, at any cost, and without regard to the quality of life, or *theist*, thinking that it is a mortal sin to play God regarding the manner of one's death.[95]

CONCLUSION

Medical futility in the ICU is very expensive on multiple levels. Economically, it is one of the leading drivers of rapidly rising healthcare costs in the United States. As the "baby boomers" age and medical technology advances, this will become unsustainable financially in the next few decades. There is also a personal toll with this type of care that involves patients, families, physicians, nurses, and the ICU staff.

There are multiple reasons for this type of care being done. From a patient and family standpoint, crucial conversations and advanced care planning are essential. Once considered taboo, these discussions need to occur more frequently, and healthcare providers need to find ways to facilitate this. From a healthcare perspective, more education is required in death and dying communication and ethics. Although once considered "touchy, feely" topics, these must be regarded as essential for our patient's health and the healthcare system.

The third section discussed the importance of effective communication between physicians, patients, and their surrogates. For these conversations to be successful, they should include the elements of foreseeing and foretelling. Foreseeing involves looking at the prognosis based on the patient's illness and evaluating their previous comorbidities. The foretelling entails communicating this information to families to make decisions based on the patient's values.

Two technologically advanced forms of life support, ECMO and LVADs, were explored in light of the potential issues of futility and ethics that they impose. Future research on futility will look at institutional and organizational problems with this bioethical dilemma.

Additionally, the institutional issues regarding financial and legal matters were explored. Although reimbursement may decrease when attempting to decrease futile care and shorten LOS, the institution's cost savings offset this. New payment models such as ACOs and VBPs should encourage healthcare systems to decrease futile ICU care.

Lastly, legal concerns with attempting to decrease futile ICU care were addressed. Although once problematic, DFLST should not be deterred because of worries of legal prosecution. Both the Quinlan case and the Herbert case set clear precedence for the validity of this procedure. The judicial system in the United

States distinctly gives physicians the responsibility of making ethical decisions regarding ICU care appropriateness.

TAKE-HOME POINTS

- Although the intensive care units (ICUs) may only have a small fraction of the beds in an average American hospital, they are responsible for a significant amount of the hospital's budget. It is also where a high percentage of hospital deaths occur.
- Medical futility refers to actions that are unlikely to make the patient well. Terminology, such as inappropriate or potentially inappropriate, is also gaining favor among academicians as it is less judgmental.
- Autonomy allows the patient or their surrogates to make healthcare decisions. Often, the patient is too ill to make decisions, and the family may make choices that conflict with the patient's previous wishes.
- Beneficence is also of concern when providing medically inappropriate care.
- Distributive justice is an ethical concern concerning futile care in the ICU. These beds are a limited resource that needs appropriate use. Improper ICU bed utilization can lead to delays or denial for patients who could benefit from such care.
- Family members often lack the essential information to make end-of-life decisions. These discussions are complicated, and it is usually easier to avoid them.
- Physicians list many reasons for providing futile care. These include the feeling that physicians are trained to treat, often are inexperienced with death and dying, do not want to give up hope, feel death is the enemy, worry about legal consequences, are poor communicators, are compelled to do everything possible, may have an emotional attachment to patients, goes against their personality, may have had personal experiences with dying family members, or believe that their religion demands it.
- While most physicians accept that patients could decline treatment, many still insist that once treatment has been started, it cannot be stopped if doing so would result in a patient's death. This feeling is even though medical ethicists have clarified that withholding and withdrawing life-sustaining treatment were morally equal.
- The decision to forgo life-sustaining treatment should not be deterred because of worries of legal prosecutions, as multiple legal cases in the US have set clear precedence for the validity of this procedure.
- From a healthcare perspective, more education is required in death-and-dying communication skills and healthcare ethics.

NOTES

1 J. Randall Curtis et al., "End-of-Life Care in the Intensive Care Unit: Can We Simultaneously Increase Quality and Reduce Costs?," *American Journal of Respiratory and Critical Care Medicine* 186, no. 7 (October 1, 2012): 587–592, https://doi.org/10.1164/rccm.201206-1020CP.

2 Paul E. Marik, "The Cost of Inappropriate Care at the End of Life," *American Journal of Hospice & Palliative Medicine* 32, no. 7 (November 2015): 703–8, https://doi.org/10.1177/1049909114537399.

3 Cynthia Hsu-Kim et al., "Integrating Palliative Care into Critical Care," *Journal of Intensive Care Medicine (Sage Publications Inc.)* 30, no. 6 (September 2015): 358–364, https://doi.org/10.1177/0885066614523923.

4 Merriam-Webster, *Merriam-Webster's Intermediate Dictionary* (Springfield, MA: Merriam-Webster, 2020).

5 James L. Bernat, "Medical Futility: Definition, Determination, and Disputes in Critical Care," *Neurocritical Care* 2, no. 2 (2005): 198, https://doi.org/10.1385/ncc:2:2:198.

6 Barry R. Masters, "Principles of Biomedical Ethics, Seventh Edition Eds: Tom L. Beauchamp and James F. Childress Oxford University Press, 2013. XVI, 459 Pages, US$66.95, ISBN-13: 978-0-19–992458-5," *Graefe's Archive for Clinical and Experimental Ophthalmology: Incorporating German Journal of Ophthalmology* 252, no. 9 (2014): 1523, https://doi.org/10.1007/s00417-014-2676-5.

7 Tom L. Beauchamp and James F. Childress, *Principles of Biomedical Ethics.*, 7th ed. (Oxford University Press, 2013).

8 Salimah H. Meghani and Pamela S. Hinds, "Policy Brief: The Institute of Medicine Report Dying in America: Improving Quality and Honoring Individual Preferences near the End of Life," *Nursing Outlook* 63, no. 1 (January 1, 2015): 51–59.

9 Thanh N. Huynh et al., "The Frequency and Cost of Treatment Perceived to Be Futile in Critical Care," *JAMA Internal Medicine* 173, no. 20 (November 11, 2013): 1887–1894, https://doi.org/10.1001/jamainternmed.2013.10261.

10 James L. Bernat, "Medical Futility: Definition, Determination, and Disputes in Critical Care," *Neurocritical Care* 2, no. 2 (2005): 198, https://doi.org/10.1385/ncc:2:2:198.

11 Thanh N. Huynh et al., "The Frequency and Cost of Treatment Perceived to Be Futile in Critical Care," *JAMA Internal Medicine* 173, no. 20 (November 11, 2013): 1887–1894, https://doi.org/10.1001/jamainternmed.2013.10261.

12 Thanh N. Huynh et al., "The Opportunity Cost of Futile Treatment in the ICU," *Critical Care Medicine* 42, no. 9 (September 2014): 1977–1982, https://doi.org/10.1097/CCM.0000000000000402.

13 M. Hoffmann et al., "Psychological Symptoms in Relatives of Critically Ill Patients (ICU Families): A Prospective Multicenter Study," *Intensive Care Medicine* 46, no. 5 (May 2020): 1060–1062, https://doi.org/10.1007/s00134-020-05997-5.

14 Azoulay E et al., "Risk of Post-Traumatic Stress Symptoms in Family Members of Intensive Care Unit Patients," *American Journal of Respiratory & Critical Care Medicine* 171, no. 9 (May 2005): 987–994, https://doi.org/10.1164/rccm.200409-1295oc.

15 Trevor M. Bibler, Myrick C. Jr. Shinall, and Devan Stahl, "Responding to Those Who Hope for a Miracle: Practices for Clinical Bioethicists," *American Journal of Bioethics* 18, no. 5 (2018): 40–51.

16 Leili Yekefallah et al., "Nurses' Experiences of Futile Care at Intensive Care Units: A Phenomenological Study," *Global Journal of Health Science* 7, no. 4 (January 14, 2015): 235–242, https://doi.org/10.5539/gjhs.v7n4p235.
17 Ralf J. Jox et al., "Medical Futility at the End of Life: The Perspectives of Intensive Care and Palliative Care Clinicians," *Journal of Medical Ethics* 38, no. 9 (2012): 540.
18 Betty R. Ferrell, "Understanding the Moral Distress of Nurses Witnessing Medically Futile Care," *Oncology Nursing Forum* 33, no. 5 (January 1, 2006): 922–930, https://doi.org/10.1188/06.ONF.922-930.
19 David F. Kelly, Gerard Magill, and H. ten Have, *Contemporary Catholic Health Care Ethics.*, Second edition. (Georgetown University Press, 2013).
20 Cynthia Hsu-Kim et al., "Integrating Palliative Care into Critical Care," *Journal of Intensive Care Medicine (Sage Publications Inc.)* 30, no. 6 (September 2015): 358–364, https://doi.org/10.1177/0885066614523923.
21 Lindy Willmott et al., "Reasons Doctors Provide Futile Treatment at the End of Life: A Qualitative Study," *Journal of Medical Ethics* 42, no. 8 (August 2016): 496.
22 Thanh N. Huynh et al., "The Opportunity Cost of Futile Treatment in the ICU," *Critical Care Medicine* 42, no. 9 (September 2014): 1977–1982, https://doi.org/10.1097/CCM.0000000000000402.
23 Lindy Willmott et al., "Reasons Doctors Provide Futile Treatment at the End of Life: A Qualitative Study," *Journal of Medical Ethics* 42, no. 8 (August 2016): 496.
24 Dale F. Whelehan, Kevin C. Conlon, and Paul F. Ridgway, "Medicine and Heuristics: Cognitive Biases and Medical Decision-Making," *Irish Journal of Medical Science*, May 14, 2020, https://doi.org/10.1007/s11845-020-02235-1.
25 Derek Doyle, *Oxford Textbook of Palliative Medicine.*, third edition (Oxford: Oxford University Press, 2004).
26 Derek Doyle, *Oxford Textbook of Palliative Medicine.*, third edition (Oxford: Oxford University Press, 2004).
27 Dragana Bolcic-Jankovic et al., "Exploring Determinants of Surrogate Decision-Maker Confidence : An Example From the ICU," *Journal of Empirical Research on Human Research Ethics: An International Journal* 9, no. 4 (2014): 76.
28 Erwin J. O. Kompanje, Ruth D. Piers, and Dominique D. Benoit, "Causes and Consequences of Disproportionate Care in Intensive Care Medicine," *Current Opinion in Critical Care* 19, no. 6 (December 2013): 630–635, https://doi.org/10.1097/MCC.0000000000000026.
29 Dale F. Whelehan, Kevin C. Conlon, and Paul F. Ridgway, "Medicine and Heuristics: Cognitive Biases and Medical Decision-Making," *Irish Journal of Medical Science*, May 14, 2020, https://doi.org/10.1007/s11845-020-02235-1.
30 Qian Yang, Jin Long Du, and Feng Shao, "Mortality Rate and Other Clinical Features Observed in Open vs Closed Format Intensive Care Units: A Systematic Review and Meta-Analysis," *Medicine* 98, no. 27 (July 2019): e16261, https://doi.org/10.1097/MD.0000000000016261.
31 J. Randall Curtis and Burt Robert A., "Why Are Critical Care Clinicians So Powerfully Distressed by Family Demands for Futile Care?," *Journal of Critical Care* 18, no. 1 (March 1, 2003): 22–24.
32 J. M. Luce, "Making Decisions about the Forgoing of Life-Sustaining Therapy," *American Journal of Respiratory and Critical Care Medicine* 156, no. 6 (December 1997): 1715–1718.

33 Nicholas A. Christakis and Robert Wood Johnson, "Extent and Determinants of Error in Physicians' Prognoses in Terminally Ill Patients: Prospective Cohort Study," *Western Journal of Medicine* 172, no. 5 (May 2000): 310.

34 Lindy Willmott et al., "Reasons Doctors Provide Futile Treatment at the End of Life: A Qualitative Study," *Journal of Medical Ethics* 42, no. 8 (2016): 496.

35 J. Randall Curtis et al., "End-of-Life Care in the Intensive Care Unit: Can We Simultaneously Increase Quality and Reduce Costs?," *American Journal of Respiratory and Critical Care Medicine* 186, no. 7 (October 1, 2012): 587–592, https://doi.org/10.1164/rccm.201206-1020CP.

36 Lindy Willmott et al., "Reasons Doctors Provide Futile Treatment at the End of Life: A Qualitative Study," *Journal of Medical Ethics* 42, no. 8 (2016): 496. Dale F. Whelehan, Kevin C. Conlon, and Paul F. Ridgway, "Medicine and Heuristics: Cognitive Biases and Medical Decision-Making," *Irish Journal of Medical Science*, May 14, 2020, https://doi.org/10.1007/s11845-020-02235-1. Dragana Bolcic-Jankovic et al., "Exploring Determinants of Surrogate Decision-Maker Confidence : An Example From the ICU," *Journal of Empirical Research on Human Research Ethics: An International Journal* 9, no. 4 (2014): 76.

37 Stephen D Brown, "Is There a Place for CPR and Sustained Physiological Support in Brain-Dead Non-Donors?," *Journal of Medical Ethics* 43, no. 10 (October 2017): 679–683, https://doi.org/10.1136/medethics-2015–103106.

38 Kristen G. Schaefer and Susan D. Block, "Physician Communication with Families in the ICU: Evidence-Based Strategies for Improvement," *Current Opinion in Critical Care* 15, no. 6 (December 2009): 569–577, https://doi.org/10.1097/MCC.0b013e328332f524.

39 Amalie M. Hauge, "One Last Round of Chemo? Insights from Conversations between Oncologists and Lung Cancer Patients about Prognosis and Treatment Decisions," *Social Science & Medicine* 266 (December 1, 2020).

40 Ralf J. Jox et al., "Medical Futility at the End of Life: The Perspectives of Intensive Care and Palliative Care Clinicians," *Journal of Medical Ethics* 38, no. 9 (2012): 540.

41 Bert Musschenga, "Is There a Problem With False Hope?," *The Journal of Medicine and Philosophy* 44, no. 4 (July 29, 2019): 423–441, https://doi.org/10.1093/jmp/jhz010.

42 Carla C. Braxton, Celia N. Robinson, and Samir S. Awad, "Escalation of Commitment in the Surgical ICU," *Critical Care Medicine* 45, no. 4 (April 2017): e433–e436, https://doi.org/10.1097/CCM.0000000000002261.

43 Margaret L. Campbell and Jorge A. Guzman, "Impact of a Proactive Approach to Improve End-of-Life Care in a Medical ICU," *Chest* 123, no. 1 (January 2003): 266–271, https://doi.org/10.1378/chest.123.1.266.

44 Jorge I. F. Salluh and Márcio Soares, "ICU Severity of Illness Scores: APACHE, SAPS and MPM," *Current Opinion in Critical Care* 20, no. 5 (October 2014): 557–565, https://doi.org/10.1097/MCC.0000000000000135.

45 Sally A. Norton et al., "Proactive Palliative Care in the Medical Intensive Care Unit: Effects on Length of Stay for Selected High-Risk Patients," *Critical Care Medicine* 35, no. 6 (June 2007): 1530–1535.

46 Margaret L. Campbell and Jorge A. Guzman, "Impact of a Proactive Approach to Improve End-of-Life Care in a Medical ICU," *Chest* 123, no. 1 (January 2003): 266–271, https://doi.org/10.1378/chest.123.1.266.

47 Margaret L. Campbell and Jorge A. Guzman, "A Proactive Approach to Improve End-of-Life Care in a Medical Intensive Care Unit for Patients with Terminal Dementia:,"

Critical Care Medicine 32, no. 9 (September 2004): 1839–1843, https://doi.org/10.1097/01.CCM.0000138560.56577.88.
48 Alexia M. Torke, G. Caleb Alexander, and John Lantos, "Substituted Judgment: The Limitations of Autonomy in Surrogate Decision Making," *Journal of General Internal Medicine* 23, no. 9 (September 2008): 1514–1517, https://doi.org/10.1007/s11606-008-0688-8.
49 Amy B. Petrinec and Barbara J. Daly, "Post-Traumatic Stress Symptoms in Post-ICU Family Members: Review and Methodological Challenges," *Western Journal of Nursing Research* 38, no. 1 (January 2016): 57–78, https://doi.org/10.1177/0193945914544176.
50 Kristen G. Schaefer and Susan D. Block, "Physician Communication with Families in the ICU: Evidence-Based Strategies for Improvement," *Current Opinion in Critical Care* 15, no. 6 (December 2009): 569–577, https://doi.org/10.1097/MCC.0b013e328332f524.
51 Mark King, Larry Novik, and Charles Citrenbaum, *Irresistible Communication: Creative Skills for the Health Professional* (Philadelphia: Saunders, 1983).
52 Lindy Willmott et al., "Reasons Doctors Provide Futile Treatment at the End of Life: A Qualitative Study," *Journal of Medical Ethics* 42, no. 8 (2016): 496.
53 Kristen G. Schaefer and Susan D. Block, "Physician Communication with Families in the ICU: Evidence-Based Strategies for Improvement," *Current Opinion in Critical Care* 15, no. 6 (December 2009): 569–577, https://doi.org/10.1097/MCC.0b013e328332f524.
54 Kristen G. Schaefer and Susan D. Block, "Physician Communication with Families in the ICU: Evidence-Based Strategies for Improvement," *Current Opinion in Critical Care* 15, no. 6 (December 2009): 569–577, https://doi.org/10.1097/MCC.0b013e328332f524.
55 Douglas B. White et al., "Expanding the Paradigm of the Physician's Role in Surrogate Decision-Making: An Empirically Derived Framework*:," *Critical Care Medicine* 38, no. 3 (March 2010): 743–750, https://doi.org/10.1097/CCM.0b013e3181c58842.
56 Dennis Rosen, Vital Conversations : Improving Communication Between Doctors and Patients. (Columbia University Press, 2014).
57 Cynthia Hsu-Kim et al., "Integrating Palliative Care into Critical Care," *Journal of Intensive Care Medicine (Sage Publications Inc.)* 30, no. 6 (September 2015): 358–364, https://doi.org/10.1177/0885066614523923.
58 Alexia M. Torke, G. Caleb Alexander, and John Lantos, "Substituted Judgment: The Limitations of Autonomy in Surrogate Decision Making," *Journal of General Internal Medicine* 23, no. 9 (September 2008): 1514–1517, https://doi.org/10.1007/s11606-008-0688-8.
59 Daniel P. Sulmasy and Lois Snyder, "Substituted Interests and Best Judgments: An Integrated Model of Surrogate Decision Making," *JAMA* 304, no. 17 (November 3, 2010): 1946, https://doi.org/10.1001/jama.2010.1595.
60 Zachary Obinna Enumah, Joseph Carrese, and Chun Woo Choi, "The Ethics of Extracorporeal Membrane Oxygenation: Revisiting the Principles of Clinical Bioethics," *The Annals of Thoracic Surgery*, October 2020, S0003497520317379, https://doi.org/10.1016/j.athoracsur.2020.08.045.
61 Kollengode Ramanathan, "Ethical Challenges of Adult ECMO," *Indian Journal of Thoracic and Cardiovascular Surgery*, February 17, 2020, https://doi.org/10.1007/s12055-020-00922-3.
62 Esther S. Pak, Christopher A. Jones, and Paul J. Mather, "Ethical Challenges in Care of Patients on Mechanical Circulatory Support at End-of-Life," *Current Heart Failure Reports* 17, no. 4 (August 2020): 153–160, https://doi.org/10.1007/s11897-020-00460-4.

63 Anna Joong et al., "Providing Compassionate End of Life Care in the Setting of Mechanical Circulatory Support," *Current Pediatrics Reports* 7, no. 4 (December 2019): 168–175, https://doi.org/10.1007/s40124-019-00206-4.

64 Thanh N. Huynh et al., "The Frequency and Cost of Treatment Perceived to Be Futile in Critical Care," *JAMA Internal Medicine* 173, no. 20 (November 11, 2013): 1887–1894, https://doi.org/10.1001/jamainternmed.2013.10261.

65 Nita Khandelwal et al., "Evaluating the Economic Impact of Palliative and End-of-Life Care Interventions on Intensive Care Unit Utilization and Costs from the Hospital and Healthcare System Perspective," *Journal of Palliative Medicine* 20, no. 12 (December 2017): 1314–1320, https://doi.org/10.1089/jpm.2016.0548.

66 Dereddi Raja S. Reddy, John C. O'Horo, and Sumedh S. Hoskote, "Judgment of Futile Care in the ICU," *Critical Care Medicine* 43, no. 5 (May 2015): e151.

67 Dereddi Raja S. Reddy, John C. O'Horo, and Sumedh S. Hoskote, "Judgment of Futile Care in the ICU," *Critical Care Medicine* 43, no. 5 (May 2015): e151.

68 Nita Khandelwal et al., "Evaluating the Economic Impact of Palliative and End-of-Life Care Interventions on Intensive Care Unit Utilization and Costs from the Hospital and Healthcare System Perspective," *Journal of Palliative Medicine* 20, no. 12 (December 2017): 1314–1320, https://doi.org/10.1089/jpm.2016.0548.

69 Anjali P. Dogra and Todd Dorman, "Critical Care Implications of the Affordable Care Act:," *Critical Care Medicine* 44, no. 3 (March 2016): e168–e173, https://doi.org/10.1097/CCM.0000000000001431.

70 Hannah Wunsch, Hayley Gershengorn, and Damon C. Scales, "Economics of ICU Organization and Management," *Critical Care Clinics* 28, no. 1 (January 2012): 25–37, https://doi.org/10.1016/j.ccc.2011.09.004.

71 Nita Khandelwal et al., "Evaluating the Economic Impact of Palliative and End-of-Life Care Interventions on Intensive Care Unit Utilization and Costs from the Hospital and Healthcare System Perspective," *Journal of Palliative Medicine* 20, no. 12 (December 2017): 1314–1320, https://doi.org/10.1089/jpm.2016.0548.

72 Anjali P. Dogra and Todd Dorman, "Critical Care Implications of the Affordable Care Act:," *Critical Care Medicine* 44, no. 3 (March 2016): e168–e173, https://doi.org/10.1097/CCM.0000000000001431.

73 Amy S. Kelley et al., "Determinants of Medical Expenditures in the Last 6 Months of Life," *Annals of Internal Medicine* 154, no. 4 (February 15, 2011): 235, https://doi.org/10.7326/0003–4819-154-4–201102150-00004.

74 David Crippen, End-of-Life Communication in the ICU : A Global Perspective (New York: Springer, 2008).

75 Kenneth R. White et al., "Nonclinical Outcomes of Hospital-Based Palliative Care," *Journal of Healthcare Management* 51, no. 4 (August 2006): 260–273; discussion 273–274. Caroline M. Quill et al., "Variation in Decisions to Forgo Life-Sustaining Therapies in US ICUs," *Chest* 146, no. 3 (September 2014): 573–582, https://doi.org/10.1378/chest.13–2529. Alexander Capron, "Looking Back at Withdrawal of Life-Support Law and Policy to See What Lies Ahead for Medical Aid-in-Dying," *Yale Journal of Biological Medicine* 92.4 (December 20, 2019): 781–791.

76 J. Randall Curtis et al., "End-of-Life Care in the Intensive Care Unit: Can We Simultaneously Increase Quality and Reduce Costs?," *American Journal of Respiratory and*

Critical Care Medicine 186, no. 7 (October 1, 2012): 587–592, https://doi.org/10.1164/rccm.201206-1020CP.

77 Caroline M. Quill et al., "Variation in Decisions to Forgo Life-Sustaining Therapies in US ICUs," *Chest* 146, no. 3 (September 2014): 573–582, https://doi.org/10.1378/chest.13–2529.

78 Lindy Willmott et al., "Reasons Doctors Provide Futile Treatment at the End of Life: A Qualitative Study," *Journal of Medical Ethics* 42, no. 8 (2016): 496.

79 Lewis Cohen et al., "Accusations of Murder and Euthanasia in End-of-Life Care," *Journal of Palliative Medicine* 8, no. 6 (December 2005): 1096–1104, https://doi.org/10.1089/jpm.2005.8.1096.

80 Lewis Cohen et al., "Accusations of Murder and Euthanasia in End-of-Life Care," *Journal of Palliative Medicine* 8, no. 6 (December 2005): 1096–1104, https://doi.org/10.1089/jpm.2005.8.1096.

81 Janice Knebl, personal communication.

82 Alexander Capron, "Looking Back at Withdrawal of Life-Support Law and Policy to See What Lies Ahead for Medical Aid-in-Dying," *Yale Journal of Biological Medicine* 92.4 (December 20, 2019): 781–791.

83 Tom L. Beauchamp and James F. Childress, *Principles of Biomedical Ethics.*, 7th ed. (Oxford University Press, 2013).

84 Alexander Capron, "Looking Back at Withdrawal of Life-Support Law and Policy to See What Lies Ahead for Medical Aid-in-Dying," *Yale Journal of Biological Medicine* 92.4 (December 20, 2019): 781–791.

85 David F. Kelly, Gerard Magill, and H. ten Have, *Contemporary Catholic Health Care Ethics.*, Second edition. (Georgetown University Press, 2013).

86 Jeremy Sugarman and Daniel P. Sulmasy, eds., *Methods in Medical Ethics*, 2nd ed (Washington, D.C: Georgetown University Press, 2010).

87 Alexander Capron, "Looking Back at Withdrawal of Life-Support Law and Policy to See What Lies Ahead for Medical Aid-in-Dying," *Yale Journal of Biological Medicine* 92.4 (December 20, 2019): 781–791.

88 Ronald Crook, "Criminal Law—Homicide—Removal of Intravenous Feeding Line from Vegetative, Comatose Patient at Family's Request Is Not Murder," *Cumberland Law Review 15*, 1984, 225–238.

89 John R. Connery, 'The Clarence Herbert Case: Was Withdrawal of Treatment Justified?" In *Artificial Nutrition and Hydration and the Permanently Unconscious Patient: The Catholic Debate*, edited by Ronald P. Hamel and James J. Walter (Washington, DC: Georgetown University Press, 2007), 257–264.

90 Ronald Crook, "Criminal Law—Homicide—Removal of Intravenous Feeding Line from Vegetative, Comatose Patient at Family's Request Is Not Murder," *Cumberland Law Review 15*, 1984, 225–238.

91 Alexander Capron, "Looking Back at Withdrawal of Life-Support Law and Policy to See What Lies Ahead for Medical Aid-in-Dying," *Yale Journal of Biological Medicine* 92.4 (December 20, 2019): 781–791.

92 Ronald Crook, "Criminal Law—Homicide—Removal of Intravenous Feeding Line from Vegetative, Comatose Patient at Family's Request Is Not Murder," *Cumberland Law Review 15*, 1984, 225–238.

93 M. L. Campbell, K. S. Bizek, and M. Thill, "Patient Responses during Rapid Terminal Weaning from Mechanical Ventilation: A Prospective Study," *Critical Care Medicine* 27, no. 1 (January 1999): 73–77.

94 Amy S. Kelley et al., "Determinants of Medical Expenditures in the Last 6 Months of Life," *Annals of Internal Medicine* 154, no. 4 (February 15, 2011): 235, https://doi.org/10.7326/0003-4819-154-4-201102150-00004.

95 Lewis M. Cohen, "Murder and Euthanasia Accusations Against Physicians," *Mayo Clinic Proceedings* 87, no. 9 (September 2012): 814–816, https://doi.org/10.1016/j.mayocp.2012.05.016.

BIBLIOGRAPHY

Azoulay, E., et al. "Risk of Post-Traumatic Stress Symptoms in Family Members of Intensive Care Unit Patients." *American Journal of Respiratory & Critical Care Medicine* 171, no. 9 (May 2005): 987–994. https://doi.org/10.1164/rccm.200409-1295oc.

Beauchamp, Tom L., and James F. Childress. *Principles of Biomedical Ethics.* 7th ed. Oxford University Press, 2013.

Bernat, James L. "Medical Futility: Definition, Determination, and Disputes in Critical Care." *Neurocritical Care* 2, no. 2 (2005): 198. https://doi.org/10.1385/ncc:2:2:198.

Bibler, Trevor M., Myrick C. Jr. Shinall, and Devan Stahl. "Responding to Those Who Hope for a Miracle: Practices for Clinical Bioethicists." *American Journal of Bioethics* 18, no. 5 (2018): 40–51.

Bolcic-Jankovic, Dragana, Clarridge Brian R., LeBlanc Jessica L., Mahmood Rumel S., Roman Anthony M., and Freeman Bradley D. "Exploring Determinants of Surrogate Decision-Maker Confidence : An Example From the ICU." *Journal of Empirical Research on Human Research Ethics: An International Journal* 9, no. 4 (2014): 76.

Braxton, Carla C., Celia N. Robinson, and Samir S. Awad. "Escalation of Commitment in the Surgical ICU." *Critical Care Medicine* 45, no. 4 (April 2017): e433–e436. https://doi.org/10.1097/CCM.0000000000002261.

Brown, Stephen D. "Is There a Place for CPR and Sustained Physiological Support in Brain-Dead Non-Donors?" *Journal of Medical Ethics* 43, no. 10 (October 2017): 679–683. https://doi.org/10.1136/medethics-2015-103106.

Campbell, M L, K S Bizek, and M Thill. "Patient Responses during Rapid Terminal Weaning from Mechanical Ventilation: A Prospective Study." *Critical Care Medicine* 27, no. 1 (January 1999): 73–77.

Campbell, Margaret L., and Jorge A. Guzman. "A Proactive Approach to Improve End-of-Life Care in a Medical Intensive Care Unit for Patients with Terminal Dementia:" *Critical Care Medicine* 32, no. 9 (September 2004): 1839–1843. https://doi.org/10.1097/01.CCM.0000138560.56577.88.

Campbell, Margaret L., and Jorge A. Guzman. "Impact of a Proactive Approach to Improve End-of-Life Care in a Medical ICU." *Chest* 123, no. 1 (January 2003): 266–271. https://doi.org/10.1378/chest.123.1.266.

Capron, Alexander. "Looking Back at Withdrawal of Life-Support Law and Policy to See What Lies Ahead for Medical Aid-in-Dying." *Yale J Biol Med.* 92.4 (December 20, 2019): 781–791.

Christakis, Nicholas A., and Robert Wood Johnson. "Extent and Determinants of Error in Physicians' Prognoses in Terminally Ill Patients: Prospective Cohort Study." *Western Journal of Medicine* 172, no. 5 (May 2000): 310.

Cohen, Lewis, Linda Ganzini, Christine Mitchell, Stephen Arons, Elizabeth Goy, and James Cleary. "Accusations of Murder and Euthanasia in End-of-Life Care." *Journal of Palliative Medicine* 8, no. 6 (December 2005): 1096–1104. https://doi.org/10.1089/jpm.2005.8.1096.

Cohen, Lewis M. "Murder and Euthanasia Accusations Against Physicians." *Mayo Clinic Proceedings* 87, no. 9 (September 2012): 814–816. https://doi.org/10.1016/j.mayocp.2012.05.016.

Connery, John R. 'The Clarence Herbert Case: Was Withdrawal of Treatment Justified?" In *Artificial Nutrition and Hydration and the Permanently Unconscious Patient: The Catholic Debate*, Edited by Hamel Ronald P. and Walter James J., 257–264. Washington, DC: Georgetown University Press, 2007.

Crippen, David. *End-of-Life Communication in the ICU : A Global Perspective.* New York: Springer, 2008.

Crook, Ronald. "Criminal Law—Homicide—Removal of Intravenous Feeding Line from Vegetative, Comatose Patient at Family's Request Is Not Murder." *Cumberland Law Review 15*, 1984, 225–238.

Curtis, J. Randall, and Robert A. Burt. "Why Are Critical Care Clinicians So Powerfully Distressed by Family Demands for Futile Care?" *Journal of Critical Care* 18, no. 1 (March 1, 2003): 22–24.

Curtis, J. Randall, Ruth A. Engelberg, Mark E. Bensink, and Scott D. Ramsey. "End-of-Life Care in the Intensive Care Unit: Can We Simultaneously Increase Quality and Reduce Costs?" *American Journal of Respiratory and Critical Care Medicine* 186, no. 7 (October 1, 2012): 587–592. https://doi.org/10.1164/rccm.201206-1020CP.

Dogra, Anjali P., and Todd Dorman. "Critical Care Implications of the Affordable Care Act:" *Critical Care Medicine* 44, no. 3 (March 2016): e168–e173. https://doi.org/10.1097/CCM.0000000000001431.

Doyle, Derek. *Oxford Textbook of Palliative Medicine.* 3rd edition. Oxford: Oxford University Press, 2004.

Enumah, Zachary Obinna, Joseph Carrese, and Chun Woo Choi. "The Ethics of Extracorporeal Membrane Oxygenation: Revisiting the Principles of Clinical Bioethics." *The Annals of Thoracic Surgery*, October 2020, S0003497520317379. https://doi.org/10.1016/j.athoracsur.2020.08.045.

Ferrell, Betty R. "Understanding the Moral Distress of Nurses Witnessing Medically Futile Care." *Oncology Nursing Forum* 33, no. 5 (January 1, 2006): 922–930. https://doi.org/10.1188/06.ONF.922-930.

Hauge, Amalie M. "One Last Round of Chemo? Insights from Conversations between Oncologists and Lung Cancer Patients about Prognosis and Treatment Decisions." *Social Science & Medicine* 266 (December 1, 2020).

Hoffmann, M., M.-M. Jeitziner, R. Riedl, P. Eller, K. Amrein, ICU-Families Study Group, J. C. Schefold, et al. "Psychological Symptoms in Relatives of Critically Ill Patients (ICU Families): A Prospective Multicenter Study." *Intensive Care Medicine* 46, no. 5 (May 2020): 1060–1062. https://doi.org/10.1007/s00134-020-05997-5.

Hsu-Kim, Cynthia, Tara Friedman, Edward Gracely, and James Gasperino. "Integrating Palliative Care into Critical Care." *Journal of Intensive Care Medicine (Sage Publications Inc.)* 30, no. 6 (September 2015): 358–364. https://doi.org/10.1177/0885066614523923.

Huynh, Thanh N., Eric C. Kleerup, Prince P. Raj, and Neil S. Wenger. "The Opportunity Cost of Futile Treatment in the ICU." *Critical Care Medicine* 42, no. 9 (September 2014): 1977–1982. https://doi.org/10.1097/CCM.0000000000000402.

Huynh, Thanh N., Kleerup Eric C., Wiley Joshua F., Savitsky Terrance D., Guse Diana, Garber Bryan J., and Wenger Neil S. "The Frequency and Cost of Treatment Perceived to Be Futile in Critical Care." *JAMA Internal Medicine* 173, no. 20 (November 11, 2013): 1887–1894. https://doi.org/10.1001/jamainternmed.2013.10261.

Jox, Ralf J., Andreas Schaider, Georg Marckmann, and Gian Domenico Borasio. "Medical Futility at the End of Life: The Perspectives of Intensive Care and Palliative Care Clinicians." *Journal of Medical Ethics* 38, no. 9 (2012): 540.

Joong, Anna, Sabrina F. Derrington, Angira Patel, Philip T. Thrush, Kiona Y. Allen, and Bradley S. Marino. "Providing Compassionate End of Life Care in the Setting of Mechanical Circulatory Support." *Current Pediatrics Reports* 7, no. 4 (December 2019): 168–175. https://doi.org/10.1007/s40124-019-00206-4.

Kelley, Amy S., Susan L. Ettner, R. Sean Morrison, Qingling Du, Neil S. Wenger, and Catherine A. Sarkisian. "Determinants of Medical Expenditures in the Last 6 Months of Life." *Annals of Internal Medicine* 154, no. 4 (February 15, 2011): 235. https://doi.org/10.7326/0003-4819-154-4-201102150-00004.

Kelly, David F., Gerard Magill, and H. ten Have. *Contemporary Catholic Health Care Ethics*. Second edition. Georgetown University Press, 2013.

Khandelwal, Nita, Lyndia C. Brumback, Scott D. Halpern, Norma B. Coe, Babette Brumback, and J. Randall Curtis. "Evaluating the Economic Impact of Palliative and End-of-Life Care Interventions on Intensive Care Unit Utilization and Costs from the Hospital and Healthcare System Perspective." *Journal of Palliative Medicine* 20, no. 12 (December 2017): 1314–1320. https://doi.org/10.1089/jpm.2016.0548.

King, Mark, Larry Novik, and Charles Citrenbaum. *Irresistible Communication: Creative Skills for the Health Professional*. Philadelphia: Saunders, 1983.

Kompanje, Erwin J. O., Ruth D. Piers, and Dominique D. Benoit. "Causes and Consequences of Disproportionate Care in Intensive Care Medicine." *Current Opinion in Critical Care* 19, no. 6 (December 2013): 630–635. https://doi.org/10.1097/MCC.0000000000000026.

Luce, J. M. "Making Decisions about the Forgoing of Life-Sustaining Therapy." *American Journal of Respiratory and Critical Care Medicine* 156, no. 6 (December 1997): 1715–1718.

Marik, Paul E. "The Cost of Inappropriate Care at the End of Life." *American Journal of Hospice & Palliative Medicine* 32, no. 7 (November 2015): 703–708. https://doi.org/10.1177/1049909114537399.

Masters, Barry R. "Principles of Biomedical Ethics, Seventh Edition Eds: Tom L. Beauchamp and James F. Childress Oxford University Press, 2013. XVI, 459 Pages, US$66.95, ISBN-13: 978-0-19–992458-5." *Graefe's Archive for Clinical and Experimental Ophthalmology: Incorporating German Journal of Ophthalmology* 252, no. 9 (2014): 1523. https://doi.org/10.1007/s00417-014-2676-5.

Meghani, Salimah H., and Pamela S. Hinds. "Policy Brief: The Institute of Medicine Report Dying in America: Improving Quality and Honoring Individual Preferences near the End of Life." *Nursing Outlook* 63, no. 1 (January 1, 2015): 51–59.

Merriam-Webster. *Merriam-Webster's Intermediate Dictionary*. Springfield, MA: Merriam-Webster, 2020.

Musschenga, Bert. "Is There a Problem With False Hope?" *The Journal of Medicine and Philosophy* 44, no. 4 (July 29, 2019): 423–441. https://doi.org/10.1093/jmp/jhz010.

Norton, Sally A, Laura A Hogan, Robert G Holloway, Helena Temkin-Greener, Marcia J Buckley, and Timothy E Quill. "Proactive Palliative Care in the Medical Intensive Care Unit: Effects on Length of Stay for Selected High-Risk Patients." *Critical Care Medicine* 35, no. 6 (June 2007): 1530–1535.

Pak, Esther S., Christopher A. Jones, and Paul J. Mather. "Ethical Challenges in Care of Patients on Mechanical Circulatory Support at End-of-Life." *Current Heart Failure Reports* 17, no. 4 (August 2020): 153–160. https://doi.org/10.1007/s11897-020-00460-4.

Petrinec, Amy B., and Barbara J. Daly. "Post-Traumatic Stress Symptoms in Post-ICU Family Members: Review and Methodological Challenges." *Western Journal of Nursing Research* 38, no. 1 (January 2016): 57–78. https://doi.org/10.1177/0193945914544176.

Quill, Caroline M., Sarah J. Ratcliffe, Michael O. Harhay, and Scott D. Halpern. "Variation in Decisions to Forgo Life-Sustaining Therapies in US ICUs." *Chest* 146, no. 3 (September 2014): 573–582. https://doi.org/10.1378/chest.13-2529.

Ramanathan, Kollengode. "Ethical Challenges of Adult ECMO." *Indian Journal of Thoracic and Cardiovascular Surgery*, February 17, 2020. https://doi.org/10.1007/s12055-020-00922-3.

Reddy, Dereddi Raja S., John C. O'Horo, and Sumedh S. Hoskote. "Judgment of Futile Care in the ICU." *Critical Care Medicine* 43, no. 5 (May 2015): e151.

Rosen, Dennis. *Vital Conversations : Improving Communication Between Doctors and Patients*. Columbia University Press, 2014.

Salluh, Jorge I.F., and Márcio Soares. "ICU Severity of Illness Scores: APACHE, SAPS and MPM." *Current Opinion in Critical Care* 20, no. 5 (October 2014): 557–565. https://doi.org/10.1097/MCC.0000000000000135.

Schaefer, Kristen G, and Susan D Block. "Physician Communication with Families in the ICU: Evidence-Based Strategies for Improvement." *Current Opinion in Critical Care* 15, no. 6 (December 2009): 569–577. https://doi.org/10.1097/MCC.0b013e328332f524.

Sugarman, Jeremy, and Daniel P. Sulmasy, eds. *Methods in Medical Ethics*. 2nd ed. Washington, D.C: Georgetown University Press, 2010.

Sulmasy, Daniel P., and Lois Snyder. "Substituted Interests and Best Judgments: An Integrated Model of Surrogate Decision Making." *JAMA* 304, no. 17 (November 3, 2010): 1946. https://doi.org/10.1001/jama.2010.1595.

Torke, Alexia M, G Caleb Alexander, and John Lantos. "Substituted Judgment: The Limitations of Autonomy in Surrogate Decision Making." *Journal of General Internal Medicine* 23, no. 9 (September 2008): 1514–1517. https://doi.org/10.1007/s11606-008-0688-8.

Whelehan, Dale F, Kevin C Conlon, and Paul F Ridgway. "Medicine and Heuristics: Cognitive Biases and Medical Decision-Making." *Irish Journal of Medical Science*, May 14, 2020. https://doi.org/10.1007/s11845-020-02235-1.

White, Douglas B., Grace Malvar, Jennifer Karr, Bernard Lo, and J. Randall Curtis. "Expanding the Paradigm of the Physician's Role in Surrogate Decision-Making: An Empirically Derived Framework." *Critical Care Medicine* 38, no. 3 (March 2010): 743–750. https://doi.org/10.1097/CCM.0b013e3181c58842.

White, Kenneth R., Kristie G. Stover, J. Brian Cassel, and Thomas J. Smith. "Nonclinical Outcomes of Hospital-Based Palliative Care." *Journal of Healthcare Management / American College of Healthcare Executives* 51, no. 4 (August 2006): 260–273; discussion 273–274.

Willmott, Lindy, Benjamin White, Cindy Gallois, Malcolm Parker, Nicholas Graves, Sarah Winch, Leonie Kaye Callaway, Nicole Shepherd, and Eliana Close. "Reasons Doctors Provide Futile Treatment at the End of Life: A Qualitative Study." *Journal of Medical Ethics* 42, no. 8 (2016): 496.

Wunsch, Hannah, Hayley Gershengorn, and Damon C. Scales. "Economics of ICU Organization and Management." *Critical Care Clinics* 28, no. 1 (January 2012): 25–37. https://doi.org/10.1016/j.ccc.2011.09.004.

Yang, Qian, Jin Long Du, and Feng Shao. "Mortality Rate and Other Clinical Features Observed in Open vs Closed Format Intensive Care Units: A Systematic Review and Meta-Analysis." *Medicine* 98, no. 27 (July 2019): e16261. https://doi.org/10.1097/MD.0000000000016261.

Yekefallah, Leili, Tahereh Ashktorab, Houman Manoochehri, and Alavi Majd Hamid. "Nurses' Experiences of Futile Care at Intensive Care Units: A Phenomenological Study." *Global Journal of Health Science* 7, no. 4 (January 14, 2015): 235–242. https://doi.org/10.5539/gjhs.v7n4p235.

Chapter 7

A Patient-Centered Palliative Approach to End-of-life Care

INTRODUCTION

This chapter will explore and expand upon some of the themes already discussed. Albert Einstein, the father of modern physics, has lamented, "It has become appallingly obvious that our technology has exceeded our humanity!"[1] The premise is that technology does an abysmal job of dealing with end-of-life care. Physicians and other healthcare workers are inundated by the science involved in the medical profession. These innovations have been instrumental in treating patients using a disease-centered model.[2] However, technology does poorly in the patient-centered model, especially with end-of-life care. Too often, the focus on science and technology leads to medically ineffective care, significant expenses, and increased suffering.[3] Unfortunately, this has only worsened in the United States over time.[4] However, Palliative care may provide some answers, and this chapter will explore that theme.

It was not always like this; years ago, care for the dying had its roots in the religious community. In the middle of the last century, Dame Cicely Saunders and others looked to make this type of care part of the medical mainstream.[5] Dr. Saunders added aggressive and competent symptom control to this type of care. She also looked beyond physical symptoms with her concept of "total pain." Some spiritual components were perhaps lost, but the emphasis was still on patient-focused care.[6]

Unfortunately, beginning in the last century and extending into this century, the emphasis is now on disease-centered care. This approach is helpful in some circumstances, especially with curable and reversible illnesses;[7] however, it has shown to be, at best, inadequate when it comes to the care of the dying. At worst, it can increase suffering and cost and lead to poorer outcomes. When

DOI: 10.4324/9781003654124-8

the emphasis is on the disease and not the patient, there is more treatment and suffering with little change in the result.[8]

Some clinicians are also reluctant to eliminate patients' suffering for fear of causing early death. This hesitation could include the removal of life-sustaining therapies when they are no longer beneficial.[9] It also could mean palliative sedation and aggressive pain management.[10] Although these two therapies have not been shown to diminish life expectancy, many in the field still believe that the only technology is appropriate when patients are very ill despite suffering.[11]

Modern medicine has made great strides over the last several decades concerning support for failing organs. Besides organ transplantation, machines support people if their hearts, lungs, and kidneys have failed. However, if the native organs do not improve, then a decision must be made to continue these therapies. Even though most patients would choose not to remain on machines to sustain their lives, removing these treatments becomes problematic, especially as these therapies evolve. Many clinicians are troubled by the thought of removing these devices, as they will most certainly cause the death of the person. Although most clinicians would say that quality of life is essential, having these discussions with patients and families is challenging. When these talks occur, it is often very late in the disease process, if they occur at all.[12]

Palliative care is the medical specialty that looks to help with some of these dilemmas. It does this by putting the emphasis back on the patient and their family. As technologies fail to provide the intended results, the focus is on controlling the patient's symptoms and suffering.[13] Communication with the patient and their families is also stressed. These can help with the difficult decisions that need to be made. By emphasizing the patient, palliative care tries to deal with end-of-life care in the matter Cecily Saunders once endeavored. Palliative care fills the gap that technology cannot provide.

PATIENT-CENTERED VS. DISEASE-CENTERED CARE

Eric Cassell writes:

> *To manage the physical symptoms that lead to suffering, doctors must not only "think pathophysiology" and "think body," they must "think person" as well. This will allow them to track the symptom from its origin in the disease to its association with the characteristics of the sick person that causes suffering. When they do this, they will find that modern medicine has provided them*

> *with effective tools to intervene in almost any symptom at virtually any stage in its development.*[14]

Nevertheless, one of the debates in our healthcare system is whether we should focus on treating diseases or patients. A patient-centered focus "Is *about* the patients, *with* the patients, and *for* the patients, to ensure current and future doctors remain sensitive to all of the needs of the people they care for."[15]

Unfortunately, many organizations have failed to understand that patient-centeredness is the overarching aim that encompasses the rest. The *raison d'etre* for healthcare and healthcare systems is to better the health and well-being of individuals and populations. This paradigm requires the patient to partner with and co-design all improvement activities, a concept many leaders and clinicians still find threatening or unnecessary. In addition to co-designing care, attaining a patient-centered healthcare system requires an organizational focus on leadership values and human resources policies that recruit and retain staff with aptitudes for service and empathy. These same foundational strategies create high-performing organizations that are safe, excellent workplaces, and financially strong.[16] This focus is essential for end-of-life care, where the patient's and their family's goals may differ from a disease-centered model.

CLINICAL SETTINGS

Disease-centered approaches are appropriate when individuals have a single predominant disease, and everyone with the illness desires the same outcome, such as prolonged survival or cure. However, this disease-centered framework is ill-suited for persons with multiple chronic conditions, including most older adults with cardiovascular diseases and most adult healthcare users of all ages. Disease-centered decision-making for this population results in treatment burden when patients must adhere to multiple guidelines and harm when guideline recommendations conflict. Furthermore, disease-centered proposals may not address what matters most to these patients who vary in their health priorities.[17] For example, preventing cardiovascular events in the future may have little value to someone with a limited lifespan.

One outcomes-based approach quickly gaining popularity involves an open-ended assessment of patients' valued outcomes. Rather than starting with healthcare decisions, it consists of asking, "What matters most to you?" and having the patient identify the specific goals they would like to achieve. Frequently, individuals respond with statements about taking care of themselves and participating in meaningful activities.

This approach has excellent theoretical appeal. Individuals are encouraged to think broadly about what matters to them—beginning with values and goals rather than treatment options can improve decision-making by not prespecifying these options.[18] In practice, patient goal-directed care starts with a skilled clinician eliciting patients' health outcome goals and care preferences. Clinically feasible methods are available to help patients move from general values or unrealistic goals to specific, measurable, achievable, realistic, and time-bound goals that integrate an understanding of prognosis, clinical course, and objective outcomes as essential for use in clinical decision-making.[19]

Therefore, there is a need to develop an approach that meets the particular needs of vulnerable older patients and builds on each approach described above. Centering the approach to identifying and exploring trade-offs will emphasize to patients and physicians that there are options for managing chronic disease and that disease-directed therapy may not match patients' priorities. Understanding patients' goals can help shape an overall care plan. It will move the approach from considering every step in chronic disease management as a separate decision. The critical challenge is reducing the complexity of the many individual choices faced by patients with different chronic diseases, conditions, and symptoms into meaningful categories that can help guide decision-making.[20]

Patient goal-directed care may initially seem overwhelming and time-consuming. However, experience with this approach will stimulate efforts to simplify the process within demanding clinical workflows. Focusing all care on a unified set of individualized patient outcome goals, rather than disparate disease-specific outcomes, should reduce fragmentation among and demands on overwhelmed clinicians while raising patient trust and satisfaction with their healthcare. Patient goal-directed care may benefit persons with multiple chronic conditions for whom many often contradictory and burdensome care options are available.[21] This shift is essential as a focus on more comfort care develops as the person nears death.[22]

While this task is daunting, there are potential ways to move forward. One is to identify "classes" of decisions that share a standard set of trade-offs. Among older persons with multiple chronic conditions, primary or secondary prevention medications have common trade-offs between future reductions in risk and current potential for direct adverse effects, complex medication regimens, and risks of polypharmacy. Understanding how a patient values present vs. future health risks can help to inform an overall approach to preventative medications.[23] For example, it makes no sense for a hospice patient to continue taking cholesterol-lowering medicine no matter their cardiac status! Cardiology uses trial-derived evidence to inform its decisional guidelines. Unfortunately, older adults with multiple co-morbidities have largely been excluded from these evidence-generating trials, leading to therapeutic uncertainty for this large segment of the clinical population. A disease treatment in an otherwise healthy adult may not have the same benefit to a patient who has multiple diseases. Interest in the movement from disease-based to patient goals-directed care will hopefully fuel the generation of evidence linking cardiovascular and other treatments to patient outcome goals.[24]

ONCOLOGY

The *Cambridge Academic Dictionary* defines an oncologist as "a medical practitioner qualified to diagnose and treat tumors."[25] One could argue that a more accurate description would be "a medical practitioner qualified to diagnose and treat *patients* with tumors." As was discussed in a previous section, the emphasis should be on the patient, not the disease. Treating cancer is a technology-based task of matching appropriate medications, treatments, and protocols to findings seen on physical exams, laboratory, and imaging studies. Patients complain, get sick, vomit, cry, lose their jobs, and some even die. Perhaps that is why there is an attraction for some oncologists to focus on the disease and not the patient. However, most oncologists will admit the need for high-quality communication and shared decision-making between themselves and patients concerning the goals of care.[26]

Costs for new cancer medicines are high and, at best, only weakly associated with clinical benefits. The strength of this relationship nevertheless varied across countries. Some new cancer drugs—particularly in the US—may be neither affordable nor clinically beneficial over existing treatments. While all countries can benefit from strategies that more robustly align price with therapeutic benefit in cancer drugs, the US stands out in its emphasis on improving both affordability and value in cancer drug treatment. US payers and patients consistently pay more for recently licensed cancer drugs than in other countries, yet do so without necessarily leading to more significant health benefits. While all countries share the opportunity to improve value-for-money in cancer drug spending, the US may benefit the most from a re-imagined approach to drug pricing. As the US seeks to contain drug costs while improving patient outcomes, other countries may offer lessons on better ensuring affordability and value for money in oncology.[27] The US tends to use these drugs more frequently and may pay almost twice as much as other countries, a double-whammy to the healthcare budget.

Oncologists in one study reported that a patient's desire to undergo chemotherapy is a leading factor in their decision to offer it. However, many physicians believe that older adults with an end-stage disease are less likely to want treatment and more likely to stop it when compared with younger patients. Furthermore, they believe that the following factors explain the decreased desire for treatment among older adults: older patients are more accepting of their cancer diagnosis and its consequences, are more satisfied with the lives they have lived, and prefer to preserve their quality of life rather than experience the adverse effects of aggressive treatments.[28] On the other hand, younger patients are likely to receive aggressive therapy because the potential to extend their lives is more significant.[29] However, what about cancer patients who are not at the extremes of age? This situation is where decision-making becomes problematic.

When oncologists and patients discuss goals of care, patients are more likely to get care consistent with their personal choices and have a better quality of life near death. Best clinical practices include eliciting decision-making preferences and understanding the patient's goals of care. In addition, professional guidelines recommend that goals of care and end-of-life (EOL) discussions begin during periods of relative medical stability, preferably when the patient is initially diagnosed with metastatic cancer. Research has shown that early discussions about goals of care are associated with better quality of life, reduced use of non-beneficial medical care near death, and positive family outcomes after death.[30]

However, other studies have shown that conversations about goals of care often fail to provide patients with sufficient information about prognosis to allow for appropriate decisions. It usually occurs so late in the patient's illness that their effect on care processes is reduced.[31] The increasing use of expensive cancer treatments close to the patient's death is often explained by oncologists' failure to communicate to patients how close to dying they are, implying that patients are usually ill-prepared and over-treated when they die.[32] In one study, a moderate (but not strong) relationship between the goals of care oncologists assumed that patients wanted and the goals of care expressed by patients. That observation indicates a lack of oncologists' understanding of a patient's goals of care, reflecting a lack of high-quality communication and decision-making.[33]

Some oncologists will state that cancer treatment results are often difficult to predict. This type of reasoning is similar to what we discussed with ICU medicine. As stated before, this could include an *anchoring* heuristic, "I once had a patient that was like and did well," or a *bandwagon* where one team member pushes to keep going, especially if that person is the oncologist.[34] With the rapid development of new cancer therapies, prognostic uncertainty has made decision-making more complex for patients and providers. The difficulty of prognostic uncertainty near death, or the lack of a "crystal ball," is not new. However, exceptional responders with advanced cancer who exhibit a "Lazarus effect," or a durable response that extends life and occasionally even cures the underlying illness with complete remission, are increasing. (Exceptional responders are the focus of a new National Cancer Institute Initiative and include patients who respond uniquely to treatments that are not effective for most other patients with the same illness.[35])

Is prognostic uncertainty alone enough to justify chemotherapy when the patient is close to death? Research is notable for elucidating factors that influence oncologists when prescribing chemotherapy near death. In one analysis of 17 in-depth interviews with oncologists who practice in various settings, participants noted dealing with two types of prognostic uncertainty. The first uncertainty was predicting the time of death, and the second was knowing whether chemotherapy would ultimately help. Notably, all seemed to be able to call to mind cases of the rare patient who improved against all odds after late chemotherapy. While physicians may avoid difficult conversations or interactions with patients without realizing it, this research suggests otherwise. Oncologists acknowledged the emotionally draining nature of communication specific to the cessation of chemotherapy or not starting it and a staggering sense of responsibility for life-and-death decisions.[36]

Patient factors influencing oncologists' decisions around prescribing chemotherapy near death were also notable. Some acknowledged chemotherapy might be used as a form of "palliation for emotional symptoms." Others noted it could be used as "a means to preserve hope" for patients' wishes regarding the pursuit of treatment. Also, the patient's ability to weigh trade-offs was an important patient-level factor identified in this and other studies. For example, one oncologist interviewed noted:

> *If there is even a 2% chance of a long-term remission with an immunologic, many patients and families are willing to take those odds, and I worry that more patients are spending their final moments undergoing aggressive therapy in the hospital and clinical setting rather than focusing on the quality of the end of their life at home.*[37]

Modes of prognosticating serve to negotiate treatment decisions and future scenarios. Two elements tightly intertwined in terminal cancer, where decisions on treatment withdrawal often coincide with the transition to palliative care for many patients, signifying imminent death. The analysis shows how oncologists employ four situated modes of prognosticating, which mediate the prognostic uncertainty in interaction with the patient. They *hint* (i.e., provide clues that the patient can unpack or not); they *inform* (i.e., offer relatively detailed information to patients open to hearing this); they *calibrate* (i.e., work to adjust or transform a patient's current expectations); or they *organize* (i.e., make arrangements about the patient's remaining life, including referrals to specialized, palliative care).[38]

Ultimately, the oncologist makes a palliative care referral after discussing it with the patient and their family.[39] Sometimes, this referral is made early in the disease course, but often it is made very late. The oncologist's view of EOL care is a significant determining factor. A qualitative study of 18 academic oncologists reported that they varied in their approaches to EOL care. In an accompanying editorial, von Gunten expanded on this concept and labeled the oncologists as either type I or II. Type I oncologists "viewed their role as encompassing both biomedical and psychosocial aspects of cancer care [and] reported a straightforward method of communication about end-of-life care and an ability to influence patient and family coping with death positively … In contrast, type II oncologists described a biomedical role primarily. They reported a more distant relationship with the patient, a sense of failure at being unable to change disease progression, and an absence of collegial support …"[40]

Other American oncologists perceived palliative care referral as a loss of control and interference in the care process.[41] Data from one review suggested that oncologists felt that the beliefs and expectations of patients and families hindered palliative care referral. Unrealistic expectations of cure, unwillingness to discuss prognosis, and non-curative and reluctance to discuss palliative care referral were certain attitudes that hindered palliative care referral.[42] As a result, patients with hematological cancer are referred to palliative care services less often than those with solid tumors despite higher inpatient mortality and a shorter interval between the first consultation and death. The complexity of individual prognostication, ongoing therapeutic goals of cure, the technical nature and complications of treatment, the intensity of medical care even when approaching the end of life, and the speed of change to a terminal event all pose difficulties and hinder referral.[43] Oncologists also have to deal with label avoidance stigma or choose not to pursue a management line due to the stigma associated with the language used concerning the illness or treatment.

French oncologists believe that the term palliative care has the potential to induce fear, and American lung cancer specialists believe that patients and their families get alarmed when mentioning palliative care.[44] Nevertheless, many oncologists recognize the benefits of palliative care. Pain and symptom management and psychosocial support are the well-known benefits of palliative care referral. In many studies, oncologists and hematologists subscribe to the notable benefits of palliative care referral.[45] However, only a few studies elucidated the lesser-known benefits of palliative care, such as facilitating goals of care discussion and shared decision-making.[46]

Innovative approaches can facilitate an earlier palliative care consult by oncologists. A modified palliative care model is an unmet need in oncology. Ideally, palliative care is introduced early and provided alongside care of curative or life-prolonging intent.[47] Some American oncologists feel that oncology and palliative care have complementary roles and prefer palliative care teams to be embedded in oncology clinics.[48] Outpatient palliative care clinics are the ideal model for early incorporation alongside oncology. This model uses a multidisciplinary palliative care team that operates out of an independent clinic space within the hospital. Often, these clinics are located in tertiary cancer centers and provide same-day appointments, in-person follow-ups, a telephone callback system for urgent symptoms, and after-hours support.[49]

The first in-person randomized control trial (RCT) of early palliative care occurred in the USA. In 2010, Temel et al. reported a study of early-on palliative care versus standard oncologic care (with palliative care involvement as needed) for newly diagnosed metastatic non-small-cell lung cancer patients.[50] The palliative care involvement was provided by palliative care physicians and advanced practice nurses, working to improve the patient's mood and quality of life. Unexpectedly, more prolonged survival was also reported.[51] Effective trials used specialized palliative care teams embedded in the oncology clinic or free-standing. While these RCTs have all been based on early routine involvement of palliative care in the disease course, this model is resource-intensive and may be impractical, where oncologist-initiated referral still predominates. However, models of automatic referral based on symptoms or other triggers are currently being tested in clinical trials.[52]

For oncologists, comfort with EOL care is associated with enhanced access to palliative care. However, ironically, oncologists who are less comfortable with EOL care reported delivering less supportive care and referring fewer patients to specialist palliative care, resulting in lower access to palliative care. Thus, it is imperative to ensure that oncology specialists have adequate training and support for delivering EOL care and a supportive environment to build a collaborative relationship with the specialist palliative care team.[53]

In conclusion, oncologists need to continue to work on communication skills when dealing with patients with advanced cancers. This action will facilitate better and earlier goals of care discussions with their patients and their families. Palliative care must explore innovative care delivery models for earlier and seamless collaboration with their oncology colleagues. Although technology has provided us with novel therapies for cancer care, these medications are often expensive and offer limited benefits over existing treatments. These newer treatments are exciting but often overhyped. Therefore, two things need articulating—how well a regimen works and how much it costs—at the center of discussion.[54] Palliative care may be helpful in these discussions, and different models are being explored.

MEDICAL EDUCATION

Changing how we treat chronically ill patients needs to occur, starting with how physicians are trained. Currently, medical training is too focused on hospital and specialty-based education. This system has resulted in a physician workforce with too many specialists and too few doctors who are prepared to work in primary care. In addition, hospital-based training leaves many physicians unprepared to practice in ambulatory care settings where many of them will work.[55] Although the United States does well at limiting hospital admissions and lengths of stays in cancer patients with a life expectancy of six months or less,[56] it still leads most other countries in Intensive Care Unit admissions during this same time period.[57] Learning should also involve settings outside the hospital, including primary care offices, community health centers, and patients' homes. The experiences from these locations can introduce some of the complexities of content and relationships that may be missing when limited to patients in a hospital bed.[58] Since most end-of-life care is not done in the hospital setting,[59] experience in treating patients in these locations is essential.[60]

Medical students usually enter medical school with the desire, as Virgil put it, "to understand the cause of things" in the world of science and technology. They want to use this knowledge to help others. Still, at some point, they will realize that helping others is different from just solving medical problems.[61] Many institutions are moving from a traditional two years of "basic" or "preclinical" sciences and two years of "clinical" sciences to earlier clinical experiences in the form of modules or blocks that provide education through a patient-based approach as opposed to a subject or disease-based approach. It is unclear if this change will lead physicians to help students focus more on patients and less on diseases.[62] However, medical schools should provide students with opportunities for early patient contact that increases as the student progresses, follows patients through care pathways, and learns about the role of the patient narratives and values in health and healthcare.[63] Such integration will be diverse and dependent on the local socio-cultural context, and it will develop as the population base changes and the trainee's expertise matures.[64]

This early relationship between patients and students is crucial for learning. As patients increasingly become recognized as experts in their own diseases, there has been greater patient involvement in medical curricula, including teaching clinical skills, assessing learners, and contributing to curriculum development.[65] Care for the dying needs to be an integral part of this learning.

In closing, patient-centered care is pivotal for healthcare and learning institutions. As our society's interactions become increasingly distant and technical with each generation, clinicians must redouble their efforts to ensure the humanity of their work is not diminished and that the physician-patient relationship remains grounded in reality—at the bedside. The importance is evident: Ensuring that healthcare professionals can bridge the divide between themselves and their patients is imperative to restoring the public's faith in our profession.[66] A focus on patient-centeredness is associated with better health status and more efficient care. Studies have found that health systems with more patient-centered goals had better overall outcomes than those without such focus. Patients with fulfilled expectations tend to be more satisfied with their healthcare encounters. Others have suggested that patient-centeredness is intrinsically essential regardless of its effect on clinical outcomes, on moral grounds alone.[67]

HOSPICE AND PALLIATIVE CARE

Palliative care boldly and optimistically asserts that suffering can and must be relieved despite overwhelming illness. This assertion is derived from a right ethos. There may be individual barriers that patients or families bring to the clinical setting or, more prominent, pragmatic, economic, geopolitical, or social reasons that make it challenging to provide palliative care. However, none of these concerns undermine the duty to prioritize the relief of suffering for people with incurable illnesses and the families that support them.[68] This audacious statement appears in the preface of the *Oxford Textbook of Palliative Medicine.* Modern medicine has come far in treating illnesses, but we have yet to conquer death (and most likely never will!) Technology has its limits and will not be the solution to EOL care. One thing we have done is to learn to treat diseases that once killed people very quickly.

Nevertheless, the challenge is having all patients have better lives, regardless of their medical status. EOL care is very challenging, and many have considered technology the solution. The remaining sections of this chapter will look at the origins of hospice and palliative medicine, discuss the current status, and finally, comment on what needs to be done.

Origins

Palliative care and its "older sister" hospice arose from the need to treat these patients, even when the medical options were limited. The "right ethos" derives from the determination to relieve suffering, whether the patient is living with or dying from a disease. Hospices arose in the fourth century when Christianity became the Roman Empire's official religion. The word *hospes* originally meant *host,* but it gradually changed its meaning to refer to strangers or guests. The derivative word *hospitium* came to mean a feeling of relationship between them and the place in which it occurred. Hospices, originally for pilgrims and travelers, also cared for the sick, and hospitals developed from them.[69]

The Christian background was fundamental to the origins of hospices, and a degree persists even today. However, the religious impetus also produced a humanitarian response of care for the sick and dying, which was fundamental throughout the East and West. Respect for the suffering in the Middle East in the early centuries, the foundation of hospitals in the Byzantine period, the monastic care of the sick in the Middle Ages, nursing orders such as the French Sisters of Charity founded by Vincent de Paul in the seventeenth century, and the Lutheran order of nursing deaconesses founded by Pastor Fliedner at Kaiserswerth in Germany in the nineteenth century: all were the results of profound faith. Kaiserswerth, for example, carried out all the works of mercy, including care for the dying. Indeed, Elizabeth Fry, whose faith led her to do so much to revolutionize English prisons, was visited by Pastor Fliedner. She visited Kaiserswerth and, in 1840, made plans to develop a similar institution to train nurses in England. Moreover, this revivalist faith led to changes in the care of the sick and dying in the nineteenth century, mainly through Florence Nightingale, who also trained at Kaiserswerth.[70]

Cicely Saunders

Things did not change much for hospices until the middle of the last century when a nurse turned doctor in England began her legacy. Cicely Saunders started the first modern hospice and was more responsible for instituting the discipline and the palliative care culture than anybody else. Saunders was initially an agnostic, but she discovered she believed in God while on holiday in Cornwall with some Christian friends. It was, she said, "as if a switch had flipped." In fact, it was noted that she became a "bubbly, enthusiastic convert"[71] and soon afterward joined John Stott's congregation in London. Saunders was later advised by a surgeon that people would not listen to her as a nurse, that doctors desert the dying, and that she could best help dying patients by becoming a doctor.

She was accepted as a medical student at St Thomas' Hospital at 33. After qualifying, she obtained a research scholarship at St Mary's Hospital, Paddington, where she studied pain management in the incurably ill, and at the same time, worked at St Joseph's, a hospice for the dying poor in Bayswater, run by nuns. Here, she used her medical expertise and research findings to help the nuns improve their standard of care.[72]

Dr. Saunders coined the term "total pain" and suggested that pain has physical, psychological, social, emotional, and spiritual components. These factors combined cause "total pain" that is personal and specific to each patient. The "total pain" concept is critical for nurses and other healthcare professionals caring for hospice patients. An accurate picture of the patient's situation cannot be obtained without a complete and thorough assessment of these dimensions.[73] Dr. Saunders insisted that hospice patients be treated with dignity, compassion, respect, and rigorous scientific methodology in testing treatments for poorly controlled symptoms.[74] With this approach, Saunders established effective pain and symptom management protocols for hospice patients.

Dr. Saunders studied some existing hospices in England. The Roman Catholic Irish Sisters of Charity began an early hospice, St. Joseph's, an order founded by Mother Mary Aikenhead in Dublin. The order started caring for patients in their homes in the East End of London at the beginning of the 20th century. Another hospice, St Joseph's, was a Methodist foundation caring for the dying poor in West London.[75] Due to the efforts of Dr. Saunders, St. Christopher's Hospice opened in South London in 1967.[76]

The concept of hospices significantly changed with Dr. Saunders's founding of St. Christophers. No longer just a charitable place run by a religious community, hospices began to provide medical care to the dying. This idea was both unique and controversial at the time. Should the hospice be in the Church of England community, the Christian in general, or completely secular? Dr. Saunders wrote, "We have decided that it shall be an interdenominational foundation, although we will have something in the documents stating as firmly as possible that it must be carried out as a Christian work as well as a medical one."[77] Therefore, although her hospice had religious roots, there was also an emphasis on the medical side. Cicely Saunders was motivated by a Christian calling to examine the scientific foundations for caring for the dying. She saw this as complementary, not contradictory. In the 1950s, she began studying medicine to translate her Christian commitment.

Many new drugs were available for mood, anxiety, depression, agitation, joint and bone pain, and further pain control techniques. There were also writings on home care from social work and psychiatric overviews of the problems of the bereaved. She writes, "It was a call to the openness of all kinds and to skill and to understand alongside the friendship of the heart."[78] In fact, the Almoner (church official in charge of funding) stated, "To the outside world, you must be first and foremost a medical concern ... You are a Christian doctor, not a spiritual leader with a medical vision."[79]

So, was the idea that hospices leave the church community and become part of the medical community bad? This so-called "secularization" of hospice did have its critics. In her article "The Spiritual Dimension of Hospice: The Secularization of an Ideal," Ann Bradshaw uses a Max Weber quote early on to illustrate this. Even though it was written about nursing, it clearly expresses some sociologists' concerns over this transformation.[80] However, Dr. Saunders was steadfast in her devotion to the hospice movement. Although secular, she still maintained its vocational and spiritual basis. Dr. Saunders brought together the highest medical care with compassion. She believed it was vital that these were not separated because care for the dying was not *care* if it did not use the most up-to-date medical knowledge to alleviate pain and symptoms; neither care was genuine if it used only medicine as a technique without compassion.[81]

Her study and writings regarding pain treatment, especially cancer pain, show her dedication to hospice care's medical aspect. In 1958, she wrote, "The key to this approach seems to lie in two principles: an orientation to the prevention rather than the alleviation of pain; and a complete understanding of available pain-relieving drugs. Each of these areas receives frequent attention in publications throughout the period."[82] These recommendations are still used today.[83] She also championed the concept of "total pain," which, as Armstrong wrote in 1987, "Indeed became a central element in the emergent field of terminal care, which rapidly gained momentum after the opening by Cicely Saunders of St. Christopher's Hospice in 1967. In the intervening years, 'total pain' has remained a fundamental notion within what is now referred to as palliative care."[84]

PALLIATIVE CARE

In 1976, Balfour Mount, a urologist at Royal Victoria Hospital in Montreal, Canada, asked to come to London to study Dr. Saunder's hospice techniques. He felt these procedures could also be used for the sick and suffering patients in his tertiary acute care hospital. When he returned, Dr. Mount trained a team of clinicians to provide this type of care, which he called "palliative."[85] The word is derived from the Latin *palliatus*, which means to cloak for protection or comfort.[86] From there, St. Thomas' Hospital in London began a program in 1977. The United States also started programs in the 1970s and secured Medicare funding in 1982.[87] As a result, the delivery of palliative care is seen increasingly as a global health issue. In 2014, the World Health Assembly passed a declaration calling upon all governments to integrate palliative care into their health plans.[88]

Current and Future Utilization

In Eric Cassell's book *The Nature of Suffering and the Goals of Medicine*, he states:

> *The test of a system of medicine should be its adequacy in the face of suffering; this book starts from the premise that modern medicine fails that test. In fact, the central assumptions on which twentieth-century medicine is founded provide no basis for understanding suffering. For pain, difficulty in breathing, or other afflictions of the body, superbly yes; for suffering, no. Suffering must inevitably involve the person; bodies do not suffer, persons suffer.*[89]

This statement illustrates physicians' difficulty in treating pain and other symptoms. He further states that science is not only a way of uncovering nature's truths; it also promotes an ideal of knowledge. From a scientific point of view, acceptable knowledge is objective, reproducible, and predictable. Numerical data seem to meet the standard best, but other items such as X-rays, CT scans, electrocardiograms, spirometric tracings, and tissue slides are also acceptable. In medicine, we call such information *hard* data.

On the other hand, information that is subjective, value-laden, or cannot be measured is considered unscientific and believed to be of lesser value. It is often called *soft*. Unfortunately, symptoms are always *soft*, subjective (in that they have to do with a subject), value-laden, and nonmeasurable. Medical scientists believe hard data should always replace soft data."[90] This idea brings to mind Max Weber's statement regarding secularization in medicine; some clinicians have become "Specialists without spirit, sensualists without heart." Medicine needs to return to the idea of treating patients and not diseases. Cassell concludes that palliative care attempts to put the emphasis back on the patients and often their families. It also tries to utilize Dame Cicely Saunders' teachings that understood that even the most advanced treatments were not genuine if they used "medicine as a technique without compassion."[91]

Although palliative care is vital in EOL care, other specialists must also recognize its role. There are not enough palliative care specialists to go around, and this type of care would be limited to a minority of patients suffering. This concept has to be accepted and utilized by the medical community in its entirety. Dr. Gawande is a surgeon and not a palliative care physician. However, he eloquently puts it in his book *Being Mortal*:

> *The problem with medicine and the institutions it has spawned for the care of the sick and the old is not that they have had an incorrect view of what makes life significant. The problem is that they have had almost no view at all. Medicine's focus is narrow. Medical professionals concentrate on the repair of health, not the sustenance of the soul. However—and this is the painful paradox—we have decided that they should be the ones who largely define how we live in our waning days.*[92]

We can do better if we recognize this disparity and place the focus back on the patient!

This chapter has tried to show that palliative care is valuable in ICU and oncology. However, problems in these two realms still remain. As long as palliative care is seen as "what you do" and curing diseases "is what we do," problems will persist. Integrating palliative care, not just as a consulting service but also as a care philosophy, will be essential as the needs of the imminently dying mount. Technology has a role but has also shown false promises, which only complicates EOL care.

CONCLUSION

B. J. Miller is the founder of a hospice in California called Zen Hospice. His personal story is intriguing. While a college student, he and several friends decided to do something stupid one night. They found a railroad car and thought it would be fun to climb to the top. Miller got up there first and raised his arms in victory. Unfortunately, 11,000 volts went through his body. After a lengthy hospitalization, losing an arm and both legs, he was discharged and attended medical school. In a TED talk, he described his hospice's practice with respect to EOL care:

> *When one of our residents dies, the mortuary men come. And as we're wheeling the body out through the garden headed for the gate, we pause—anyone who wants to share a story or a song or silence as we sprinkle the body with flower petals to usher in grief with warmth. Contrast that with the typical experience in the hospital setting. Floodlit room lined with tubes and beeping machines and blinking lights that don't stop even when the patient's life has. Cleaning crew swoops in, the body is whisked away. It feels as though that person had never really existed.*[93]

A study with patients with advanced cancer showed that simply conversing with their physicians improved their quality of death and lowered their healthcare expenditures. In addition, there was no survival difference associated with healthcare expenditures, and patients whose insured healthcare costs were higher had a worse quality of life in their final week of life.[94]

We have discussed EOL quality and the impact of palliative care. It is clear that higher healthcare costs in the ICU and cancer care were not associated with better outcomes. Significant evidence supports that suffering was often made worse for the patients and their families. Having the focus placed more on the patient and less on the disease is critically important. This reality is now seen in many medical schools' curricula. Finally, hospice and palliative care medicine continue to make inroads as healthcare systems realize that a change is needed. EOL care is crucial in focusing on patients rather than their diseases and the technology to fix them. As Cicely Saunders said, "You matter because you are you, and you matter to the end of your life. We will do all we can to help you die peacefully and live until you die."[95] Healthcare professionals can better understand the patient's experience and provide more effective treatments to relieve suffering by focusing on the patient. This reason is why many clinicians went into healthcare in the first place.

TAKE-HOME POINTS

- The disease-centered approach to medical care is helpful in some circumstances, especially with curable and reversible illnesses; however, it has shown to be, at best, inadequate when it comes to the care of the dying.
- Palliative care is the medical specialty that puts the emphasis back on the patient and their family. As technologies fail to provide the intended results, the focus is on controlling the patient's symptoms and suffering.
- Patient goal-directed care may benefit persons with multiple chronic conditions for whom many often contradictory and burdensome care options are available.
- When oncologists and patients discuss goals of care, patients are more likely to get care consistent with their personal choices and have a better quality of life near death. However, other studies have shown that conversations about goals of care often fail to provide patients with sufficient information about prognosis to allow for appropriate decisions.
- Patient-centered care is pivotal for healthcare and learning institutions. As our society's interactions become increasingly distant and technical with each generation, clinicians must redouble their efforts to ensure the humanity of their work is not diminished and that the physician-patient relationship remains grounded in reality—at the bedside.

- Palliative care boldly and optimistically asserts that suffering can and must be relieved despite overwhelming illness.
- Hospice care is palliative care when the prognosis is six months or less and curative treatment is no longer available or desired.
- Cicely Saunders, the founder of the modern hospice movement, coined the term "total pain" and suggested that pain has physical, psychological, social, emotional, and spiritual components. These factors combined cause "total pain" that is personal and specific to each patient. The "total pain" concept is critical for nurses and other healthcare professionals caring for hospice patients.
- Hospice and palliative care medicine continue to make inroads as healthcare systems realize that a change is needed. EOL care is crucial in focusing on patients rather than their diseases and the technology to fix them.

NOTES

1 Alice Calaprice, *The Ultimate Quotable Einstein* (Princeton, NJ: Princeton University Press, 2010).
2 Mary E. Tinetti, Aanand D. Naik, and John A. Dodson, "Moving From Disease-Centered to Patient Goals-Directed Care for Patients With Multiple Chronic Conditions: Patient Value-Based Care," *JAMA Cardiology* 1, no. 1 (April 1, 2016): 9, https://doi.org/10.1001/jamacardio.2015.0248.
3 J. Randall Curtis et al., "End-of-Life Care in the Intensive Care Unit: Can We Simultaneously Increase Quality and Reduce Costs?," *American Journal of Respiratory and Critical Care Medicine* 186, no. 7 (October 1, 2012): 587–592, https://doi.org/10.1164/rccm.201206-1020CP.
4 J. Randall Curtis et al., "End-of-Life Care in the Intensive Care Unit: Can We Simultaneously Increase Quality and Reduce Costs?," *American Journal of Respiratory and Critical Care Medicine* 186, no. 7 (October 1, 2012): 587–592, https://doi.org/10.1164/rccm.201206-1020CP.
5 Philip Yancey, "Angel to the Dying: The Founder of the Modern Hospice Movement, Cicely Saunders, Has Made It Possible for Thousands to Die with Dignity," *Christianity Today*, December 17, 1990, www.christianitytoday.com/1990/12/profile-angle-to-dying.
6 Cicely Saunders, "Pain and Impending Death," in *Selected Writings 1958–2004*, edited by David Clark (Oxford: Oxford University Press, 2006), https://doi.org/10.1093/acprof:oso/9780198570530.003.0027.
7 Mary E. Tinetti, Aanand D. Naik, and John A. Dodson, "Moving From Disease-Centered to Patient Goals-Directed Care for Patients With Multiple Chronic Conditions: Patient Value-Based Care," *JAMA Cardiology* 1, no. 1 (April 1, 2016): 9, https://doi.org/10.1001/jamacardio.2015.0248.
8 James L. Bernat, "Medical Futility: Definition, Determination, and Disputes in Critical Care," *Neurocritical Care* 2, no. 2 (2005): 198, https://doi.org/10.1385/ncc:2:2:198.
9 J. Randall Curtis and Robert A. Burt, "Why Are Critical Care Clinicians So Powerfully Distressed by Family Demands for Futile Care?," *Journal of Critical Care* 18, no. 1 (March 1, 2003): 22–24.

10 Guy Schofield et al., "Palliative Opioid Use, Palliative Sedation and Euthanasia: Reaffirming the Distinction," *Journal of Medical Ethics* 46, no. 1 (January 2020): 48–50, https://doi.org/10.1136/medethics-2018–105256.

11 Henk ten Have and Jos V. M. Welie, "Palliative Sedation Versus Euthanasia: An Ethical Assessment," *Journal of Pain and Symptom Management* 47, no. 1 (January 1, 2014): 123–136.

12 David Crippen, *End-of-Life Communication in the ICU: A Global Perspective* (New York: Springer, 2008).

13 Cynthia Hsu-Kim et al., "Integrating Palliative Care into Critical Care," *Journal of Intensive Care Medicine (Sage Publications Inc.)* 30, no. 6 (September 2015): 358–364, https://doi.org/10.1177/0885066614523923.

14 Eric J. Cassell, *The Nature of Suffering. [Electronic Resource] : And the Goals of Medicine*. (Oxford University Press, 1991).

15 Jasmine Hearn et al., "Patient-Centered Medical Education: A Proposed Definition," *Medical Teacher* 41, no. 8 (August 2019): 934–938.

16 Susan Edgman-Levitan and Stephen C. Schoenbaum, "Patient-Centered Care: Achieving Higher Quality by Designing Care through the Patient's Eyes," *Israel Journal of Health Policy Research* 10, no. 1 (March 5, 2021): 1–5.

17 Mary E. Tinetti, Aanand D. Naik, and John A. Dodson, "Moving From Disease-Centered to Patient Goals-Directed Care for Patients With Multiple Chronic Conditions: Patient Value-Based Care," *JAMA Cardiology* 1, no. 1 (April 1, 2016): 9, https://doi.org/10.1001/jamacardio.2015.0248.

18 Terri R. Fried, Richard L. Street, and Andrew B. Cohen, "Chronic Disease Decision Making and 'What Matters Most'," *Journal of the American Geriatrics Society* 68, no. 3 (March 2020): 474–477.

19 Mary E. Tinetti, Aanand D. Naik, and John A. Dodson, "Moving From Disease-Centered to Patient Goals-Directed Care for Patients With Multiple Chronic Conditions: Patient Value-Based Care," *JAMA Cardiology* 1, no. 1 (April 1, 2016): 9, https://doi.org/10.1001/jamacardio.2015.0248.

20 Terri R. Fried, Richard L. Street, and Andrew B. Cohen, "Chronic Disease Decision Making and 'What Matters Most'," *Journal of the American Geriatrics Society* 68, no. 3 (March 2020): 474–477.

21 Mary E. Tinetti, Aanand D. Naik, and John A. Dodson, "Moving From Disease-Centered to Patient Goals-Directed Care for Patients With Multiple Chronic Conditions: Patient Value-Based Care," *JAMA Cardiology* 1, no. 1 (April 1, 2016): 9, https://doi.org/10.1001/jamacardio.2015.0248.

22 Eric J. Cassell, *The Healer's Art : A New Approach to the Doctor-Patient Relationship*. (Penguin Books, 1979).

23 Terri R. Fried, Richard L. Street, and Andrew B. Cohen, "Chronic Disease Decision Making and 'What Matters Most'," *Journal of the American Geriatrics Society* 68, no. 3 (March 2020): 474–477.

24 Mary E. Tinetti, Aanand D. Naik, and John A. Dodson, "Moving From Disease-Centered to Patient Goals-Directed Care for Patients With Multiple Chronic Conditions: Patient Value-Based Care," *JAMA Cardiology* 1, no. 1 (April 1, 2016): 9, https://doi.org/10.1001/jamacardio.2015.0248.

25 Cambridge University Press, *Cambridge Academic Content Dictionary*, 1st ed (New York: Cambridge University Press, 2009).

26 S. L. Douglas et al., "Patient–Physician Discordance in Goals of Care for Patients with Advanced Cancer," *Current Oncology* 26, no. 6 (December 2019): 370–379.

27 Sebastian Salas-Vega, Emily Shearer, and Elias Mossialos, "Relationship between Costs and Clinical Benefits of New Cancer Medicines in Australia, France, the UK, and the US," *Social Science & Medicine* 258 (August 1, 2020).

28 Minnie Bluhm et al., "Oncologists' End of Life Treatment Decisions," *Journal of Applied Gerontology* 36, no. 4 (April 2017): 416–440, https://doi.org/10.1177/0733464815595510.

29 Minnie Bluhm et al., "Oncologists' End of Life Treatment Decisions," *Journal of Applied Gerontology* 36, no. 4 (April 2017): 416–440, https://doi.org/10.1177/0733464815595510.

30 S. L. Douglas et al., "Patient–Physician Discordance in Goals of Care for Patients with Advanced Cancer," *Current Oncology* 26, no. 6 (December 2019): 370–379.

31 S. L. Douglas et al., "Patient–Physician Discordance in Goals of Care for Patients with Advanced Cancer," *Current Oncology* 26, no. 6 (December 2019): 370–379.

32 Amalie M. Hauge, "One Last Round of Chemo? Insights from Conversations between Oncologists and Lung Cancer Patients about Prognosis and Treatment Decisions," *Social Science & Medicine* 266 (December 1, 2020).

33 S. L. Douglas et al., "Patient–Physician Discordance in Goals of Care for Patients with Advanced Cancer," *Current Oncology* 26, no. 6 (December 2019): 370–379.

34 Nicholas A. Christakis and Robert Wood Johnson, "Extent and Determinants of Error in Physicians' Prognoses in Terminally Ill Patients: Prospective Cohort Study," *Western Journal of Medicine* 172, no. 5 (May 2000): 310.

35 Chithra R. Perumalswami, Reshma Jagsi, and Susan Dorr Goold, "Predicting a 'Lazarus Effect' in Patients With Advanced Cancer Near the End of Life: Prognostic Uncertainty, Oncologists' Emotions, and Ethical Questions," *The American Journal of Bioethics : AJOB* 19, no. 12 (December 2019): 57–60, https://doi.org/10.1080/15265161.2019.1675799.

36 Amalie M. Hauge, "One Last Round of Chemo? Insights from Conversations between Oncologists and Lung Cancer Patients about Prognosis and Treatment Decisions," *Social Science & Medicine* 266 (December 1, 2020).

37 Chithra R. Perumalswami, Reshma Jagsi, and Susan Dorr Goold, "Predicting a 'Lazarus Effect' in Patients With Advanced Cancer Near the End of Life: Prognostic Uncertainty, Oncologists' Emotions, and Ethical Questions," *The American Journal of Bioethics : AJOB* 19, no. 12 (December 2019): 57–60, https://doi.org/10.1080/15265161.2019.1675799.

38 Amalie M. Hauge, "One Last Round of Chemo? Insights from Conversations between Oncologists and Lung Cancer Patients about Prognosis and Treatment Decisions," *Social Science & Medicine* 266 (December 1, 2020).

39 Naveen Salins et al., "How Views of Oncologists and Haematologists Impacts Palliative Care Referral: A Systematic Review," *BMC Palliative Care* 19, no. 1 (2020), https://doi.org/10.1186/s12904-020-00671-5.

40 David Hui et al., "Impact of Oncologists' Attitudes Toward End-of-Life Care on Patients' Access to Palliative Care," *The Oncologist* 21, no. 9 (September 2016): 1149–1155, https://doi.org/10.1634/theoncologist.2016–0090.

41 Naveen Salins et al., "How Views of Oncologists and Haematologists Impacts Palliative Care Referral: A Systematic Review," *BMC Palliative Care* 19, no. 1 (2020), https://doi.org/10.1186/s12904-020-00671-5.

42 Naveen Salins et al., "How Views of Oncologists and Haematologists Impacts Palliative Care Referral: A Systematic Review," *BMC Palliative Care* 19, no. 1 (2020), https://doi.org/10.1186/s12904-020-00671-5.

43 Hon Wai Benjamin Cheng and Ka On Lam, "Supportive and Palliative Care in Hemato-Oncology: How Best to Achieve Seamless Integration and Subspecialty Development?," *Annals of Hematology* 100, no. 3 (2021): 601, https://doi.org/10.1007/s00277-020-04386-8.

44 Naveen Salins et al., "How Views of Oncologists and Haematologists Impacts Palliative Care Referral: A Systematic Review," *BMC Palliative Care* 19, no. 1 (2020), https://doi.org/10.1186/s12904-020-00671-5.

45 Naveen Salins et al., "How Views of Oncologists and Haematologists Impacts Palliative Care Referral: A Systematic Review," *BMC Palliative Care* 19, no. 1 (2020), https://doi.org/10.1186/s12904-020-00671-5.

46 Naveen Salins et al., "How Views of Oncologists and Haematologists Impacts Palliative Care Referral: A Systematic Review," *BMC Palliative Care* 19, no. 1 (2020), https://doi.org/10.1186/s12904-020-00671-5.

47 Hon Wai Benjamin Cheng and Ka On Lam, "Supportive and Palliative Care in Hemato-Oncology: How Best to Achieve Seamless Integration and Subspecialty Development?," *Annals of Hematology* 100, no. 3 (2021): 601, https://doi.org/10.1007/s00277-020-04386-8.

48 Naveen Salins et al., "How Views of Oncologists and Haematologists Impacts Palliative Care Referral: A Systematic Review," *BMC Palliative Care* 19, no. 1 (2020), https://doi.org/10.1186/s12904-020-00671-5.

49 Jean Mathews, Breffni Hannon, and Camilla Zimmermann, "Models of Integration of Specialized Palliative Care with Oncology," *Current Treatment Options in Oncology* 22, no. 5 (2021), https://doi.org/10.1007/s11864-021-00836-1.

50 Jennifer S. Temel et al., "Early Palliative Care for Patients with Metastatic Non-Small-Cell Lung Cancer," *New England Journal of Medicine* 363 (2010): 733–742.

51 Jean Mathews, Breffni Hannon, and Camilla Zimmermann, "Models of Integration of Specialized Palliative Care with Oncology," *Current Treatment Options in Oncology* 22, no. 5 (2021), https://doi.org/10.1007/s11864-021-00836-1.

52 Jean Mathews, Breffni Hannon, and Camilla Zimmermann, "Models of Integration of Specialized Palliative Care with Oncology," *Current Treatment Options in Oncology* 22, no. 5 (2021), https://doi.org/10.1007/s11864-021-00836-1.

53 David Hui et al., "Impact of Oncologists' Attitudes Toward End-of-Life Care on Patients' Access to Palliative Care," *The Oncologist* 21, no. 9 (September 2016): 1149–1155, https://doi.org/10.1634/theoncologist.2016–0090.

54 Audrey A. Tran, Milos Miljković, and Vinay Prasad, "Analysis of Estimated Clinical Benefit of Newly Approved Drugs for US Patients with Acute Myeloid Leukemia," *Leukemia Research* 96 (September 1, 2020).

55 Michael McCarthy, "US Panel Calls for Sweeping Changes to Funding of Graduate Medical Education," *BMJ: British Medical Journal* 349 (August 1, 2014).

56 Justin E. Bekelman et al., "Comparison of Site of Death, Health Care Utilization, and Hospital Expenditures for Patients Dying With Cancer in 7 Developed Countries," *JAMA: Journal of the American Medical Association* 315, no. 3 (January 19, 2016): 272–283.

57 J. Randall Curtis et al., "End-of-Life Care in the Intensive Care Unit: Can We Simultaneously Increase Quality and Reduce Costs?," *American Journal of Respiratory and Critical Care Medicine* 186, no. 7 (October 1, 2012): 587–592, https://doi.org/10.1164/rccm.201206-1020CP.

58 Tim Swanwick, *Understanding Medical Education: Evidence, Theory and Practice*, second edition (Malden, MA: Wiley-Blackwell, 2014), page 216.

59 Justin E. Bekelman et al., "Comparison of Site of Death, Health Care Utilization, and Hospital Expenditures for Patients Dying With Cancer in 7 Developed Countries," *JAMA: Journal of the American Medical Association* 315, no. 3 (January 19, 2016): 272–283.

60 Michael McCarthy, "US Panel Calls for Sweeping Changes to Funding of Graduate Medical Education," *BMJ: British Medical Journal* 349 (August 1, 2014).

61 Tim Swanwick, *Understanding Medical Education : Evidence, Theory and Practice.* Page 213

62 Kent J. DeZee et al., "Medical Education in the United States of America," *Medical Teacher* 34, no. 7 (July 2012): 521–525.

63 Jasmine Hearn et al., "Patient-Centered Medical Education: A Proposed Definition," *Medical Teacher* 41, no. 8 (August 2019): 934–938.

64 Jasmine Hearn et al., "Patient-Centered Medical Education: A Proposed Definition," *Medical Teacher* 41, no. 8 (August 2019): 934–938.

65 Shannon Fong et al., "Patient-Centred Education: How Do Learners' Perceptions Change as They Experience Clinical Training?," *Advances in Health Sciences Education* 24, no. 1 (March 2019): 15–32.

66 Michael Shamoon, "'Future-Proofing' Communication Skills for Future Physician Learners," *Journal of Graduate Medical Education* 11, no. 1 (February 2019): 106, https://doi.org/10.4300/JGME-D-18-00858.1.

67 Shannon Fong et al., "Patient-Centred Education: How Do Learners' Perceptions Change as They Experience Clinical Training?," *Advances in Health Sciences Education* 24, no. 1 (March 2019): 15–32.

68 Nathan Cherny et al., *Oxford Textbook of Palliative Medicine*, fifth edition, Oxford Textbooks in Anaesthesia (Oxford: Oxford University Press, 2015), Preface.

69 A. Bradshaw, "The Spiritual Dimension of Hospice. The Secularization of an Ideal," *Social Science & Medicine*, August 1996, 409–419.

70 A. Bradshaw, "The Spiritual Dimension of Hospice. The Secularization of an Ideal," *Social Science & Medicine*, August 1996, 409–419.

71 Philip Yancey, "Angel to the Dying: The Founder of the Modern Hospice Movement, Cicely Saunders, Has Made It Possible for Thousands to Die with Dignity," *Christianity Today*, December 17, 1990, www.christianitytoday.com/1990/12/profile-angle-to-dying.

72 Philip Yancey, "Angel to the Dying: The Founder of the Modern Hospice Movement, Cicely Saunders, Has Made It Possible for Thousands to Die with Dignity," *Christianity Today*, December 17, 1990, www.christianitytoday.com/1990/12/profile-angle-to-dying.

73 Cicely Saunders, Mary Baines, and Robert Dunlop, "Control of Symptoms Other than Pain," in *Living with Dying: A Guide to Palliative Care* (Oxford: Oxford University Press, 1995), https://doi.org/10.1093/acprof:oso/9780192625144.003.0005.

74 Nathan Cherny et al., *Oxford Textbook of Palliative Medicine*, fifth edition, Oxford Textbooks in Anaesthesia (Oxford: Oxford University Press, 2015), page 3.

75 A. Bradshaw, "The Spiritual Dimension of Hospice. The Secularization of an Ideal," *Social Science & Medicine*, August 1996, 409–419.

76 Nathan Cherny et al., *Oxford Textbook of Palliative Medicine*, fifth edition, Oxford Textbooks in Anaesthesia (Oxford: Oxford University Press, 2015), page 3.

77 David Clark, "Religion, Medicine, and Community in the Early Origins of St. Christopher's Hospice," *Journal of Palliative Medicine* Volume 4, Number 3, (2001): 353–360.

78 A. Bradshaw, "The Spiritual Dimension of Hospice. The Secularization of an Ideal," *Social Science & Medicine*, August 1996, 409–419.

79 David Clark, "Religion, Medicine, and Community in the Early Origins of St. Christopher's Hospice," *Journal of Palliative Medicine* Volume 4, Number 3, (2001): 353–360.

80 A. Bradshaw, "The Spiritual Dimension of Hospice. The Secularization of an Ideal," *Social Science & Medicine*, August 1996, 409–419.

81 A. Bradshaw, "The Spiritual Dimension of Hospice. The Secularization of an Ideal," *Social Science & Medicine*, August 1996, 409–419.

82 David Clark, "Religion, Medicine, and Community in the Early Origins of St. Christopher's Hospice," *Journal of Palliative Medicine* Volume 4, Number 3, (2001): 353–360.

83 Nathan Cherny et al., *Oxford Textbook of Palliative Medicine*, fifth edition, Oxford Textbooks in Anaesthesia (Oxford: Oxford University Press, 2015), page 3.

84 David Clark, "'Total Pain', Disciplinary Power and the Body in the Work of Cicely Saunders, 1958–1967," *Social Science & Medicine* 19 (1999): 727–736.

85 Nathan Cherny et al., *Oxford Textbook of Palliative Medicine*, fifth edition, Oxford Textbooks in Anaesthesia (Oxford: Oxford University Press, 2015).

86 Merriam-Webster, *Merriam-Webster's Intermediate Dictionary* (Springfield, MA: Merriam-Webster, 2020).

87 Nathan Cherny et al., *Oxford Textbook of Palliative Medicine*, fifth edition, Oxford Textbooks in Anaesthesia (Oxford: Oxford University Press, 2015).

88 David Clark, "Mapping Levels of Palliative Care Development in 198 Countries: The Situation in 2017," *Journal of Pain and Symptom Management* 59, no. 4 (April 2020): 794–807.

89 Eric J. Cassell, *The Nature of Suffering and the Goals of Medicine*. 2nd ed. (Oxford University Press, 2004), Preface.

90 Eric J. Cassell, *The Nature of Suffering and the Goals of Medicine*. 2nd ed. (Oxford University Press, 2004), page 90.

91 A. Bradshaw, "The Spiritual Dimension of Hospice. The Secularization of an Ideal," *Social Science & Medicine*, August 1996, 409–419.

92 Atul Gawande, *Being Mortal : Illness, Medicine and What Matters in the End* (London: Wellcome Collection, 2014).

93 B. J. Miller, "How Can We Prepare For A Graceful Death?," *TED Radio Hour (NPR)*, January 29, 2016, TED Talk extract transcript at www.npr.org/transcripts/464455068.

94 Baohui Zhang et al., "Health Care Costs in the Last Week of Life: Associations With End-of-Life Conversations," *Archives of Internal Medicine* 169, no. 5 (March 9, 2009): 480–488, https://doi.org/10.1001/archinternmed.2008.587.

95 David Clark (ed.), *Cicely Saunders—Founder of the Hospice Movement: Selected Letters 1959–1999* (Oxford: Oxford University Press, 2002).

BIBLIOGRAPHY

Bekelman, Justin E., Scott D. Halpern, Carl Rudolf Blankart, Julie P. Bynum, Joachim Cohen, Robert Fowler, Stein Kaasa, et al. "Comparison of Site of Death, Health Care Utilization, and Hospital Expenditures for Patients Dying With Cancer in 7 Developed Countries." *JAMA: Journal of the American Medical Association* 315, no. 3 (January 19, 2016): 272–283.

Bernat, James L. "Medical Futility: Definition, Determination, and Disputes in Critical Care." *Neurocritical Care* 2, no. 2 (2005): 198. https://doi.org/10.1385/ncc:2:2:198.

Bluhm, Minnie, Cathleen M. Connell, Nancy Janz, Kathleen Bickel, Raymond DeVries, and Maria Silveira. "Oncologists' End of Life Treatment Decisions." *Journal of Applied Gerontology* 36, no. 4 (April 2017): 416–440. https://doi.org/10.1177/0733464815595510.

Bradshaw., A. "The Spiritual Dimension of Hospice. The Secularization of an Ideal." *Social Science & Medicine*, August 1996, 409–419.

Calaprice, Alice. *The Ultimate Quotable Einstein*. Princeton, NJ: Princeton University Press, 2010.

Cambridge University Press. *Cambridge Academic Content Dictionary*. 1st ed. New York: Cambridge: Cambridge University Press, 2009.

Cassell, Eric J. *The Healer's Art : A New Approach to the Doctor-Patient Relationship.* London: Penguin Books, 1979.

Cassell, Eric J. *The Nature of Suffering and the Goals of Medicine.* 2nd ed. Oxford: Oxford University Press, 2004.

Cheng, Hon Wai Benjamin, and Ka On Lam. "Supportive and Palliative Care in Hemato-Oncology: How Best to Achieve Seamless Integration and Subspecialty Development?" *Annals of Hematology* 100, no. 3 (2021): 601. https://doi.org/10.1007/s00277-020-04386-8.

Cherny, Nathan, Marie Fallon, Stein Kaasa, Russell K. Portenoy, and David C. Currow. *Oxford Textbook of Palliative Medicine*. Vol. Fifth edition. Oxford Textbooks in Anaesthesia. Oxford: OUP Oxford, 2015.

Christakis, Nicholas A., and Robert Wood Johnson. "Extent and Determinants of Error in Physicians' Prognoses in Terminally Ill Patients: Prospective Cohort Study." *Western Journal of Medicine* 172, no. 5 (May 2000): 310.

Clark, David (ed.). *Cicely Saunders—Founder of the Hospice Movement: Selected Letters 1959–1999*. Oxford: Oxford University Press, 2002.

Clark, David. "'Total Pain', Disciplinary Power and the Body in the Work of Cicely Saunders, 1958–1967." *Social Science & Medicine* 19 (1999): 727–736.

Clark, David. "Mapping Levels of Palliative Care Development in 198 Countries: The Situation in 2017." *Journal of Pain and Symptom Management* Volume 59 Number 4 (April 2020): 794–807.

Clark, David. "Religion, Medicine, and Community in the Early Origins of St. Christopher's Hospice." *Journal of Palliative Medicine* Volume 4, Number 3, (2001): 353–360.

Crippen, David. *End-of-Life Communication in the ICU: A Global Perspective.* New York: Springer, 2008.

Curtis, J. Randall, and Robert A. Burt. "Why Are Critical Care Clinicians So Powerfully Distressed by Family Demands for Futile Care?" *Journal of Critical Care* 18, no. 1 (March 1, 2003): 22–24.

Curtis, J. Randall, Ruth A. Engelberg, Mark E. Bensink, and Scott D. Ramsey. "End-of-Life Care in the Intensive Care Unit: Can We Simultaneously Increase Quality and Reduce Costs?"

American Journal of Respiratory and Critical Care Medicine 186, no. 7 (October 1, 2012): 587–592. https://doi.org/10.1164/rccm.201206-1020CP.

DeZee, Kent J., Anthony R. Artino, D. Michael Elnicki, Paul A. Hemmer, and Steven J. Durning. "Medical Education in the United States of America." *Medical Teacher* 34, no. 7 (July 2012): 521–525.

Douglas, S. L., B. J. Daly, N. J. Meropol, and A. R. Lipson. "Patient-Physician Discordance in Goals of Care for Patients with Advanced Cancer." *Current Oncology* 26, no. 6 (December 2019): 370–79.

Edgman-Levitan, Susan, and Stephen C. Schoenbaum. "Patient-Centered Care: Achieving Higher Quality by Designing Care through the Patient's Eyes." *Israel Journal of Health Policy Research* 10, no. 1 (March 5, 2021): 1–5.

Fong, Shannon, Amy Tan, Joanna Czupryn, and Anna Oswald. "Patient-Centred Education: How Do Learners' Perceptions Change as They Experience Clinical Training?" *Advances in Health Sciences Education* 24, no. 1 (March 2019): 15–32.

Fried, Terri R., Richard L. Street, and Andrew B. Cohen. "Chronic Disease Decision Making and 'What Matters Most'." *Journal of the American Geriatrics Society* 68, no. 3 (March 2020): 474–477.

Gawande, Atul. *Being Mortal : Illness, Medicine and What Matters in the End*. Wellcome. London: Wellcome Collection, 2014.

Hauge, Amalie M. "One Last Round of Chemo? Insights from Conversations between Oncologists and Lung Cancer Patients about Prognosis and Treatment Decisions." *Social Science & Medicine* 266 (December 1, 2020).

Hearn, Jasmine, Mohamed Dewji, Claire Stocker, and Greg Simons. "Patient-Centered Medical Education: A Proposed Definition." *Medical Teacher* 41, no. 8 (August 2019): 934–938.

Hsu-Kim, Cynthia, Tara Friedman, Edward Gracely, and James Gasperino. "Integrating Palliative Care into Critical Care." *Journal of Intensive Care Medicine (Sage Publications Inc.)* 30, no. 6 (September 2015): 358–364. https://doi.org/10.1177/0885066614523923

Hui, David, Maria Agustina Cerana, Minjeong Park, Kenneth Hess, and Eduardo Bruera. "Impact of Oncologists' Attitudes Toward End-of-Life Care on Patients' Access to Palliative Care." *The Oncologist* 21, no. 9 (September 2016): 1149–1155. https://doi.org/10.1634/theoncologist.2016-0090.

Mathews, Jean, Breffni Hannon, and Camilla Zimmermann. "Models of Integration of Specialized Palliative Care with Oncology." *Current Treatment Options in Oncology* 22, no. 5 (2021). https://doi.org/10.1007/s11864-021-00836-1.

McCarthy, Michael. "US Panel Calls for Sweeping Changes to Funding of Graduate Medical Education." *BMJ: British Medical Journal* 349 (August 1, 2014).

Merriam-Webster. *Merriam-Webster's Intermediate Dictionary*. Springfield, MA: Merriam-Webster, 2020.

Perumalswami, Chithra R, Reshma Jagsi, and Susan Dorr Goold. "Predicting a 'Lazarus Effect' in Patients With Advanced Cancer Near the End of Life: Prognostic Uncertainty, Oncologists' Emotions, and Ethical Questions." *The American Journal of Bioethics : AJOB* 19, no. 12 (December 2019): 57–60. https://doi.org/10.1080/15265161.2019.1675799.

Salas-Vega, Sebastian, Emily Shearer, and Elias Mossialos. "Relationship between Costs and Clinical Benefits of New Cancer Medicines in Australia, France, the UK, and the US." *Social Science & Medicine* 258 (August 1, 2020).

Salins, Naveen, Arunangshu Ghoshal, Sean Hughes, and Nancy Preston. "How Views of Oncologists and Haematologists Impacts Palliative Care Referral: A Systematic Review." *BMC Palliative Care* 19, no. 1 (2020). https://doi.org/10.1186/s12904-020-00671-5.

Saunders, Cicely. "Pain and Impending Death." In *Selected Writings 1958–2004*. Edited by David Clark. Oxford: Oxford University Press, 2006. https://doi.org/10.1093/acprof:oso/9780198570530.003.0027.

Saunders, Cicely, Mary Baines, and Robert Dunlop. "Control of Symptoms Other than Pain." In *Living with Dying: A Guide to Palliative Care*. Oxford: Oxford University Press, 1995. https://doi.org/10.1093/acprof:oso/9780192625144.003.0005.

Schofield, Guy, Idris Baker, Rachel Bullock, Hannah Clare, Paul Clark, Derek Willis, Craig Gannon, and Rob George. "Palliative Opioid Use, Palliative Sedation and Euthanasia: Reaffirming the Distinction." *Journal of Medical Ethics* 46, no. 1 (January 2020): 48–50. https://doi.org/10.1136/medethics-2018-105256.

Shamoon, Michael. "'Future-Proofing' Communication Skills for Future Physician Learners." *Journal of Graduate Medical Education* 11, no. 1 (February 2019): 106. https://doi.org/10.4300/JGME-D-18-00858.1.

Swanwick, Tim. *Understanding Medical Education : Evidence, Theory and Practice*. Vol. Second edition. Malden, MA: Wiley-Blackwell, 2014.

Ten Have, Henk, and Jos V. M. Welie. "Palliative Sedation Versus Euthanasia: An Ethical Assessment." *Journal of Pain and Symptom Management* 47, no. 1 (January 1, 2014): 123–136.

Tinetti, Mary E., Aanand D. Naik, and John A. Dodson. "Moving From Disease-Centered to Patient Goals-Directed Care for Patients With Multiple Chronic Conditions: Patient Value-Based Care." *JAMA Cardiology* 1, no. 1 (April 1, 2016): 9. https://doi.org/10.1001/jamacardio.2015.0248.

Tran, Audrey A., Milos Miljković, and Vinay Prasad. "Analysis of Estimated Clinical Benefit of Newly Approved Drugs for US Patients with Acute Myeloid Leukemia." *Leukemia Research* 96 (September 1, 2020).

Yancey, Philip. "Angel to the Dying: The Founder of the Modern Hospice Movement, Cicely Saunders, Has Made It Possible for Thousands to Die with Dignity." *Christianity Today*, December 17, 1990. www.christianitytoday.com/1990/12/profile-angle-to-dying.

Zhang, Baohui, Alexi A. Wright, Haiden A. Huskamp, Matthew E. Nilsson, Matthew L. Maciejewski, Craig C. Earle, Susan D. Block, Paul K. Maciejewski, and Holly G. Prigerson. "Health Care Costs in the Last Week of Life: Associations With End-of-Life Conversations." *Archives of Internal Medicine* 169, no. 5 (March 9, 2009): 480–488. https://doi.org/10.1001/archinternmed.2008.587.

Chapter 8

The Organization of Healthcare as a Sustainable Resource

INTRODUCTION

In 1991, veteran auto journalist Angus Makenzie wrote this about an expensive American luxury car, the 1991 Lincoln Town Car:

> *It wasn't merely that the Lincoln wallowed around the track like a drunken water buffalo, the asthmatic V-8 wheezing away under the hood. It was the depressingly cynical debasing of the American Dream it represented. Successful Germans could buy a Mercedes S-Class. Successful Brits could buy a Bentley. But successful Americans were offered a fat, frumpy old Ford in a nylon prom dress.*[1]

In a very real sense, much the same can be said about the United States' healthcare system. It is expensive, underperforms, and cannot compete well with other countries. In 2021, the *Detroit Free Press* reported that the Lincoln Motor Company announced it would no longer make luxury sedans (it will continue to make SUVs). It is reasonable to ask whether our healthcare system is doomed to the same fate.

INFLUENCING FACTORS

In Ezekiel Emanuel's book, *Which Country Has the World's Best Health Care?*, he examined healthcare in eleven countries in twenty-two categories. These categories included details regarding affordability, availability, and quality. The United States ranked among the best in six categories and the worst in twelve. He goes on to say:

> *For all that money, the US healthcare system performs poorly on many dimensions, including ones that Americans prize highly, such as patient choice*

DOI: 10.4324/9781003654124-9

> *in hospitals and physicians with Canada, France, Germany, the Netherlands, Switzerland, Taiwan, and other countries excelling and outperforming the United States on this very dimension. Moreover, there is ample data that quality in the United States is—to put it charitably—inconsistent; it ranks poorly in many areas amenable to healthcare interventions, such as infant and maternal mortality. As a result, US healthcare is not in the top 10 in many dimensions.*[2]

This section will explore the factors influencing US healthcare, including economic, legal, and administrative features.

Economic

From an economic standpoint, three things about the US healthcare system should be discussed: cost, availability, and sustainability. Simply put, how much does it cost, whom does it cover now, and can it continue to cover us in the future? The US pays more for healthcare than any other country by a significant amount, and it is not just the dollar amount.[3] If it was that, we could argue that everything is more expensive in the US, so why should healthcare be any different? Nevertheless, it is also high based on our gross domestic product (GDP) percentage and continues to rise. If everything is expensive here, then the percentage of GDP should be flat, but it is not, and it is getting worse. US health spending is by far the highest globally when expressed as a percentage of GDP or per capita income. In 2016, US healthcare spending was $3.4 trillion, which is 18.1% of the US GDP or $10,700 per capita.[4] That outrageous price is predicted to reach 20% by 2025, with no other nation coming close to that percentage of GDP for healthcare.[5] Switzerland is the next country on the list for total spending, with 12.2% of GDP and $9700 per capita. At the other end of the spectrum, China pays 6.2% of its GDP for healthcare or $960 per capita.[6]

Furthermore, what do we get for all this money? Unfortunately, the US still does not have universal healthcare, which separates us from most industrial countries. About 10% of Americans are not currently covered.[7] While this percentage is lower than the 25% uninsured before Medicare and Medicaid and the 16% uninsured before enacting the Affordable Care Act, the United States remains unique among other industrialized countries by having a sizable minority of individuals who lack insurance for basic healthcare needs. Although access to medical treatment in the United States is more equitable than it would be in a purely competitive market economy, it is less fair than in all other high-income nations. Thus, 22.3% of the US population reported missing a medical consultation because of cost, compared to a mean of 9.4% for ten other high-income countries studied.[8] Also, the US has the least financial protection for families with children. Private health insurance premiums for such families are usually not subsidized, placing an enormous burden on families. Frequently, families have out-of-pocket expenditures for deductibles and co-pays for tertiary-level pediatric care.[9]

The third item regarding the US healthcare system is whether or not it is sustainable. The United States pays the most and still has many uninsured citizens compared to other countries. Nevertheless, it still may not have enough money to stay afloat at current spending levels. What is not usually realized is that roughly half of all US health spending runs directly through the government under Medicare, Medicaid, Tricare for the military, VA care, and public health. Therefore, the US health system ceased to be mainly privately funded long ago.[10]

Since it began in 1965, Medicare has provided such a safety net in the form of a single-payer, national health insurance program for Americans over 65. In 2016, Medicare comprised 15% of the federal budget— $678.7 billion—and covered 56.8 million Americans (roughly 18%). Although healthcare costs remain a significant financial strain on elderly patients and disabled people, lawmakers have sought to alleviate that burden through a series of Medicare programs. These benefit programs are paid out of trusts primarily funded by general tax revenue, payroll taxes, and premiums associated with Medicare plans.[11] Clearly, Medicare is an enormous benefit to the population segment that needs healthcare the most. Nevertheless, unfortunately, good intentions will not be enough to keep Medicare solvent.[12]

Let us look more deeply at how the government pays for Medicare. Two separate trusts fund Medicare: the Hospital Insurance (HI) trust fund and the Supplementary Medical Insurance (SMI) trust fund. The SMI trust fund covers Parts B and D of Medicare. Part B covers physicians, outpatient hospital treatment, and home health services, while Part D covers prescription drugs. The Board of Trustees project will remain financially balanced for the foreseeable future. That is the good news. However, the HI trust fund is estimated to be depleted by 2029, and that covers Part A of Medicare, which helps pay for costs associated with hospital stays, home health services post-hospital discharge, skilled nursing facilities, and hospice care. Therefore, the Medicare section pays for the care of the sickest individuals who will be bankrupt in less than a decade.[13]

Why is this occurring? Mainly because the HI is based on workers' contributions. Because of the aging baby-boom generation, fewer workers per retiree will contribute to the Medicare Hospital Insurance Trust Fund in the coming decades. Projected growth in Medicare expenditures will deplete the reserves in this fund in the coming decade unless some action is taken to increase contributions (raising employee withhold amount) or reduce the draw from the fund(cutting services,) both of which are vastly unpopular.[14] The very nature of the funding of Part A does not have a clear plan to adjust to this changing demographic, which is a significant cause for alarm. Part A, or the HI trust fund (whose total revenue in 2016 was $290.8 billion), as previously stated, is funded primarily by payroll taxes (87.2% of total HI trust fund revenue). It is also supported by interest on trust assets (2.6%), taxation on social security benefits (8%), premiums (1.1%), and general revenue, which is money from the US Treasury (4%),[15] assets (2.6%), taxation on social security benefits (8%), premiums (1.1%), and general revenue, which is money from the US Treasury, (4%).[16] Because many Part A factors— such as future wages, labor participation rates, and death rates—are more difficult to predict many years in advance, budgeting Part A out of the general revenue is less practicable. Furthermore, tax rates on employees and employers are not adjusted annually to meet the trust fund's demands.[17]

So let us assume that US citizens wake up one morning and realize that we are already spending too much on healthcare, and then the only solution is to cut spending. Of course, this decision will be difficult since, for one thing, coverage for all Americans still does not exist. In addition, not all spending is the same. Therefore, identifying and protecting expenditures in which dollars should not be cut (e.g., prevention, immunizations, ensuring equity) is an integral part of that roadmap, along with efforts to continue to create universal coverage.[18] So, where will these cuts be made? The following section will look at one possible area where the United States also leads the world (and not in a good way!).

Legal

There is an urgent need to bring US healthcare costs down to a sustainable range for both public and private payers. Existing programs to cut costs often include reductions in payment levels, benefit structures, and eligibility. A better strategy would reduce waste, not value-added care.[19] One item on the list of things to cut would be the high cost of malpractice insurance and its direct and indirect costs on total US healthcare spending. According to a 2008 Manhattan Institute's Center for Legal Policy report, US litigation expenses are at least twice those in other developed countries. Experts have estimated US medical liability claims to be roughly 10% of all tort litigation, with at least half of related expenses going to legal costs rather than compensating patients.[20] Some experts have argued that high malpractice expenses are a significant driver of prices in the US system. However, academic research has failed to support this argument. For example, Mello et al. (2010) conclude, "Overall annual medical liability system costs, including defensive medicine, are estimated to be $55.6 billion in 2008 dollars or 2.4% of total healthcare spending."[21] Though not trivial, such figures can explain only a tiny fraction of the US and other countries' cost differences.[22]

Nevertheless, the practice of medicine has changed dramatically in the past decade. Therefore, the discussion of the cost of our medical liability system should also be updated. Previously, independent physicians provided medical care; hospitals and healthcare systems generally had limited liability, and negligence was assessed on an individual physician level.[23] In contrast, contemporary medical care occurs in a complex environment with multiple physicians within more extensive healthcare organizations. Recognizing that our current system does a poor job of promoting physicians' or patients' interests, some organizations are looking at malpractice reform to address system inefficiencies. These changes could neutralize the "deny and defend" stance that impairs patient-physician communication, discourages reporting medical errors, adapts to the changing landscape of medicine centered on patient outcomes, and requires collective accountability.[24] Many physicians would welcome the change in handling medical liability, although some would complain about the loss of autonomy. However, whether this would lead to significant healthcare savings is still unclear. The costs of adjudicating malpractice claims and payouts and the premiums from insuring against these costs are substantial. However, the medical malpractice tort system's direct costs likely pale compared to the indirect costs of defensive medicine.[25]

Defensive medicine is the practice of using excessive tests and treatments to reduce a healthcare provider's risk of malpractice suits, even when it is felt that these items will most likely not help.[26] This activity is widely believed to exist throughout American healthcare due to fears of malpractice litigation. It is thought to be an enormous waste of healthcare dollars.[27] One study from the UK stated that the US spends a staggering 2% of GDP on diagnostics, compared to only 0.54% in the UK, and similarly low values in other advanced economies such as France and Germany. They reasoned that this is caused by the high cost of medical education, which makes the physician wage much higher than the alternative (UK physician wages), and the high level of malpractice risk. These factors incentivize physicians to order excessive diagnostics to reduce malpractice risk.[28] Would lowering physician's salaries in the US really decrease the number of tests ordered and make them less worried about losing their careers? However, reducing the number of diagnostics to 1% of GDP would save over 200 billion dollars, which is significant!

Allowing the fear of litigation to be a reason for ordering more tests, procedures, and treatment is very problematic; however, changing the US's medical litigation system may fail to fix that. The survey, which had a 62% response rate, revealed that physicians with fewer than five years of practice had a much higher subjective fear of malpractice litigation than those with more than five years of practice experience, suggesting more experienced physicians had less fear of malpractice suits. The authors found that fear of malpractice did not significantly change in response to malpractice reforms. Overall, whether a state was a riskier malpractice environment or had higher malpractice insurance premiums did not considerably affect the subjective fear of malpractice experienced by that state's physicians.[29]

Although needed for many reasons, malpractice reform is not likely to lower costs significantly, at least in the short run. Significant tort reform has occurred in the last two decades, a sign of progress. It is encouraging to see changes focusing more on patient safety and outcomes and less on disciplinary issues. Finally, the reason for and the cost of "defensive medication" was explored. In this chapter, the focus was on the financial cost of this type of practice. However, there are non-financial costs as well. These practices cause damage to patients in ways that cannot be easily measured just based on price. There is the time involved, sometimes involving hospital stays. Safety issues concern the morbidity and mortality of unneeded invasive procedures. Finally, these unneeded diagnostics are anxiety-provoking to patients and their families.[30]

Administrative

The former president of Egypt, Gamal Abdel Nasser, once said this about the US, "The genius of you Americans is that you never make clear-cut stupid moves, only complicated stupid moves, which make the rest of us wonder at the possibility that we might be missing something."[31] This statement is harsh but also true. Two facts about the US healthcare system cannot be disputed: it is expensive and complicated. As a percentage of GDP or per capita income, US health spending is by far the highest globally, even though the US population is among the youngest among the developed nations.[32] In 2016, total national health spending in the United States amounted to $3.4 trillion, a claim of 18.1% of the US GDP, which then was $18.5 trillion. That claim is projected to reach 20% by 2025. No nation even comes close to ceding that large a slice of its GDP to its healthcare sector. Compared with other high-income countries, the US is first in healthcare spending but last in life expectancy, infant mortality, and other healthcare aims.[33] Moreover, to add even more shame, the US spends more on administrative costs than any other country, accounting for 25–30% of the total healthcare budget.[34] This section will look at these problems, how we got there, and possibly what can be done to reverse this unhealthy condition.

US hospitals spend 25.3% on administrative costs, and that percentage continues to rise. The next highest was the Netherlands (19.8%) and England (15.5%). Scotland and Canada, whose single-payer systems pay hospitals global operating budgets with separate grants for capital, had the lowest administrative costs.[35] Costs were intermediate in France and Germany (which bill per patient but pay separately for capital projects) and Wales. Reducing the US per capita spending for hospital administration to Scottish or Canadian levels would have saved more than $150 billion in 2011.[36]

Put another way, a Commonwealth Fund comparison of health insurance administrative costs showed that the US spent $737 per capita on administration, compared to $94 per capita in the median OECD country. The next-highest-spending country after the US (Switzerland) had administrative costs of only $280.[37] So, not only is the US spending more on healthcare than anyone else, but it is also spending it on items that do not directly affect patient care. So what does this money purchase?

Much of the expense is mandated by the current reimbursement system, which requires that charges for each of the 1.6 billion hospital admissions and physician visits each year be attributed to a specific patient. Additional costs result from efforts by hospitals and insurers to gain financially by identifying and marketing lucrative services.[38] This practice is what is called the fee-for-service (FFS) system. When a patient is hospitalized, everything (and I mean everything!) is billed to their insurance company separately. Think of going to a restaurant and ordering a nice meal. Under the FFS, you would be billed separately for each individual ingredient in the meal, plus separate fees for preparing it, cooking it, plating it, serving it, removing it when you are finished, cleaning it up, etc. This practice creates a complex billing, coding, and documenting system for maximum reimbursement from insurers, thus adding to the high administrative costs that plague the system. The focus on micromanagement has obscured the fundamentally inefficient structure required to implement such policies.[39]

The United States is in a crisis as it grapples with how to pay for healthcare. FFS, the most common billing practice, is commonly identified as the single biggest hurdle to improving healthcare; it rewards the quantity but not the quality of healthcare.[40] More nonclinical workers are needed to maintain this system. Applying data from the Bureau of Labor Statistics (BLS) and the American Medical Association, from 1990 to 2012, the number of workers in the US health system grew by nearly 75%. Almost 95% of this growth was in non-physician employees. Based on BLS median wages, this equates to $823,000 in labor costs per physician.[41] Billing and insurance-related activities account for 62% of US administrative costs.[42] Billing costs are expensive in the US; for example, in a primary care practice, these services cost nearly four times more than similar services in Canada.[43]

Besides the cost, the other downside of hospital systems' growing administrative costs is that it perpetuates bad behavior. Increasingly, administrators are focused on the profit motive rather than improving the healthcare for the community they serve. This activity concerns how insurers pay the hospitals, causing a destructive symbiotic relationship between hospital administration and payers. The way hospitals are reimbursed is insidious. It rewards bad behavior and, in some ways, expects it from hospital leaders. Administrators are often and sometimes only judged by their ability to increase revenue and profitability. This solitary emphasis has the damaging effect of suppressing other valuable skills and the better angels of their nature.[44]

The US healthcare system's administrative structure is increasingly less efficient than Canada's national health program.[45] Current health policies to improve care efficiency have imposed substantial new bureaucratic costs and burdens.[46] So, how do hospitals stay profitable? Hospitals win the profit game by raising prices, not improving care. Praiseworthy clinical community services that provide care for more Medicaid or uninsured patients are undesirable for hospitals because they can drain hospital resources. So-called "losers" care for a disproportionate share of publicly insured patients or have the misfortune of being in rural America. As a result, public hospitals lagged, while not-for-profits grew their profits even faster than for-profits. Becoming part of an extensive hospital system, or "chaining up," was a winning strategy, presumably because it increased hospitals' ability to negotiate with insurers, allowing them to demand higher prices. One could, therefore, conclude that the bureaucracy created a need for more bureaucracy.[47] Regarding increasing efficiency, doctors, patients, and nurses perform before an enlarging audience of utilization reviewers, efficiency experts, and cost managers. A cynic viewing the uninflected curve of rising healthcare spending might wonder whether the cost-containment experts cost more than they contain; one is reminded of the Chinese proverb, "There is no use going to bed early to save candles if the result is twins."[48]

Putting doctors, patients, and nurses in a "spectator" position concerning healthcare has been shown to have a harmful effect. In too many hospitals, the administration is monopolized by non-clinicians. Other factors include the ongoing consolidation of hospital systems, with ever-more administrative layers, and the rapidly growing number of employed non-physicians.[49] In addition, There was a strong association between leadership quality and burnout and the satisfaction level of individual physicians. Organizational factors that impact physician well-being include the efficiency of the practice environment, the level of flexibility/autonomy provided to physicians, and workload expectations. Extensive research indicates that physicians' well-being and professional satisfaction profoundly affect the quality of care and patient adherence to treatment recommendations and medical care.[50] These effects on quality of care, combined with the impact of satisfaction and burnout on turnover and associated costs, underscore the critical importance of physician satisfaction and burnout to healthcare organizations' long-term success.[51]

A physician who identifies as burned out "is angry, irritable, impatient, has increased absenteeism, decreased productivity and decreased quality of care." The most significant incidence of burnout (50%) was among physicians 45–54 years old, in which productivity should be at its highest and practices should be economically stable. When the study was repeated in 2019, the findings had not significantly changed, with a 44% "feeling burned out" rate and an alarming 14% report of suicidal thoughts. Compared with doctoral-level professionals in other fields, physicians work more extended hours, are less satisfied with their work–life balance, and experience burnout symptoms at significantly higher rates.[52] An economic analysis shows that about $4.6 billion in costs are attributable to burnout each year in the United States.[53] At an organizational level, $7600 per employed physician annually is associated with burnout-associated outcomes such as turnover and reduced clinical hours.[54]

Traditionally, the case for alleviating physician burnout has been made primarily on ethical grounds. However, evidence now shows a significant cost impact as well. Healthcare administration has grown significantly over the past several decades, focusing on increasing revenues and improving efficiency. However, analyses show that despite the massive increase in administrative costs, it fails at both tasks. Further studies also show that the rise of administrative burden on healthcare systems can also harm the providers that the system needs.

DESIGNATED ORGANIZATIONAL ELEMENTS

This section will examine the inefficiencies associated with high costs in healthcare systems, insurance, and pharmaceutical companies. Most of these costs are based on our current FFS billing system and the need to keep these entities profitable. Profit-seeking, as a single goal, does not just weaken efficiency and equity; it also advances corruption. For-profit hospitals have frequently been charged with some terrible activities, paying billions to resolve fraud and abuse allegations. However, the waning significance of ethical issues for non-profit and public hospital leaders has an even more substantial impact because they control 80% of local hospitals and almost all university medical centers.[55] Insurance companies also pay a high price to counteract hospital systems' aggressive billing practices. Considering the healthcare system and the insurance company's overuse of funds for administration services and their growing co-dependency on each other, methods that would cut costs, simplify, and make these systems more efficient need to be examined. Finally, the role of pharmaceutical companies concerning healthcare costs and sustainability needs to be studied.

When it comes to drug prices and drug price regulations, the United States is remarkable, but in the wrong way. With less than 4.5% of the world's population, the United States accounts for over 40% of all drug expenditures.[56] Our healthcare system accounts for by far the most significant portion of the nearly one trillion worldwide annual pharmaceutical spending. Prescription drug spending has become the fastest-growing component of total health spending in the United States.[57]

Healthcare Systems

Even though it is common knowledge that the US spends more on healthcare than anyone else, why this occurs is unknown. The conventional wisdom is that the commonly used fee-for-service system is the main reason for uncertainty and underinvestment in the items that could prevent healthcare waste and poor outcomes. Previous findings have found that the US underinvests in supportive social programs. However, other data suggest that higher prices, especially for medications, are also to blame for the high cost of healthcare.[58]

However, there have been some helpful changes in US healthcare as well. The rise of computer technology and artificial intelligence has enhanced healthcare. These breakthroughs have partly led healthcare to change from "passive and hospital-centric to preventative and personalized and from disease-centric to health-centric."[59] There has also been a trend in the US for end-of-life care to be less hospital-centric.[60] For example, between 82.6% and 88.7% of patients who died in the last six months were hospitalized in Belgium, Canada, England, and Norway, while less than 77% were hospitalized in the US. During this time, the US had the fewest mean per capita hospital days at 10.7 while Belgium had 27.7 and Norway had 24.8 per capita hospital days.[61]

However, despite this low hospital rate for most dying patients, 40.3% of US cancer patients were admitted to the ICU in the last six months of life compared with less than 18% in other reporting countries. Likewise, the average length of stay in the ICU in the US was 3.6 days, while it was less than 1.5 days in other reporting countries.[62] 40.3% of US cancer patients had an ICU admission in the last 180 days compared with less than 18% in other reporting countries.

Although the prevalence and price of critical illness are increasing in the United States, there is a focus both on limiting the rising costs of healthcare and improving the quality of end-of-life care. Over 25% of all US healthcare costs are spent in the last year of a person's life, and about 20% of these patients will die in the intensive care unit (ICU).[63] However, although hospice has consistently demonstrated a superior ability to manage symptoms, reduce costs, and maintain high satisfaction levels, concerns about underutilization remain. In 2015, only 46% of US deaths involved hospice.[64]

The US spends 32% of its healthcare budget on hospital care. The *2015 Comparative Price Report,* published by the International Federation of Health Plans, examines hospital prices by country. According to the report, charges per day for a medical admission were as follows at the research time: Spain, $424; South Africa, $631; Australia, $765; New Zealand, $2142; Switzerland, $4781. The United States topped them all at an alarming $5220![65]

Acute care surgery (ACS) patients comprise 20% of the inpatient population. However, 25% of total inpatient costs in the US ACS include Trauma, Surgical Critical Care, and Emergency General Surgery (EGS), including both operative and non-operative conditions. In addition to being costly, they have higher healthcare utilization and worse outcomes. Therefore, there is an opportunity to improve the clinical trajectory for ACS patients, affecting the overall US healthcare costs. Emergency general surgery (EGS) comprises 70–80% of ACS activities and 70% of ACS costs; the most significant impact may be improved care for the EGS population.[66] Which hospitals perform the surgery should be considered and compared to similar hospitals to identify possible overutilization tendencies.

Large hospital systems that have taken on smaller hospitals can use shared knowledge and organized cooperative improvement strategies to assist poorly performing hospitals in becoming better-performing "Honor Roll" hospitals. Indeed, the practices of high-performing partners, such as training staff to identify and adequately manage complications, should be shared with the other hospitals. Networks can also use this strategy to recommend investments in personnel and resources to increase safety and reduce variation across their member hospitals. Greater attention to these details may help hospitals improve the clinical potential of their associated hospitals and achieve better quality with the consolidations.[67]

The amount of surgery and what type also needs scrutiny? Compared to other countries, the US has higher than average levels of some surgeries, such as coronary artery bypass procedures, at 79 per 100,000 compared with about 54 per 100,000 in similar countries. Likewise, there are higher than average knee replacements at 226 per 100,000 population compared to 163 and coronary angioplasties at 248 per 100,000 population compared with 217 in other countries.[68] However, obesity in the United States is a critical problem that may also contribute to the higher rate of these specific procedures.

Despite increased hospitalizations due to surgical procedures, the US's inpatient utilization is comparable with other countries studied. The number of US hospital discharges, at 125 per 1,000 population per year, was just below half of the distribution (ranging from 84 per 1,000 in Canada to 255 per 1,000 in Germany, with a mean of 150 per 1,000 in all 11 countries). When specific diagnoses were studied, the numbers were also favorable. For example, acute myocardial infarction had a rate of 192 per 100,000 population compared with a mean of 190 for other studied countries. Likewise, pneumonia 365 compared with 352 and chronic obstructive pulmonary disease 230 compared with 206, rated similarly to the standards of all 11 countries. With discharges for mental and behavioral conditions, the US was below the mean of all 11 countries at 679 per 100,000 compared with a mean of 736 per 100,000 population.[69] Therefore, the high cost of hospitalization in the US cannot be attributed to a high admission rate.

The higher hospitalization costs in the US are also evidently not due to more extended stays. The average length of stay in seven European countries was 8.1 days, whereas, in the United States, it was 6.1. What should be noted is the enormous variation in charges among hospitals in the United States. For example, though the average total cost (hospital and physician) for an appendectomy was $15,930, the 25th percentile was $9332, and the 95th was an incredible $33,250—and this is for a simple procedure generally requiring no particular expertise. For a total knee replacement, the 25th percentile charge was $18,577, and the 95th charge was $55,579. For coronary artery bypass grafting, the 25th percentile charge was $50,859, and the 95th was $161,148.[70]

Why this vast variation? The McKinsey Global Institute (2008) attributed the "excess" costs to the "judgment-based nature of physician care." (Some doctors order more tests than others).[71] Other factors include technological innovation that drives prices higher rather than lower and demand growth that appears to be due to greater supply availability. (The more we have, the harder we try to sell it!) Add to this the relatively price-insensitive patients with limited out-of-pocket costs. The excessive costs produced by these factors "ripple through the supply chain" because payers are " unwilling or unable to push back" on price increases. While insurers and employers ostensibly negotiate prices on behalf of consumers, they may not always have the incentive to get the best deal, a health economist told Bloomberg News, because "They're negotiating with somebody else's money."[72] So, as long as the patients are not complaining and the hospital and insurance administrators are happy, there is little incentive to lower costs. Transparency is essential here. Studies show that clients are still interested in total costs, even if their out-of-pocket costs are unaffected.[73] Poor-performing and expensive hospitals need further scrutiny for the US healthcare system to survive.

Finally, what happens outside the hospital can also impact hospital costs. Primary care and outpatient services can decrease inpatient utilization. A strong relationship exists between higher levels of physician-level continuity, a core principle of primary care, and lower total healthcare costs and hospitalizations. Higher continuity, measured at the patient, was significantly associated with reducing emergency care for elderly patients.[74] "Usual care" for people with advanced illness in the United States is often episodic, crisis-driven, and hospital-based.[75] High-impact primary care practices that include continuity and comprehensiveness could simultaneously serve as quality and resource use standards, given their demonstrated relationship to substantial cost/utilization reductions.[76] Long-term care reform and community-based support can also impact hospital utilization.

Residential programs use "aging in place" programs where elderly residents can remain in one dwelling even as their care needs increase. Innovative, "non-institutional," homelike settings still need to be developed. The extension of community-based care and short-term respite care services for developing community-based long-term care still relies on some hospital-based care to assist it.[77] Our healthcare system should be adept at providing care to elderly patients in multiple settings, including one's own home or nursing home, that enables a patient's choices to be respected. For example, a nursing home resident may want some measures to prolong life and increase comfort but not go to the emergency department or hospital. This plan can only be honored if the facility can provide these services.[78]

In conclusion, hospitalizations account for almost a third of the United States Healthcare costs. However, the admission rate and length of stay are comparable, if not lower, than in many countries.[79] The surgical rate may be slightly higher, but the variability of a procedure's costs is excessive, as is the success rate.[80] There exists an opportunity for improvement to correct this inconsistency. Primary care must also be promoted, as this type of care is essential for an affordable and quality healthcare system.[81] Finally, end-of-life and long-term care need better coordination. The US system has an excess of ICU admissions for cancer patients and those with six months or less to live. 25% of the total cost is spent on patients in their final year of life. Hospice services could help lower these costs while providing better care for the dying.[82]

Insurance Companies

Insurance coverage for healthcare in the United States is a complex system that includes employer-sponsored private insurance, Medicare, Medicaid, Affordable Care Act (ACA) based plans, the Children's Health Insurance Programs (CHIP), the Veteran's Administration (VA), the Indian Health Service (IHS), Tricare (for military families), and multiple programs to cover other individuals not covered by different plans. However, approximately 10% of the population remains uninsured.[83] As stated in the previous section, the rise in hospital administrators is due, at least in part, to an attempt to maximize insurance reimbursement.[84] However, the insurance companies themselves also have high operating costs. According to a paper by America's Health Insurance Plans (AHIP), private health insurers, on average, take a loss of about 17.8% of the insurance payments for "operating costs," which means marketing and administration. Another 2.7% goes to profits. That cost was as high as 45% pre-Obamacare (ACA) for smaller insurers selling policies in the (nongroup) market for individually purchased insurance.[85]

Many would argue that the only way to solve this dilemma is for the US to convert to a single-payer system. Examples of a radical restructuring of US healthcare include a government-sponsored, single-payer system of universal coverage with generous benefits; a system of means-tested tax credits providing health insurance premium support, with an expanded emphasis on high-deductible health plans and associated health savings accounts; or implementation of a national health system of universal coverage (whether single-payer or insurance-based) modeled after another country.[86] However, Germany does not have a single-payer system, and it does pretty well. Statutory Health Insurance (SHI) covers approximately 87% of the population, including privately employed workers and their dependents, the unemployed, and retired workers. The SHI is not a single-payer system; patients are covered by over 100 sickness funds, with the five largest covering 33 million members or 47% of the SHI market. Private health insurance covers about 11% of the population. Overall, the system is self-governed by the payers, hospitals, physicians, and patients. There is a free choice among hospitals and physicians with excellent access and low co-pays with this system. Although many sickness funds are associated with inefficiencies, their cost is 11.5% of GDP or $6200 per capita compared to 17.9% or $10,700 for the US.[87]

So, it is possible to keep our current system if we simplify it and make it more efficient. Most billing and insurance-related (BIR) administrative costs in the United States are due to the claims-based health insurance transactions that have become the backbone of our healthcare industry. Whether the insurer is a private health insurance company or a government program, detailed information is needed to satisfy their interest in ensuring that the service for which a payment is requested is medically necessary and that the codes used for billing purposes are justified by clinical documentation. In addition, Medicare and Medicaid are increasingly being served by Medicare Advantage and Medicaid Managed Care (i.e., by private insurers). While these insurers receive capitated payments from the government, they generally contract medical services (physician and hospital) on a fee-for-service basis. Thus, the insurance-based, fee-for-service payment structure and associated BIR administrative costs are becoming even more entrenched.[88] So, even a single-payer government-based system may not necessarily solve the complexity problem.

If fee-for-service is the problem, alternative payment systems must be implemented. As stated previously in this book, if restaurants used the fee-for-service model, the billing would be ridiculous. For almost all types of products and services, customers pay a single amount for the whole package that meets their needs. For example, you purchase a meal at a restaurant and decide if you want appetizers, drinks, or desserts. These items have a single cost, and the billing is relatively simple and straightforward.

In limited cases like organ transplantation, bundled payments have existed in healthcare.[89] They are commonly seen for procedures such as plastic surgery, Lasik eye surgery, and in vitro fertilization that patients pay for directly. Rather than the complicated and inefficient system that we have today of billing for every item separately, a bundled payment system would emphasize achieving the best patient outcomes at a low cost. This action could unleash a new kind of competition that improves patients' value, informs and increases patient choice, reshapes provider strategy, lowers system cost, and alters industry structure for the better.[90]

The current system also creates an atmosphere that frustrates physicians, nurses, and patients. The value system that most healthcare professionals aspire to continues to erode and is being replaced by an inefficient system that feeds on its own inefficiency.[91] Alternative payment systems such as bundled payments are a step in the right direction, along with creative ways to fund hospitals. Change will be difficult as many have profited from the status quo.[92] However, change needs to occur as our current healthcare system will collapse under its own weight unless a change occurs.

Pharmaceuticals Companies

The US spends just under 500 billion on drugs annually, constituting approximately 17% of US healthcare spending. A total of 10% of healthcare spending is for purchasing drugs in retail pharmacies, and the other 7% is for medications administered in hospitals, nursing homes, or physicians' offices. This cost is over $14.00 per capita for prescription drugs, more than twice the per capita spending in most European countries. This high drug spending results from high drug prices, not higher American drug use. Approximately 90% of all prescriptions in the United States are for generic drugs, but they account for only 26% of drug costs. This fact represents a significant increase in generic use since Medicare began paying for drugs in 2006. The use of generic medications is significantly higher in the US than in almost any other developed country.[93]

There are stark differences in drug expenses that are not attributable to the number of drugs that Americans consume.[94] Americans are charged much higher prices for a given medication than people of other developed countries. One reason is that the US is the only country that allows drug companies to set prices, which is a pro-free market. Still, it will enable monopolies through patents and marketing exclusivity, which goes against the free market.[95] Furthermore, drug manufacturers in recent years have been able to raise prices substantially, even for long-established generic products.[96]

The rising cost of prescription drugs in the US puts an enormous strain on public and family pocketbooks. A national poll of more than 1,200 adults found that the costs of prescription drugs should be the primary concern of the President and Congress, including "making sure that high-cost drugs are affordable to those who need them" and "government action to lower prescription drug prices." In particular, 77% of adults believe that "making sure that high-cost drugs for chronic conditions, such as HIV, hepatitis, mental illness, and cancer, are affordable to those who need them" is a top priority.[97]

A study by the Department of Health and Human Services said that about 10% of the increase in drug spending in recent years was due to population growth.

Furthermore, 30% was due to increased prescriptions per person, 30% to inflation in the general economy, and 30% to price increases for drugs or changes in drug compositions that led to higher prices. This last 30%, therefore, was above the 30% already allotted for inflation. In addition, specialty drugs, such as many newer drugs for conditions such as multiple sclerosis, rheumatoid arthritis, and cancer, were significant contributors to the growth in prescription drug spending, rising from $14.5 billion in 2009 to $27.1 billion in 2015, giving an average annual growth rate of 11.0%, the report said.[98]

An outdated and complicated distribution system is a factor in this country's high cost of medicines. Insurance companies utilize prescription benefits managers or PBMs to help set drug prices. According to his book, *Priced Out: The Economic and Ethical Costs of American Healthcare,* Reinhardt states:

> *Although PBMs claim to drive "tough" bargains with drug manufacturers and retail pharmacies over prescription drug prices, they seem to have only a modest capacity to do so. First, as stated previously, Americans' drug prices are the highest globally. Second, PBMs seem unable to challenge the huge annual price increases for existing drugs that drug companies routinely manage to impose on them, even generic drugs. For example, it was widely reported that Pfizer had raised prices on ninety-one existing drugs by an average of 20 percent since the beginning of 2017. There is a good chance that the PBMs will accept and pay such increases.*[99]

Premium-cost drugs, such as those for rheumatologic diseases and cancer, need further scrutiny. Under the Medicare program, certain specialists and outpatient departments are compensated by Medicare for the drugs they provide to their patients at the average sales price (ASP) *plus* a 6% markup to administer the drugs. It would seem more sensible for Medicare to reimburse the administration of these medications based on the procedure's complexity and not the medication's cost. With some drugs costing more than $100,000 a year, this 6% markup clearly provides a strong financial incentive for physicians to favor expensive medicines. One would hope that most physicians would be unaffected by this substantial financial incentive in their clinical decisions.[100]

Often, these drugs are used based on Clinical Practice Guidelines (CPGs.) However, those who write the CPGs may have undeclared payments from the industry, including those from pharmaceutical companies that market the high-cost medications recommended in those CPGs. Unfortunately, guidelines related to these medications are threatened by authors having financial conflicts of interest since pharmaceutical companies spend a lot of money marketing their top products. Promoting these medications may lead to physician payments, which have been shown to affect their choice of recommending these drugs.[101]

The cost of these drugs is substantial. Research shows that antineoplastic expenditures in the United States had increased consistently from $26.8 billion in 2011 to $42.1 billion in 2016. More recent increases were even more significant, with an average annual rise of 13.7% compared with the previous year. Since 2011, total drug expenditures (including antineoplastics and all other drugs) across the United States have increased from $328.4 billion (in 2011) to $448.2 billion (in 2016). Antineoplastic expenditures represented 7% of US drug expenditures in 2011 and increased to 9.4% in 2016.[102]

A specific cancer type can be studied to illustrate these concerns. Acute myeloid leukemia (AML) is the most commonly seen hematologic malignancy in adults. The treatment for AML is based on those who can tolerate standard cytarabine and daunorubicin, or "7+3" chemotherapy, and those who cannot, typically older or with significant comorbidities. The minimum cost was $1,662.50 for standard 7 + 3 chemotherapy. For salvage therapy indicated for those who failed or could not tolerate standard treatment, the maximum cost for an average regimen of Enasidenib is estimated to be around $120,131 or 75 times higher. As prices for salvage therapies intended for patients remain high, their cost-effectiveness remains uncertain. Therefore, how well a regimen works and how much it costs should be central to these complicated and often emotional discussions.[103]

How the US compares to other countries also needs to be studied. Across all eligible medicines, average treatment costs were lowest in France and Australia and highest in the UK and the US. There was no surprise there, but the drugs' prices are alarming. Compared with Australia, France, and the UK, cancer medicines were, on average, between 1.2 and 1.9 times more expensive in the US, where the average total per-patient cost for treatment was $68,255.17.

Costs for new cancer medicines are high and, at best, only weakly associated with clinical benefits. The strength of this relationship nevertheless varied across countries. Some new cancer drugs—particularly in the US—may be neither affordable nor clinically beneficial over existing treatments. While all countries can benefit from strategies that more robustly align price with therapeutic benefit in cancer drugs, the US stands out in its opportunity to improve both affordability and value in cancer drug treatment. Unfortunately, this sometimes means using new and expensive medicines that lack apparent benefit over older, less expensive ones just to gain more knowledge. US payers and patients consistently pay more for recently licensed cancer drugs than in other countries, yet do so without necessarily leading to more significant health benefits.

While all countries share the opportunity to improve value-for-money in cancer drug spending, the US may benefit the most from a re-imagined approach to drug pricing. As the government seeks to contain drug costs while improving patient outcomes, other countries may offer lessons on ensuring affordability and value for money in oncology.[104] The US not only tends to use these drugs more frequently but may pay almost twice as much for the drugs as compared to other countries, a double-whammy to the healthcare budget.

Expensive medications for other diseases follow a similar pattern. First-generation disease-modifying treatments, or DMTs, used for rheumatologic diseases originally costing $8,000 to $11,000, now cost about $60,000 annually. Costs for these medications have risen at rates 5 to 7 times higher annually than overall prescription drug inflation. Newer DMTs frequently entered the market with a 25–60% higher cost than existing DMTs. Not surprisingly, DMT costs in the US are 2 to 3 times higher than in comparable countries.[105]

To cut costs, groups such as the American Society of Clinical Oncology (ASCO), Memorial Sloan Kettering Cancer Center, and the Institute for Clinical and Economic Review developed frameworks to help patients, manufacturers, providers, and payers assess the value of treatments. However, there are many inherent complexities in determining the value of treatments, including, but not limited to, an absence of any distinct theoretical basis to measure value and any empirical analyses regarding how stakeholders should make decisions based on these value metrics.[106] These decisions are complicated. It needs to calculate life expectancy with treatment and quality of life. Nevertheless, value-based guidelines, free from pharmaceutical bias, are needed.

The high cost of pharmaceuticals in the US is alarming. Most scholars agree that some regulations for pharmaceutical companies need to be implemented. America cannot continue to pay for medications at a significantly higher rate than other countries. The actual value of neoplastic and other costly drugs must be determined. This task's researchers must not be biased by the pharmaceutical companies or be compromised by other special interest groups. Among researchers, their "better angels" must come forward.

CONCLUSION

The American Health System is in dire need of change! It is expensive, lacks quality by multiple metrics, and is in real jeopardy of becoming bankrupt this decade unless significant changes are made. This chapter looked at the economics involved in delineating this dilemma. Solving the puzzle will be no easy task.

Increasing spending is obviously not the best solution, but cutting costs is also problematic, given the need to extend coverage and improve outcomes.

In 1991, the Lincoln Town Car's MSRP was $34,207 for the high-end "Cartier" trim. Although expensive, that was not the problem even by today's standards. The complaints were because it was a disappointing automobile compared to its German and British competitors.[107] Continuing with this analogy for healthcare, one must not get too overwhelmed by the cost alone. In the 1990s, the *value equation* was the topic of many healthcare discussions. It stated that value was equal to price over quality. Because "value is defined as outcomes relative to costs, it encompasses efficiency. Cost reduction without regard to the outcomes achieved is dangerous and self-defeating, leading to false 'savings' and potentially limiting effective care."[108] The gaps in US healthcare (lack of coverage, access, choice, complexity, quality) must also be considered critically.

At one time, entering the medical profession, especially in the US, had something to do with pride and indicated that the person was among the best and brightest. Unfortunately, our healthcare industry, like the American automobile industry, has significantly declined. When discussing healthcare in the US, one can use the exact phrase to describe an outdated automobile, "depressingly cynical debasing of the American Dream it represented." Fixing the health system will likewise require the same vision and innovation that the American automobile industry once had.

Take-Home Points

- The US spends more than any other country on healthcare in terms of the dollar amount and percentage of GDP, and there are still concerns about availability and sustainability.
- US litigation expenses are at least twice those in other developed countries. Experts have estimated US medical liability claims to be roughly 10% of all tort litigation, with at least half of related expenses going to legal costs rather than compensating patients.
- The US also spends the highest on administrative costs at 23.5% compared to any other country, mainly because of the compensation structure that often reflects the complex relationship between healthcare systems and insurance companies.
- Compared to other countries, the US has higher than average levels of some surgeries, such as coronary artery bypass procedures and knee replacements. However, obesity in the United States may also contribute to the higher rate of these specific procedures.

- A strong relationship exists between higher levels of physician-level continuity, a core principle of primary care, and lower total healthcare costs and hospitalizations. Primary care and outpatient services can decrease inpatient utilization.
- Most billing and insurance-related (BIR) administrative costs in the United States are due to claims-based health insurance transactions. Detailed information is needed to justify the codes used for billing purposes.
- The high cost of pharmaceuticals in the US is alarming. Most scholars agree that some regulations for pharmaceutical companies need to be implemented. America cannot continue to pay for medications at a significantly higher rate than other countries.
- The US healthcare system is expensive and has problems with sustainability, access, and quality. Innovation and ethical decision-making are required to remedy this situation.

NOTES

1 Angus MacKenzie, "The Worst Cars I Ever Tested: A Veteran Auto Journalist's List of Most Disappointing Rides," *Motortrend*, July 23, 2020.

2 Ezekiel J. Emanuel, *Which Country Has the World's Best Health Care?* (New York: PublicAffairs, 2020), chapter 13.

3 David S. Guzick, *An Introduction to the US Health Care Industry: Balancing Care, Cost, and Access* (Baltimore: Johns Hopkins University Press, 2020).

4 Ezekiel J. Emanuel, *Which Country Has the World's Best Health Care?* (New York: PublicAffairs, 2020), chapters 1 and 12.

5 Uwe E. Reinhardt, *Priced Out: The Economic and Ethical Costs of American Health Care* (Princeton, NJ: Princeton University Press, 2019), page 13.

6 Ezekiel J. Emanuel, *Which Country Has the World's Best Health Care?* (New York: PublicAffairs, 2020), chapter 12.

7 Ezekiel J. Emanuel, *Which Country Has the World's Best Health Care?* (New York: PublicAffairs, 2020), chapter 12.

8 David S. Guzick, *An Introduction to the US Health Care Industry: Balancing Care, Cost, and Access* (Baltimore: Johns Hopkins University Press, 2020).

9 Ezekiel J. Emanuel, *Which Country Has the World's Best Health Care?* (New York: PublicAffairs, 2020), chapter 13.

10 Uwe E. Reinhardt, *Priced Out: The Economic and Ethical Costs of American Health Care* (Princeton, NJ: Princeton University Press, 2019), page 63.

11 Oscar Castro, "The Medicare Problem: A Solution to Insolvency," *BYU Journal of Public Law* 33, no. 2 (June 2019): 355–379.

12 Oscar Castro, "The Medicare Problem: A Solution to Insolvency," *BYU Journal of Public Law* 33, no. 2 (June 2019): 355–379.

13 Oscar Castro, "The Medicare Problem: A Solution to Insolvency," *BYU Journal of Public Law* 33, no. 2 (June 2019): 355–379.
14 David S. Guzick, *An Introduction to the US Health Care Industry: Balancing Care, Cost, and Access* (Baltimore: Johns Hopkins University Press, 2020).
15 Oscar Castro, "The Medicare Problem: A Solution to Insolvency," *BYU Journal of Public Law* 33, no. 2 (June 2019): 355–379.
16 Oscar Castro, "The Medicare Problem: A Solution to Insolvency," *BYU Journal of Public Law* 33, no. 2 (June 2019): 355–379.
17 Office of the Actuary, *The 2017 Annual Report to the Board of Trustees Hospital Insurance and Federal Supplementary Medical Insurance Trust Funds* 7 (2017); see also Juliette Cubanski and Tricia Neuman, "The Facts on Medicare Spending and Financing," June 22, 2018, www.kff.org/medicare/issue-brief/the-facts-on-medicarespending-and-financing.
18 J. Mac McCullough et al., "Reduction in US Health Care Spending Required to Meet the Institute of Medicine's 2030 Target.," *American Journal of Public Health* 110, no. 12 (December 2020): 1735–1740.
19 Donald M. Berwick and Andrew D. Hackbarth, "Eliminating Waste in US Health Care," *JAMA: Journal of the American Medical Association* 307, no. 14 (April 11, 2012): 1513.
20 Diana Furchtgott-Roth, "The High Cost of Medical Malpractice," *Real Clear Markets*, August 6, 2009.
21 Michelle M. Mello et al., "National Costs Of The Medical Liability System," *Health Affairs* 29, no. 9 (September 2010): 1569–1577, https://doi.org/10.1377/hlthaff.2009.0807.
22 Michael P. Keane, Barry McCormick, and Gosia Popławska, "Health Care Spending in the US vs UK: The Roles of Medical Education Costs, Malpractice Risk and Defensive Medicine," *European Economic Review* 124 (May 1, 2020).
23 Michelle M. Mello et al., "National Costs Of The Medical Liability System," *Health Affairs* 29, no. 9 (September 2010): 1569–1577, https://doi.org/10.1377/hlthaff.2009.0807.
24 Jason A. Stamm et al., "Medical Malpractice: Reform for Today's Patients and Clinicians," *The American Journal of Medicine* 129, no. 1 (January 1, 2016): 20–25.
25 James D. Reschovsky and Cynthia B. Saiontz-Martinez, "Malpractice Claim Fears and the Costs of Treating Medicare Patients: A New Approach to Estimating the Costs of Defensive Medicine," *Health Services Research* 53, no. 3 (June 2018): 1498–1516.
26 Michael J. Saks and Stephan Landsman, "The Paradoxes Of Defensive Medicine," *Health Matrix: Journal of Law-Medicine* 30 (January 2020): 25–83.
27 Michael J. Saks and Stephan Landsman, "The Paradoxes Of Defensive Medicine," *Health Matrix: Journal of Law-Medicine* 30 (January 2020): 25–83.
28 Michael P. Keane, Barry McCormick, and Gosia Popławska, "Health Care Spending in the US vs UK: The Roles of Medical Education Costs, Malpractice Risk and Defensive Medicine," *European Economic Review* 124 (May 1, 2020).
29 Jason A. Stamm et al., "Medical Malpractice: Reform for Today's Patients and Clinicians," *The American Journal of Medicine* 129, no. 1 (January 1, 2016): 20–25.
30 Jason A. Stamm et al., "Medical Malpractice: Reform for Today's Patients and Clinicians," *The American Journal of Medicine* 129, no. 1 (January 1, 2016): 20–25.
31 Quoted in Miles Copeland, *The Game of Nations*, fourth edition (New York: Simon and Schuster, 1970), page 216.

32 Uwe E. Reinhardt, *Priced Out: The Economic and Ethical Costs of American Health Care* (Princeton, NJ: Princeton University Press, 2019), page 14.

33 David S. Guzick, *An Introduction to the US Health Care Industry: Balancing Care, Cost, and Access* (Baltimore: Johns Hopkins University Press, 2020), page 436.

34 Uwe E. Reinhardt, *Priced Out: The Economic and Ethical Costs of American Health Care* (Princeton, NJ: Princeton University Press, 2019), page 24.

35 D. U. Himmelstein and S. Woolhandler, "Cost without Benefit: Administrative Waste in US Health Care," *The New England Journal of Medicine* 314, no. 7 (February 13, 1986): 441–445, https://doi.org/10.1056/NEJM198602133140710.

36 David U. Himmelstein et al., "A Comparison of Hospital Administrative Costs in Eight Nations: US Costs Exceed All Others by Far," *Health Affairs (Project Hope)* 33, no. 9 (September 2014): 1586–1594, https://doi.org/10.1377/hlthaff.2013.1327.

37 Gerard F. Anderson, Peter Hussey, and Varduhi Petrosyan, "It's Still The Prices, Stupid: Why The US Spends So Much On Health Care, And A Tribute To Uwe Reinhardt," *Health Affairs (Project Hope)* 38, no. 1 (January 2019): 87–95, https://doi.org/10.1377/hlthaff.2018.05144.

38 D. U. Himmelstein and S. Woolhandler, "Cost without Benefit: Administrative Waste in US Health Care," *The New England Journal of Medicine* 314, no. 7 (February 13, 1986): 441–445, https://doi.org/10.1056/NEJM198602133140710.

39 S. Woolhandler and D. U. Himmelstein, "The Deteriorating Administrative Efficiency of the U.S. Health Care System," *The New England Journal of Medicine* 324, no. 18 (May 2, 1991): 1253–1258, https://doi.org/10.1056/NEJM199105023241805.

40 Michael E. Porter and Robert S. Kaplan, "How to Pay for Health Care," *Harvard Business Review* 94, no. 7–8 (August 2016): 88–98, 100, 134.

41 Kocher, Robert, "The Downside of Health Care Job Growth," *Harvard Business Review*, September 23, 2013.

42 D. U. Himmelstein and S. Woolhandler, "Cost without Benefit: Administrative Waste in US Health Care," *The New England Journal of Medicine* 314, no. 7 (February 13, 1986): 441–445, https://doi.org/10.1056/NEJM198602133140710.

43 Phillip Tseng et al., "Administrative Costs Associated With Physician Billing and Insurance-Related Activities at an Academic Health Care System," *JAMA* 319, no. 7 (February 20, 2018): 691, https://doi.org/10.1001/jama.2017.19148.

44 Sidney M. Wolfe, Steffie Woolhandler, and David U. Himmelstein, "It Is Time to Liberate Hospitals from Profit-Centered Care," *Journal of General Internal Medicine* 33, no. 7 (July 2018): 980–982, https://doi.org/10.1007/s11606-018-4448-0.

45 David U. Himmelstein, Terry Campbell, and Steffie Woolhandler, "Health Care Administrative Costs in the United States and Canada, 2017," *Annals of Internal Medicine* 172, no. 2 (January 21, 2020): 134, https://doi.org/10.7326/M19–2818.

46 S. Woolhandler and D. U. Himmelstein, "The Deteriorating Administrative Efficiency of the U.S. Health Care System," *The New England Journal of Medicine* 324, no. 18 (May 2, 1991): 1253–1258, https://doi.org/10.1056/NEJM199105023241805.

47 Sidney M. Wolfe, Steffie Woolhandler, and David U. Himmelstein, "It Is Time to Liberate Hospitals from Profit-Centered Care," *Journal of General Internal Medicine* 33, no. 7 (July 2018): 980–982, https://doi.org/10.1007/s11606-018-4448-0.

48 S. Woolhandler and D. U. Himmelstein, "The Deteriorating Administrative Efficiency of the U.S. Health Care System," *The New England Journal of Medicine* 324, no. 18 (May 2, 1991): 1253–1258, https://doi.org/10.1056/NEJM199105023241805.

49 Phyllis Maguire, "The White Coats vs. the Blue Suits," *Today's Hospitalist*, July 2017.

50 Scott W. Yates, "Physician Stress and Burnout," *The American Journal of Medicine* 133, no. 2 (February 1, 2020): 160–164.

51 Tait D. Shanafelt et al., "Impact of Organizational Leadership on Physician Burnout and Satisfaction," *Mayo Clinic Proceedings* 90, no. 4 (April 2015): 432–440, https://doi.org/10.1016/j.mayocp.2015.01.012.

52 Scott W. Yates, "Physician Stress and Burnout," *The American Journal of Medicine* 133, no. 2 (February 1, 2020): 160–164.

53 Phyllis Maguire, "The White Coats vs. the Blue Suits," *Today's Hospitalist*, July 2017.

54 Shasha Han et al., "Estimating the Attributable Cost of Physician Burnout in the United States.," *Annals of Internal Medicine* 170, no. 11 (June 4, 2019): 784–790, https://doi.org/10.7326/M18–1422.

55 Sidney M. Wolfe, Steffie Woolhandler, and David U. Himmelstein, "It Is Time to Liberate Hospitals from Profit-Centered Care," *Journal of General Internal Medicine* 33, no. 7 (July 2018): 980–982, https://doi.org/10.1007/s11606-018-4448-0.

56 Ezekiel J. Emanuel, *Which Country Has the World's Best Health Care?* (New York: PublicAffairs, 2020), chapter 1.

57 Uwe E. Reinhardt, *Priced Out: The Economic and Ethical Costs of American Health Care* (Princeton, NJ: Princeton University Press, 2019), page 33.

58 Irene Papanicolas, Liana R. Woskie, and Ashish K. Jha, "Health Care Spending in the United States and Other High-Income Countries," *JAMA* 319, no. 10 (March 13, 2018): 1024–1039, https://doi.org/10.1001/jama.2018.1150.

59 Teen-Hang Meen, Yusuke Matsumoto, and Kuan-Han Lee, "Special Issue on Clinical Medicine for Healthcare and Sustainability," *Journal of Clinical Medicine* 9, no. 7 (July 13, 2020), https://doi.org/10.3390/jcm9072206.

60 Justin E. Bekelman et al., "Comparison of Site of Death, Health Care Utilization, and Hospital Expenditures for Patients Dying With Cancer in 7 Developed Countries.," *JAMA: Journal of the American Medical Association* 315, no. 3 (January 19, 2016): 272–283.

61 Justin E. Bekelman et al., "Comparison of Site of Death, Health Care Utilization, and Hospital Expenditures for Patients Dying With Cancer in 7 Developed Countries.," *JAMA: Journal of the American Medical Association* 315, no. 3 (January 19, 2016): 272–283.

62 Justin E. Bekelman et al., "Comparison of Site of Death, Health Care Utilization, and Hospital Expenditures for Patients Dying With Cancer in 7 Developed Countries.," *JAMA: Journal of the American Medical Association* 315, no. 3 (January 19, 2016): 272–283.

63 J. Randall Curtis et al., "End-of-Life Care in the Intensive Care Unit: Can We Simultaneously Increase Quality and Reduce Costs?," *American Journal of Respiratory and Critical Care Medicine* 186, no. 7 (October 1, 2012): 587–592, https://doi.org/10.1164/rccm.201206-1020CP.

64 John G. Cagle et al., "Hospice Utilization in the United States: A Prospective Cohort Study Comparing Cancer and Noncancer Deaths," *Journal of the American Geriatrics Society* 68, no. 4 (April 2020): 783–793, https://doi.org/10.1111/jgs.16294.

65 Edward P. Hoffer, "America's Health Care System Is Broken: What Went Wrong and How We Can Fix It. Part 3: Hospitals and Doctors," *The American Journal of Medicine* 132, no. 8 (August 1, 2019): 907–911.

66 Lisa M. Knowlton et al., "The Economic Footprint of Acute Care Surgery in the United States: Implications for Systems Development," *The Journal of Trauma and Acute Care Surgery* 86, no. 4 (April 2019): 609–616, https://doi.org/10.1097/TA.0000000000002181.

67 Kyle H. Sheetz et al., "Variation in Surgical Outcomes Across Networks of the Highest-Rated US Hospitals," *JAMA Surgery* 154, no. 6 (June 1, 2019): 510–515, https://doi.org/10.1001/jamasurg.2019.0090.

68 Irene Papanicolas, Liana R. Woskie, and Ashish K. Jha, "Health Care Spending in the United States and Other High-Income Countries," *JAMA* 319, no. 10 (March 13, 2018): 1024–1039, https://doi.org/10.1001/jama.2018.1150.

69 Irene Papanicolas, Liana R. Woskie, and Ashish K. Jha, "Health Care Spending in the United States and Other High-Income Countries," *JAMA* 319, no. 10 (March 13, 2018): 1024–1039, https://doi.org/10.1001/jama.2018.1150.

70 Edward P. Hoffer, "America's Health Care System Is Broken: What Went Wrong and How We Can Fix It. Part 3: Hospitals and Doctors," *The American Journal of Medicine* 132, no. 8 (August 1, 2019): 907–911.

71 Joshua D. Geleris, George Shih, and Lia Logio, "Analysis of Diagnostic Test Ordering Habits Among Internal Medicine Residents," *JAMA Internal Medicine* 178, no. 12 (December 1, 2018): 1719, https://doi.org/10.1001/jamainternmed.2018.3519.

72 Jackson Williams, "Unsustainable Health Care Spending in the USA: How Will It End?," *Futures* 126 (February 1, 2021).

73 Jessica Greene and Rebecca M. Sacks, "Presenting Cost and Efficiency Measures That Support Consumers to Make High-Value Health Care Choices," *Health Services Research* 53 (August 2018): 2662–2681, https://doi.org/10.1111/1475-6773.12839.

74 Andrew Bazemore et al., "Higher Primary Care Physician Continuity Is Associated With Lower Costs and Hospitalizations," *Annals of Family Medicine* 16, no. 6 (November 2018): 492–497, https://doi.org/10.1370/afm.2308.

75 Amy S. Kelley and Diane E. Meier, *Meeting the Needs of Older Adults with Serious Illness: Challenges and Opportunities in the Age of Health Care Reform* (New York: Humana, 2014), page 48.

76 Andrew Bazemore et al., "Higher Primary Care Physician Continuity Is Associated With Lower Costs and Hospitalizations," *Annals of Family Medicine* 16, no. 6 (November 2018): 492–497, https://doi.org/10.1370/afm.2308.

77 Teen-Hang Meen, Yusuke Matsumoto, and Kuan-Han Lee, "Special Issue on Clinical Medicine for Healthcare and Sustainability," *Journal of Clinical Medicine* 9, no. 7 (July 13, 2020), https://doi.org/10.3390/jcm9072206.

78 Amy S. Kelley and Diane E. Meier, Meeting the Needs of Older Adults with Serious Illness: Challenges and Opportunities in the Age of Health Care Reform (New York: Humana, 2014), page 179.

79 Irene Papanicolas, Liana R. Woskie, and Ashish K. Jha, "Health Care Spending in the United States and Other High-Income Countries," *JAMA* 319, no. 10 (March 13, 2018): 1024–1039, https://doi.org/10.1001/jama.2018.1150.

80 Kyle H. Sheetz et al., "Variation in Surgical Outcomes Across Networks of the Highest-Rated US Hospitals," *JAMA Surgery* 154, no. 6 (June 1, 2019): 510–515, https://doi.org/10.1001/jamasurg.2019.0090.

81 Andrew Bazemore et al., "Higher Primary Care Physician Continuity Is Associated With Lower Costs and Hospitalizations," *Annals of Family Medicine* 16, no. 6 (November 2018): 492–497, https://doi.org/10.1370/afm.2308.

82 Justin E. Bekelman et al., "Comparison of Site of Death, Health Care Utilization, and Hospital Expenditures for Patients Dying With Cancer in 7 Developed Countries," *JAMA: Journal of the American Medical Association* 315, no. 3 (January 19, 2016): 272–283.

83 Ezekiel J. Emanuel, *Which Country Has the World's Best Health Care?* (New York: PublicAffairs, 2020), chapter 1.

84 S. Woolhandler and D. U. Himmelstein, "The Deteriorating Administrative Efficiency of the U.S. Health Care System," *The New England Journal of Medicine* 324, no. 18 (May 2, 1991): 1253–1258, https://doi.org/10.1056/NEJM199105023241805.

85 Uwe E. Reinhardt, *Priced Out: The Economic and Ethical Costs of American Health Care* (Princeton, NJ: Princeton University Press, 2019), page 28.

86 David S. Guzick, *An Introduction to the US Health Care Industry: Balancing Care, Cost, and Access* (Baltimore: Johns Hopkins University Press, 2020).

87 Ezekiel J. Emanuel, *Which Country Has the World's Best Health Care?* (New York: PublicAffairs, 2020), chapter 6.

88 David S. Guzick, *An Introduction to the US Health Care Industry: Balancing Care, Cost, and Access* (Baltimore: Johns Hopkins University Press, 2020), page 364.

89 Sidney M. Wolfe, Steffie Woolhandler, and David U. Himmelstein, "It Is Time to Liberate Hospitals from Profit-Centered Care," *Journal of General Internal Medicine* 33, no. 7 (July 2018): 980–982, https://doi.org/10.1007/s11606-018-4448-0.

90 Michael E. Porter and Robert S. Kaplan, "How to Pay for Health Care," *Harvard Business Review* 94, no. 7–8 (August 2016): 88–98, 100, 134.

91 David S. Guzick, *An Introduction to the US Health Care Industry: Balancing Care, Cost, and Access* (Baltimore: Johns Hopkins University Press, 2020).

92 Uwe E. Reinhardt, *Priced Out: The Economic and Ethical Costs of American Health Care* (Princeton, NJ: Princeton University Press, 2019), page 101.

93 Ezekiel J. Emanuel, *Which Country Has the World's Best Health Care?* (New York: PublicAffairs, 2020), chapter 1.

94 Ezekiel J. Emanuel, *Which Country Has the World's Best Health Care?* (New York: PublicAffairs, 2020), chapter 13.

95 Ezekiel J. Emanuel, *Which Country Has the World's Best Health Care?* (New York: PublicAffairs, 2020), chapter 1.

96 Uwe E. Reinhardt, *Priced Out: The Economic and Ethical Costs of American Health Care* (Princeton, NJ: Princeton University Press, 2019), page 32.

97 Department of Health and Human Services, Office of the Assistant Secretary for Planning and Evaluation, "Observations on Trends in Prescription Drug Spending: Mar 2016," https://aspe.hhs.gov/sites/default/files/pdf/187586/Drugspending.pdf.

98 McCarthy Michael, "Drug's 5000% Price Rise Puts Spotlight on Soaring US Drug Costs," *BMJ: British Medical Journal* 351 (September 24, 2015).

99 Uwe E. Reinhardt, *Priced Out: The Economic and Ethical Costs of American Health Care* (Princeton, NJ: Princeton University Press, 2019), page 37.

100 Uwe E. Reinhardt, *Priced Out: The Economic and Ethical Costs of American Health Care* (Princeton, NJ: Princeton University Press, 2019), pages 37–38.

101 Rishad Khan et al., "Prevalence of Financial Conflicts of Interest Among Authors of Clinical Guidelines Related to High-Revenue Medications," *JAMA Internal Medicine* 178, no. 12 (December 1, 2018): 1712–1715, https://doi.org/10.1001/jamainternmed.2018.5106.

102 Samuel J. Hong et al., "Spending on Antineoplastic Agents in the United States, 2011 to 2016," *Journal of Oncology Practice* 14, no. 11 (September 18, 2018): e683–e691, https://doi.org/10.1200/JOP.18.00069.

103 Audrey A. Tran, Milos Miljković, and Vinay Prasad, "Analysis of Estimated Clinical Benefit of Newly Approved Drugs for US Patients with Acute Myeloid Leukemia," *Leukemia Research* 96 (September 1, 2020).

104 Sebastian Salas-Vega, Emily Shearer, and Elias Mossialos, "Relationship between Costs and Clinical Benefits of New Cancer Medicines in Australia, France, the UK, and the US," *Social Science & Medicine* 258 (August 1, 2020).

105 Daniel M. Hartung et al., "The Cost of Multiple Sclerosis Drugs in the US and the Pharmaceutical Industry: Too Big to Fail?," *Neurology* 84, no. 21 (May 26, 2015): 2185–2192, https://doi.org/10.1212/WNL.0000000000001608.

106 Samuel J. Hong et al., "Spending on Antineoplastic Agents in the United States, 2011 to 2016," *Journal of Oncology Practice* 14, no. 11 (September 18, 2018): e683–e691, https://doi.org/10.1200/JOP.18.00069.

107 Data from *MotorTrend*, July 23, 2020.

108 Michael E. Porter, "What Is Value in Health Care?," *The New England Journal of Medicine* 363, no. 26 (December 23, 2010): 2477–2481, https://doi.org/10.1056/NEJMp1011024.

BIBLIOGRAPHY

Anderson, Gerard F., Peter Hussey, and Varduhi Petrosyan. "It's Still The Prices, Stupid: Why The US Spends So Much On Health Care, And A Tribute To Uwe Reinhardt." *Health Affairs (Project Hope)* 38, no. 1 (January 2019): 87–95. https://doi.org/10.1377/hlthaff.2018.05144.

Bazemore, Andrew, Stephen Petterson, Lars E. Peterson, Richard Bruno, Yoonkyung Chung, and Robert L. Phillips. "Higher Primary Care Physician Continuity Is Associated With Lower Costs and Hospitalizations." *Annals of Family Medicine* 16, no. 6 (November 2018): 492–497. https://doi.org/10.1370/afm.2308.

Bekelman, Justin E., Scott D. Halpern, Carl Rudolf Blankart, Julie P. Bynum, Joachim Cohen, Robert Fowler, Stein Kaasa, et al. "Comparison of Site of Death, Health Care Utilization, and Hospital Expenditures for Patients Dying With Cancer in 7 Developed Countries." *JAMA: Journal of the American Medical Association* 315, no. 3 (January 19, 2016): 272–283.

Berwick, Donald M., and Andrew D. Hackbarth. "Eliminating Waste in US Health Care." *JAMA: Journal of the American Medical Association* 307, no. 14 (April 11, 2012): 1513.

Cagle, John G., Joonyup Lee, Katherine A. Ornstein, and Jack M. Guralnik. "Hospice Utilization in the United States: A Prospective Cohort Study Comparing Cancer and Noncancer

Deaths." *Journal of the American Geriatrics Society* 68, no. 4 (April 2020): 783–793. https://doi.org/10.1111/jgs.16294.

Castro, Oscar. "The Medicare Problem: A Solution to Insolvency." *BYU Journal of Public Law* 33, no. 2 (June 2019): 355–379.

Curtis, J. Randall, Ruth A. Engelberg, Mark E. Bensink, and Scott D. Ramsey. "End-of-Life Care in the Intensive Care Unit: Can We Simultaneously Increase Quality and Reduce Costs?" *American Journal of Respiratory and Critical Care Medicine* 186, no. 7 (October 1, 2012): 587–592. https://doi.org/10.1164/rccm.201206-1020CP.

Ezekiel, J. Emanuel. *Which Country Has the World's Best Health Care?* New York: PublicAffairs, 2020.

Furchtgott-Roth, Diana. "The High Cost of Medical Malpractice." *Real Clear Markets*, August 6, 2009.

Geleris, Joshua D., George Shih, and Lia Logio. "Analysis of Diagnostic Test Ordering Habits Among Internal Medicine Residents." *JAMA Internal Medicine* 178, no. 12 (December 1, 2018): 1719. https://doi.org/10.1001/jamainternmed.2018.3519.

Greene, Jessica, and Rebecca M. Sacks. "Presenting Cost and Efficiency Measures That Support Consumers to Make High-Value Health Care Choices." *Health Services Research* 53 (August 2018): 2662–2681. https://doi.org/10.1111/1475-6773.12839.

Guzick, David S. *An Introduction to the US Health Care Industry : Balancing Care, Cost, and Access*. Baltimore: Johns Hopkins University Press, 2020.

Han, Shasha, Tait D Shanafelt, Christine A Sinsky, Karim M Awad, Liselotte N Dyrbye, Lynne C Fiscus, Mickey Trockel, and Joel Goh. "Estimating the Attributable Cost of Physician Burnout in the United States." *Annals of Internal Medicine* 170, no. 11 (June 4, 2019): 784–790. https://doi.org/10.7326/M18-1422.

Hartung, Daniel M., Dennis N. Bourdette, Sharia M. Ahmed, and Ruth H. Whitham. "The Cost of Multiple Sclerosis Drugs in the US and the Pharmaceutical Industry: Too Big to Fail?" *Neurology* 84, no. 21 (May 26, 2015): 2185–2192. https://doi.org/10.1212/WNL.0000000000001608.

Himmelstein, D. U., and S. Woolhandler. "Cost without Benefit. Administrative Waste in U.S. Health Care." *The New England Journal of Medicine* 314, no. 7 (February 13, 1986): 441–445. https://doi.org/10.1056/NEJM198602133140710.

Himmelstein, David U., Terry Campbell, and Steffie Woolhandler. "Health Care Administrative Costs in the United States and Canada, 2017." *Annals of Internal Medicine* 172, no. 2 (January 21, 2020): 134. https://doi.org/10.7326/M19-2818.

Himmelstein, David U., Miraya Jun, Reinhard Busse, Karine Chevreul, Alexander Geissler, Patrick Jeurissen, Sarah Thomson, Marie-Amelie Vinet, and Steffie Woolhandler. "A Comparison of Hospital Administrative Costs in Eight Nations: US Costs Exceed All Others by Far." *Health Affairs (Project Hope)* 33, no. 9 (September 2014): 1586–1594. https://doi.org/10.1377/hlthaff.2013.1327.

Hoffer, Edward P. "America's Health Care System Is Broken: What Went Wrong and How We Can Fix It. Part 3: Hospitals and Doctors." *The American Journal of Medicine* 132, no. 8 (August 1, 2019): 907–911.

Hong, Samuel J., Edward C. Li, Linda M. Matusiak, and Glen T. Schumock. "Spending on Antineoplastic Agents in the United States, 2011 to 2016." *Journal of Oncology Practice* 14, no. 11 (September 18, 2018): e683–e691. https://doi.org/10.1200/JOP.18.00069.

Keane, Michael P., Barry McCormick, and Gosia Popławska. "Health Care Spending in the US vs UK: The Roles of Medical Education Costs, Malpractice Risk and Defensive Medicine." *European Economic Review* 124 (May 1, 2020).

Kelley, Amy S. and Diane E. Meier. *Meeting the Needs of Older Adults with Serious Illness : Challenges and Opportunities in the Age of Health Care Reform*. Aging Medicine. New York: Humana, 2014.

Khan, Rishad, Michael A. Scaffidi, Amir Rumman, Alexander W. Grindal, Ian S. Plener, and Samir C. Grover. "Prevalence of Financial Conflicts of Interest Among Authors of Clinical Guidelines Related to High-Revenue Medications." *JAMA Internal Medicine* 178, no. 12 (December 1, 2018): 1712–1715. https://doi.org/10.1001/jamainternmed.2018.5106.

Knowlton, Lisa M., Joseph Minei, Lakshika Tennakoon, Kimberly A. Davis, Jay Doucet, Andrew Bernard, Adil Haider, L. R. Tres Scherer, David A. Spain, and Kristan L. Staudenmayer. "The Economic Footprint of Acute Care Surgery in the United States: Implications for Systems Development." *The Journal of Trauma and Acute Care Surgery* 86, no. 4 (April 2019): 609–616. https://doi.org/10.1097/TA.0000000000002181.

Kocher, Robert. "The Downside of Health Care Job Growth." *Harvard Business Review*, September 23, 2013.

MacKenzie, Angus. "The Worst Cars I Ever Tested: A Veteran Auto Journalist's List of Most Disappointing Rides." *Motortrend*, July 23, 2020.

Maguire, Phyllis. "The White Coats vs. the Blue Suits." *Today's Hospitalist*, July 2017.

McCarthy Michael. "Drug's 5000% Price Rise Puts Spotlight on Soaring US Drug Costs." *BMJ: British Medical Journal* 351 (September 24, 2015).

McCullough, J. Mac, Matthew Speer, Sanne Magnan, Jonathan E. Fielding, David Kindig, and Steven M. Teutsch. "Reduction in US Health Care Spending Required to Meet the Institute of Medicine's 2030 Target." *American Journal of Public Health* 110, no. 12 (December 2020): 1735–1740.

Meen, Teen-Hang, Yusuke Matsumoto, and Kuan-Han Lee. "Special Issue on Clinical Medicine for Healthcare and Sustainability." *Journal of Clinical Medicine* 9, no. 7 (July 13, 2020). https://doi.org/10.3390/jcm9072206.

Mello, Michelle M., Amitabh Chandra, Atul A. Gawande, and David M. Studdert. "National Costs Of The Medical Liability System." *Health Affairs* 29, no. 9 (September 2010): 1569–1577. https://doi.org/10.1377/hlthaff.2009.0807.

Papanicolas, Irene, Liana R. Woskie, and Ashish K. Jha. "Health Care Spending in the United States and Other High-Income Countries." *JAMA* 319, no. 10 (March 13, 2018): 1024–1039. https://doi.org/10.1001/jama.2018.1150.

Porter, Michael E. "What Is Value in Health Care?" *The New England Journal of Medicine* 363, no. 26 (December 23, 2010): 2477–2481. https://doi.org/10.1056/NEJMp1011024.

Porter, Michael E., and Robert S. Kaplan. "How to Pay for Health Care." *Harvard Business Review* 94, no. 7–8 (August 2016): 88–98, 100, 134.

Reinhardt, Uwe E. *Priced Out: The Economic and Ethical Costs of American Health Care*. Princeton, NJ: Princeton University Press, 2019.

Reschovsky, James D., and Cynthia B. Saiontz-Martinez. "Malpractice Claim Fears and the Costs of Treating Medicare Patients: A New Approach to Estimating the Costs of Defensive Medicine." *Health Services Research* 53, no. 3 (June 2018): 1498–1516.

Saks, Michael J., and Stephan Landsman. "The Paradoxes of Defensive Medicine." *Health Matrix: Journal of Law-Medicine* 30 (January 2020): 25–83.

Salas-Vega, Sebastian, Emily Shearer, and Elias Mossialos. "Relationship between Costs and Clinical Benefits of New Cancer Medicines in Australia, France, the UK, and the US." *Social Science & Medicine* 258 (August 1, 2020).

Shanafelt, Tait D., Grace Gorringe, Ronald Menaker, Kristin A. Storz, David Reeves, Steven J. Buskirk, Jeff A. Sloan, and Stephen J. Swensen. "Impact of Organizational Leadership on Physician Burnout and Satisfaction." *Mayo Clinic Proceedings* 90, no. 4 (April 2015): 432–440. https://doi.org/10.1016/j.mayocp.2015.01.012.

Sheetz, Kyle H., Andrew M. Ibrahim, Hari Nathan, and Justin B. Dimick. "Variation in Surgical Outcomes Across Networks of the Highest-Rated US Hospitals." *JAMA Surgery* 154, no. 6 (June 1, 2019): 510–515. https://doi.org/10.1001/jamasurg.2019.0090.

Stamm, Jason A., Karen A. Korzick, Kristen Beech, and Kenneth E. Wood. "Medical Malpractice: Reform for Today's Patients and Clinicians." *The American Journal of Medicine* 129, no. 1 (January 1, 2016): 20–25.

Tran, Audrey A., Milos Miljković, and Vinay Prasad. "Analysis of Estimated Clinical Benefit of Newly Approved Drugs for US Patients with Acute Myeloid Leukemia." *Leukemia Research* 96 (September 1, 2020).

Tseng, Phillip, Robert S. Kaplan, Barak D. Richman, Mahek A. Shah, and Kevin A. Schulman. "Administrative Costs Associated With Physician Billing and Insurance-Related Activities at an Academic Health Care System." *JAMA* 319, no. 7 (February 20, 2018): 691. https://doi.org/10.1001/jama.2017.19148.

Williams, Jackson. "Unsustainable Health Care Spending in the USA: How Will It End?" *Futures* 126 (February 1, 2021).

Wolfe, Sidney M., Steffie Woolhandler, and David U. Himmelstein. "It Is Time to Liberate Hospitals from Profit-Centered Care." *Journal of General Internal Medicine* 33, no. 7 (July 2018): 980–982. https://doi.org/10.1007/s11606-018-4448-0.

Woolhandler, S., and D. U. Himmelstein. "The Deteriorating Administrative Efficiency of the U.S. Health Care System." *The New England Journal of Medicine* 324, no. 18 (May 2, 1991): 1253–1258. https://doi.org/10.1056/NEJM199105023241805.

Yates, Scott W. "Physician Stress and Burnout." *The American Journal of Medicine* 133, no. 2 (February 1, 2020): 160–164.

Chapter 9

Communication Skills for Healthcare Professionals

INTRODUCTION

So, now that you have become well-informed about bioethics, how do you convey that information to others? The challenging part about ethics is that you often deal with patients, their families, and even colleagues going through a tough time. At this time, you will need to rely on your communication skills. All the knowledge about healthcare ethics in the world will not matter if you do not know how to speak to the people who need you, and this is where many falter. Although clinicians are now getting education on communication skills, many still feel uneasy about having these conversations. Admittedly, these conversations are not easy, but as you will see, communication skills are a learned ability, much like other medical procedures.

As a palliative care physician, I have attended hundreds of family meetings. I led some of them, and for others, I was there for support. Most of these discussions involved very ill patients, their families, and the clinicians caring for them. The conversations usually involved sharing very serious information and making decisions. Some clinicians, usually the doctors, felt the best way to run the meeting was to do all the talking ("Don't interrupt me until I'm finished"). Others felt that being blunt was the best course of action ("Your loved one is as good as dead!"). Still, others felt compelled to give *every* fact and detail as if all that information would be helpful to a struggling family.

Those were usually the ones who thought that these conversations were easy. Others struggled with talking to families. I had a medical resident in the ICU that I was trying to help who was very reluctant to run a family meeting because of her shyness. One day, a patient she cared for became critical, and I noticed she had developed a rapport with the family. I urged her to lead the family meeting and assured her I would be there to support her. She agreed and did well at first, but

DOI: 10.4324/9781003654124-10

after a few minutes, her voice cracked, and tears formed and fell down her face. She persevered, however, and was able to present the needed information and have the family agree on a care plan.

Afterward, during the debriefing, she asked if she had flunked because of the crying spell. I told her that she earned an A+! The resident not only shared with the family the information they needed, but she also guided them through some tough choices that also needed to be made. Why would the fact she shed a few tears be seen as detrimental? The family knew this resident was working hard to care for their loved one. The tears were not seen as a weakness by them but rather an acknowledgment that she saw their family member as someone who mattered to her and the rest of the ICU team. With all the technology we see in medicine, we sometimes forget the importance of being human when caring for patients.

For example, early in the twenty-first century, a change in medicine was arguably the most significant since the introduction of the written language. Medical offices and hospitals now had computers to document the physician-patient relationship. Electronic health records (EHRs) presence in medical offices grew exponentially in the 2000s, from 18% in 2001 to 86% in 2017.[1] No longer were medical records written in charts by a clinician with dubious penmanship skills. Now, a laptop would replace pen and paper in medical offices, hospitals, sick bays, health centers, and wherever health professionals and patients encounter each other. Not only would doctor's notes be readable, but all other professional input from nurses, physician assistants, specialists, social workers, and everyone else there to help patients would be only a keyboard click away. Also, lab and diagnostic studies would be available to the practitioner almost immediately. These technological advances promised to improve accessibility to information and enhance the medical encounter's efficiency and quality. So, what could possibly go wrong?

One problem that quickly emerged was that the time needed to document an encounter increased rather than decreased. A new system designed for efficiency took more time than the old system of handwritten notes. Clinicians found they could not keep up with patient flow and had to either decrease the number of patients seen or bring their computers home to complete their notes. EHRs touted to be user-friendly seemed written by computer experts who knew nothing about medicine, leading to frustration and physician burnout.[2] An article in the *New England Journal of Medicine* contrasted how aviation engineers would work closely with pilots when designing new systems and compared that to the EHR rollout with physicians. "In the aviation industry, there is an abiding respect, even reverence, for the wisdom of the frontline workers. Our biggest mistake lies not in adopting clunky systems but in dismissing the concerns of the people who must use them."[3] Having a health system staffed by exasperated workers is a challenge, and efforts to improve this interaction have made some progress. However, a more damaging consequence is recognized and may be more challenging to fix. The EHR has altered how clinicians interact with patients.

The time spent on the computer has to be accounted for. Unfortunately, that comes down to less time interacting with the patient. A *Journal of the American Medical Association* editorial by Cerzick and Linn in 2016 argues that the computer limits personal interactions by decreasing eye contact with the patient.[4] Other articles complain that the computer is a physical obstruction between the patient and the physician.[5]

Betty was a memorable patient of mine. She was very bright, had a sharp, sometimes biting wit, and an excellent sense of humor. Sadly, she had some severe physical ailments. In her twenties, Betty was involved in a car accident that left her with a traumatic brain injury. In a wheelchair and with a speech impediment, it was easy for many to believe that she had an intellectual disability, which was far from the truth. Betty also had metastatic breast cancer that had spread to her lungs. Several times, she was hospitalized for shortness of breath, and each time, her breathing improved, but in decreasing amounts. She eventually chose not to return to the hospital and go to hospice. In her last conversation with me, she described her encounter with the hospitalist doing her discharge. He entered her room with a computer on a wheeled stand that he kept between them. The doctor never looked at her but instead read information off the monitor, most of which she already knew: your prognosis is poor, there are no treatments left for your cancer, hospice is appropriate, etc. When the physician inquired if she had any questions, she asked, "Why didn't you look up and see my funny (pig) hat?" With that, he backed out of the room and never commented on his dying patient's silly hat.

BETTER COMMUNICATION AS A LEARNED COMPETENCY

For many in healthcare, there is an assumption that unless one is a competent communicator, nothing can be done about it! However, more and more educators realize that good communication skills are a learned competency. For example, without training, one would not expect a surgical resident to know how to remove a gallbladder. This skill requires hours of didactic and clinical education, personal instruction, and practice. A similar conclusion can be made regarding communication skills.

Multiple surgical graduate medical education societies have proposed communication skills training projects to address this. For example, the Accreditation Council for Graduate Medical Education (ACGME) and the American Board of Orthopedic Surgery developed the Orthopedic Surgery Milestones Project for orthopedic surgeon trainees as a way of testing six required core competencies, which include not only medical knowledge and patient care skills but also professionalism, interpersonal and communication skills, and practice-based learning and improvement. Within these core competencies, residents are expected to progress to the level where they can communicate competently in difficult or adversarial patient circumstances and sustain working relationships with their patients during complex and challenging situations.[6]

The Institute of Medicine report *Dying in America* called for widespread and mandatory workforce training in communication skills,[7] and an honored hospital system decided to take on this task. Cleveland Clinic has been recognized as the number 2 hospital globally by the US News and World Report best hospitals 2021 list. It has been consistently on their top ten list for decades.[8] From August 2013 to April 2014, all employed and attending physicians were mandated to participate in an 8-hour internally offered experiential communication skills training program at Cleveland Clinic.[9]

In this observational study of a robust health system, experiential, relationship-centered communication skills training effectively improved outpatient scores and one domain of inpatient scores. Physicians reported high satisfaction with the course regarding its practical use of time, teaching relevant and feasible skills to implement in their practice, changing their attitudes, and enhancing their knowledge and skills.[10] Even a world-renowned health system can improve the communication skills of its doctors with a training program. Other health systems should take note of this!

The Need for Communication Skills

The Institute of Medicine identified patient-centered care as one of six elements of high-quality healthcare.[11] A patient-centered approach to care is based on three goals: eliciting the patient's perspective on the illness, understanding the patient's psychosocial context, and reaching shared treatment goals based on the patient's values. Patient-centered care builds on discussions and decisions that involve shared information, compassionate and empowering care provision, sensitivity to patient needs, and relationship building. In contrast to a disease-focused biomedical approach, patient-centered care considers patient preferences, needs, and values, ensuring they guide all medical decisions with scientific evidence.[12]

Disease-centered approaches are appropriate when individuals have a single predominant disease, and everyone with the illness desires the same outcome, such as prolonged survival or cardiovascular protection. However, this disease-centered framework is ill-suited for persons with multiple chronic conditions, including most older adults with cardiovascular diseases and most adult healthcare users of all ages. Disease-centered decision-making for this population results in treatment burden when patients must adhere to multiple guidelines and harm when guideline recommendations conflict. Furthermore, disease-centered recommendations may not address what matters most to these patients who vary in their health priorities.[13] For example, preventing cardiovascular events in the future may have little value to someone with a limited lifespan.

Scope of the Problem in US Healthcare

The Cleveland Clinic study cited above showed that practical communication skills could be taught. ACGME is now advocating for this type of training in its residency programs.[14] This section will examine the downside of poor communication skills, particularly with surgery and cancer care.

Communication among surgeons, patients, and families about treatment goals plays an important and understudied role in determining which surgical treatment elderly patients with serious illnesses receive, and communication inadequacies may lead to nonbeneficial procedures. However, relatively little is known about how surgeons conduct conversations with high-risk patients in the emergent setting and the barriers for surgeons. These barriers include time constraints, inadequate communication training, and a belief that patients do not want to discuss death and dying. Surgeons in a crisis are even less likely to have the time and resources to undertake difficult and time-consuming discussions about end-of-life care. Unfortunately, this is when these discussions are most needed.[15]

Problems with communication are also seen in cancer care. There is a growing body of evidence that poor communication in cancer care seems unfortunately prevalent and that it exerts a significant burden.[16] For oncologists, comfort with EOL care and communication is associated with enhanced access to palliative care. Ironically, oncologists who are less comfortable with EOL care reported delivering less supportive care and referring fewer patients to specialist palliative care, resulting in lower access to palliative care. Thus, it is imperative to ensure that oncology specialists have adequate training and support for delivering EOL care and a supportive environment to build a collaborative relationship with the specialist palliative care team.[17] Poor communication exerts costs that are potentially enormous and may include economic, social, psychological, emotional, and collateral costs to the patient, the patient's support network, the clinicians, the cancer care system, and the larger society itself.[18]

Helping Patients and Families with Decision-Making

Clinicians and ethicists will often be tasked with helping patients and families make difficult decisions. Occasionally, this discussion cannot be made with the patients as they may be too ill to participate. Therefore, the conversations are often with family members and surrogates, who may not know the patient's wishes. If the patient does not have decision-making capacity, a surrogate must serve as the key decision-maker.[19] It is not unusual for family members to state that their loved ones would "want everything done!"[20] This section will discuss helping families define realistic hope and set appropriate goals.

Defining Realistic Hope

Chapter 6 of this book dealt with futile care in the ICU and defined realistic hope for that subset of patients. That discussion concentrated on prognostic tools and studies that help clinicians predict medical outcomes for seriously ill patients. It also looked at proactive programs that address ICU outcomes early on rather than taking the traditional "wait and see" approach so often used. In this section, realistic hope will be broadened to other medical issues and deal with how this task is done intellectually and empathetically. It will also address how healthcare professionals can communicate this.

Hope is an important concept not just in medicine but in life itself. Some clinicians worry that truth-telling may destroy hope and even go as far as promoting false hope.[21] Nevertheless, bad things happen to good people, and a provider must be honest to allow hope to continue. What is hope? One definition offered by Dufault and Martocchio describes hope as "a multi-dimensional dynamic life force characterized by a confident yet uncertain expectation of achieving a future good, which, to the hoping person, is realistically possible and personally significant."[22] Uncertainty is a critical word in this definition; medical professionals cannot guarantee success, and often its probability is minuscule. Multiple studies show that hope is essential when treating diseases. Even when a cure is impossible, hope for a better quality of life can still be maintained in chronically ill patients.[23]

Oncologists are especially susceptible to this problem and may have difficulty talking to their patients when the prognosis is less than rosy. Sometimes, it may be easier to suggest another treatment rather than discuss that the treatments are not working. Therefore, oncologists will recommend a different medication, even if the likelihood of success is nil. They feel anything is better than admitting that no cancer treatments are left. However, this is unfair to patients and their families.

Patients and families may also cling to false hopes. Clinicians may face a dying, incurably ill patient. Still, they or their families typically want to keep fighting because they are waiting for a miracle. These cases are generally complex for the healthcare team to deal with and usually involve a time-limited trial and multiple interventions to resolve.[24] There are also patients in denial of their illness. They will not accept the possibility of dying and keep insisting on further treatment, even against their doctors' advice.[25] So what, then, is realistic hope?

For clinicians, giving patients false hope is not the solution. Resolving this problem involves talking with patients and sometimes their families honestly. Although some patients will reject any discussion, most patients do want to have these talks with their clinicians if it is framed correctly. The goal should be to elicit what is essential to the patient and proceed from there.[26] As previously stated, hope starts with a desire, which should be explored in detail. The timing of these discussions is also a factor. Too often, physicians wait for a crisis to bring up sensitive topics such as advance directives, palliative care, and hospice. A better strategy would be to have these discussions regularly. In that way, these talks seem more normal and likely less scary for clinicians and patients. Goals can change over time, and what the patient hopes for may also shift. When patients are knowledgeable about their condition, they can make better decisions.[27]

Setting Appropriate Goals

A 2022 article, "Clinician Perspectives on How to Hold Earlier Discussions About Palliative and End-of-Life Care With Chronic Obstructive Pulmonary Disease Patients: A Qualitative Study," suggested that too often it is done superficially at the first visit, perhaps with an education pamphlet and then not until the patient is dying.[28] There are likely many reasons for this; some were discussed in the previous section. Nevertheless, this practice is widespread and harmful to patients.

Ideally, these talks should be done early on, routinely, and with any clinical changes.[29] Routine conversations throughout the disease course help educate the patient and make the discussions seem less dreadful than when done only at times of crisis.[30] Too often, physicians and patients are uncomfortable having these talks, so it is simply easier not to have them at all. However, if these talks are done regularly, a rapport can develop, making these discussions more productive and less frightening. Nurses and other healthcare professionals can facilitate these discussions with the proper training and support. Along with these routine ones, meetings should occur whenever there is a clinical change, such as worsening symptoms and hospitalizations.

Indeed, most patients with chronic illnesses prefer to be managed in their homes. Hospitalizations signal an event that is profoundly significant to the patient. These events frequently occur in older patients with multiple chronic illnesses. The treatment plan for the patient has now transitioned from outpatient only to outpatient, with hospitalizations as needed. As patients clinically change, goals may also change. Early in the disease process, the patient may prefer an aggressive, do-everything approach; later, a more palliative approach may be desired. One hospital studied the impact of GOC discussions with elderly patients that occurred routinely on the third day of admission. Their findings confirm a decrease in burdensome interventions.[31]

As the patient's condition progresses, another transition may occur; the patient may become too frail or ill to live independently at home safely (or comfortably). The following change is to an extended care facility (ECF). Although this would seem a good time to have a GOC chat, it is often not done. Perhaps the person can no longer have these discussions with their caregivers or can do so only to a limited degree. If these discussions had been held prior, with family members present, it would have eased the worry about making future decisions. If these discussions were not held prior, the task becomes more burdensome. Clinicians and non-clinicians at ECFs must be trained and comfortable with these conversations.[32]

These transitions can occur rapidly with cancer patients, yet often, these conversations are not completed or documented. A 2022 article in *Cancer* showed that GOC notes were only present in 35% of the charts. These end-of-life discussions were considered "early" if they occurred more than thirty days before the patient's death. When the notes were completed, the oncologist did 50%, 41% were done by a hospitalist, 3% by a palliative care consultant, and 6% by other clinicians.[33] It is unclear what happened to the remaining 65% of patients; some may have had a conversation, but it was not documented. Others may have occurred within 30 days of death or not at all. Programs to incentivize these conversations are being studied as a quality measure. However, there is still a long way to go.[34]

Finally, what should be included in GOC discussions? Disease-specific education is always helpful; handing out a brochure on an early visit is not likely to be sufficient. After that, educating patients and sometimes their families about end-of-life (EOL) issues is a critical duty for all healthcare providers and facilities. These discussions should include advance care planning (ACP) and choices regarding future treatments like CPR, life support, artificial nutrition and hydration (ANH), and rehospitalization. A decision-maker (or makers) should be designated, and discussion opportunities should be made available with them, the patient, and their providers. Appropriate ACP documentation should also be completed.[35]

Other topics should also be discussed according to the patient's individual needs. For example, hospice and palliative care referrals could be beneficial to patients who are suffering. Symptom management can significantly improve QOL for patients at the EOL. A simple question about how comfortable the patient wants to be is often neglected when the goal is disease-centered and not patient-centered. These discussions have a dual function; they help the patient and their family understand the disease process and what choices are available. They also help medical professionals understand what the patient feels is meaningful to them. These GOC discussions can be challenging but more challenging when they are not had at all.[36]

BASIC STRUCTURE FOR COMMUNICATION WITH ETHICS CONSULTS

In 1992, an oncologist named Robert Buckman MD wrote a book, *Breaking Bad News: A Guide for Health Care Professionals*,[37] which discusses the problem with giving this type of information and proposes a protocol to address this. This six-step protocol is called SPIKES and stands for Setting, Perception, Invitation, Knowledge, Emotions, and Strategy (or Summary.)

First, having the proper setting is vital; people should be sitting, and appropriate introductions should be made. The room should be private, quiet, and free from interruptions. Next, exploring the patient's knowledge, expectations, and hopes (step 2 of SPIKES) will allow the physician to understand where the patient is and start the discussion. The third step involves getting permission to give information. While most patients desire complete information about their diagnosis, prognosis, and illness details, some do not. When a clinician hears a patient expresses a desire for information explicitly, it may lessen the anxiety associated with divulging the bad news. The way in which the patient and their families want to receive the information can also be discussed here.[38]

The fourth step is the actual giving of the information (or bad news). A few simple techniques may improve this one-way part of the physician-patient dialogue. First, start at the patient's level of comprehension and vocabulary. Second, try not to use jargon or words the audience may not understand. Third, avoid excessive bluntness as it is likely to leave the patient isolated and later angry, with a tendency to blame the messenger for the bad news. Fourth, information should be given in small chunks, and the patient's understanding should be checked periodically. Fifth, when the prognosis is poor, avoid saying, "There is nothing more we can do for you." Instead, discuss what can be done, such as symptom control and advance care planning.[39]

The next step is "emotion." Too often, physicians want to keep talking. Many researchers have found that this is a particular difficulty for medical professionals when they have bad news. The uncertainty of the patient's and family's reactions and emotions can be distressing. Physicians may also have problems with silence, which may occur after bad news is given.[40] The final step is to plan for a future meeting to discuss strategies and follow-up appointments. Discussing what can be accomplished is reassuring and allows the patient to realize they will not be abandoned.[41] Utilizing this basic framework can benefit whoever runs the family meeting: physicians, nurses, social workers, chaplains, and even clinical ethicists.[42]

Shared Decision-Making

Making decisions for a patient who is too ill to make them for themselves can be very challenging. It is beneficial if the patient has completed an advance directive or, at the very least, discussed with their family what type of care they would want in this situation. Often, both of these helpful aids are missing, and decision-making with families can be complicated. The traditional ways to make decisions include substituted judgment, where a family member or surrogate attempts to make an appropriate decision based on what they think the patient would have wanted. Suppose the patient has never made their wishes known. In that case, the best interest standard is initiated, where a determination is made based on what a "reasonable person" would decide in a similar situation.[43]

One study examined the "substituted interest" model, where families are guided in decision-making.[44] For instance, the substituted judgment standard would ask, "In this situation, if your mother could talk, what would she choose?" Best interest would ask, what is best for your mother?" The substituted interests model says, "Tell us about your mother." A good surrogate can articulate the patient's authentic values by describing the patient's loves, beliefs, and fundamental moral commitments rather than just specific preferences. Surrogates, ideally formally designated, know the patient as a person even if they do not know their precise wishes. The substituted interests model reframes surrogate decision-making as an approach that promotes the patient as a unique person in the context of their relationships, applying the patient's authentic values, wishes, and real interests as best they can be known. It recognizes each patient as unique and provides a framework to help families make personal decisions for their loved ones.[45]

The Clinician's Role in Family Meetings

There is limited data on the role of a clinical ethicist in family meetings.[46] One article states, "Despite the interpersonal nature of family meetings and the frequency in which they occur, the clinical ethics literature is devoid of any detailed descriptions of what clinical ethicists should actually be doing during family meetings."[47] The prior sections of this essay presented an essential structure for the family meeting to help families with decision-making where the patient could not tell us their wishes. Clinical ethicists should note these strategies and use them to plan family meetings when resolving ethical dilemmas.

CONCLUSION

This chapter looked at the importance of communication skills in clinical ethics. The first two sections looked at the need for better communication in healthcare and some problems resulting from poor communication. The third section looked at the types of decisions that need to be made during these encounters. Finally, the last section examined how these challenging family meetings can be structured. There has been considerable emphasis on improving communication skills on multiple levels; however, the conclusion "More research is needed" still occurs too frequently. It is essential for those involved with resolving ethical dilemmas to keep learning, including a host of professionals, from ethics consultants to nurses, physicians, chaplains, social workers, and leadership. Being successful at communication skills is a challenge, and like any other competency, it requires knowledge, practice, and experience.

TAKE-HOME POINTS

- Good communication skills are a learned competency.
- A patient-centered approach to care is based on three goals: eliciting the patient's perspective on the illness, understanding the patient's psychosocial context, and reaching shared treatment goals based on the patient's values.
- Poor communication exerts costs that are potentially enormous and may include economic, social, psychological, emotional, and collateral costs to the

patient, the patient's support network, the clinicians, the cancer care system, and the larger society itself.

- For clinicians, giving patients false hope is not the solution. Resolving this problem involves talking with patients and sometimes their families honestly. Although some patients will reject any discussion, most patients do want to have these talks with their clinicians if it is framed correctly.
- Goals of care discussions should include disease-specific education, advance care planning, specific patient needs, and end-of-life care.
- *Breaking Bad News, A Guide for Health Care Professionals* discusses the problem with giving this type of information and proposes a protocol to address this. This six-step protocol is called SPIKES and stands for Setting, Perception, Invitation, Knowledge, Emotions, and Strategy (or Summary). This framework can be used for other serious conversations as well.
- The substituted judgment standard would ask, "In this situation, if your mother could talk, what would she choose?" Best interest would ask, what is best for your mother?"
- The substituted interests model reframes surrogate decision-making as an approach that promotes the patient as a unique person in the context of their relationships, applying the patient's authentic values, wishes, and real interests as best they can be known.

NOTES

1 Kevin B. Johnson, Michael J. Neuss, and Don Eugene Detmer, "Electronic Health Records and Clinician Burnout: A Story of Three Eras," *Journal of the American Medical Informatics Association* 28, no. 5 (April 23, 2021): 967–973, https://doi.org/10.1093/jamia/ocaa274, page 967.

2 Edward R. Melnick et al., "Perceived Electronic Health Record Usability as a Predictor of Task Load and Burnout Among US Physicians: Mediation Analysis.," *Journal of Medical Internet Research* 22, no. 12 (December 2020), page 2.

3 Lisa Rosenbaum, "Transitional Chaos or Enduring Harm? The EHR and the Disruption of Medicine.," *New England Journal of Medicine* 373, no. 17 (October 22, 2015): 1585–1588, https://doi.org/10.1056/NEJMp1509961.

4 Zuzanna Czernik and C. T. Lin, "Time at the Bedside (Computing)," *JAMA* 315, no. 22 (June 14, 2016): 2399, https://doi.org/10.1001/jama.2016.1722, page 1722.

5 Edward R. Melnick et al., "Perceived Electronic Health Record Usability as a Predictor of Task Load and Burnout Among US Physicians: Mediation Analysis.," *Journal of Medical Internet Research* 22, no. 12 (December 2020).

6 Linda Roberts et al., "Communication Skills Training for Surgical Residents: Learning to Relate to the Needs of Older Adults," *Journal of Surgical Education* 75, no. 5 (September 1, 2018): 1180–1187.

7 Institute of Medicine Committee on *Approaching Death, Addressing Key End-of-Life Issues, Dying in America: Improving Quality and Honoring Individual Preferences Near the End of Life* (Washington, DC: National Academies Press, 2015).

8 US News and World Report, "Best Hospitals by Specialty," July 28, 2020, https://health.usnews.com/best-hospitals/rankings.
9 Adrienne Boissy et al., "Communication Skills Training for Physicians Improves Patient Satisfaction," *Journal of General Internal Medicine* 31, no. 7 (July 2016): 755–761, https://doi.org/10.1007/s11606-016-3597-2.
10 Adrienne Boissy et al., "Communication Skills Training for Physicians Improves Patient Satisfaction," *Journal of General Internal Medicine* 31, no. 7 (July 2016): 755–761, https://doi.org/10.1007/s11606-016-3597-2.
11 Institute of Medicine Committee on Approaching Death, *Addressing Key End-of-Life Issues, Dying in America: Improving Quality and Honoring Individual Preferences Near the End of Life* (Washington, DC: National Academies Press, 2015).
12 M. Jawad Hashim, "Patient-Centered Communication: Basic Skills," *American Family Physician* 95, no. 1 (January 1, 2017): 29–34.
13 Mary E. Tinetti, Aanand D. Naik, and John A. Dodson, "Moving From Disease-Centered to Patient Goals-Directed Care for Patients With Multiple Chronic Conditions: Patient Value-Based Care," *JAMA Cardiology* 1, no. 1 (April 1, 2016): 9, https://doi.org/10.1001/jamacardio.2015.0248.
14 Linda Roberts et al., "Communication Skills Training for Surgical Residents: Learning to Relate to the Needs of Older Adults," *Journal of Surgical Education* 75, no. 5 (September 1, 2018): 1180–1187.
15 Zara Cooper et al., "Pitfalls in Communication That Lead to Nonbeneficial Emergency Surgery in Elderly Patients with Serious Illness: Description of the Problem and Elements of a Solution," *Annals of Surgery* 260, no. 6 (December 2014): 949–957, https://doi.org/10.1097/SLA.0000000000000721.
16 Sally E. Thorne et al., "Is There a Cost to Poor Communication in Cancer Care?: A Critical Review of the Literature," *Psycho-Oncology* 14, no. 10 (October 2005): 875–884, https://doi.org/10.1002/pon.947.
17 David Hui et al., "Impact of Oncologists' Attitudes Toward End-of-Life Care on Patients' Access to Palliative Care.," *The Oncologist* 21, no. 9 (September 2016): 1149–1155, https://doi.org/10.1634/theoncologist.2016–0090.
18 Sally E. Thorne et al., "Is There a Cost to Poor Communication in Cancer Care?: A Critical Review of the Literature," *Psycho-Oncology* 14, no. 10 (October 2005): 875–884, https://doi.org/10.1002/pon.947.
19 Nancy Berlinger, Bruce Jennings, and Susan M. Wolf, *The Hastings Center Guidelines for Decisions on Life-Sustaining Treatment and Care Near the End of Life*, revised and expanded second edition (Oxford: Oxford University Press, 2013), page 48.
20 Dragana Bolcic-Jankovic et al., "Exploring Determinants of Surrogate Decision-Maker Confidence: An Example From the ICU," *Journal of Empirical Research on Human Research Ethics: An International Journal* 9, no. 4 (2014): 76.
21 Bert Musschenga, "Is There a Problem With False Hope?," *The Journal of Medicine and Philosophy* 44, no. 4 (July 29, 2019): 423–441, https://doi.org/10.1093/jmp/jhz010.
22 Karin Dufault and Benita C. Martocchio, "Hope: Its Spheres and Dimensions," *Nursing Clinics of North America* 20, no. 2 (June 1985): 379–391, https://doi.org/10.1016/S0029–6465(22)00328-0.
23 Hamed Salimi et al., "Hope Therapy in Cancer Patients: A Systematic Review," *Supportive Care in Cancer* 30, no. 6 (June 2022): 4675–4685, https://doi.org/10.1007/s00520-022-06831-y.
24 Trevor M. Bibler, Myrick C. Jr. Shinall, and Devan Stahl, "Responding to Those Who Hope for a Miracle: Practices for Clinical Bioethicists," *American Journal of Bioethics* 18, no. 5 (2018): 40–51.
25 Bert Musschenga, "Is There a Problem With False Hope?," *The Journal of Medicine and Philosophy* 44, no. 4 (July 29, 2019): 423–441, https://doi.org/10.1093/jmp/jhz010.

26 M. Jawad Hashim, "Patient-Centered Communication: Basic Skills," *American Family Physician* 95, no. 1 (January 1, 2017): 29–34.
27 Nuno Tavares et al., "Clinician Perspectives on How to Hold Earlier Discussions About Palliative and End-of-Life Care With Chronic Obstructive Pulmonary Disease Patients: A Qualitative Study," *Journal of Hospice & Palliative Nursing* 24, no. 3 (June 2022): E101–E107, https://doi.org/10.1097/NJH.0000000000000858.
28 Nuno Tavares et al., "Clinician Perspectives on How to Hold Earlier Discussions About Palliative and End-of-Life Care With Chronic Obstructive Pulmonary Disease Patients: A Qualitative Study," *Journal of Hospice & Palliative Nursing* 24, no. 3 (June 2022): E101–E107, https://doi.org/10.1097/NJH.0000000000000858.
29 Brynn Bowman and Diane E Meier, "Palliative Care for Respiratory Disease: An Education Model of Care," *Chronic Respiratory Disease* 15, no. 1 (February 2018): 36–40, https://doi.org/10.1177/1479972317721562.
30 Nuno Tavares et al., "Clinician Perspectives on How to Hold Earlier Discussions About Palliative and End-of-Life Care With Chronic Obstructive Pulmonary Disease Patients: A Qualitative Study," *Journal of Hospice & Palliative Nursing* 24, no. 3 (June 2022): E101–E107, https://doi.org/10.1097/NJH.0000000000000858.
31 Ashwin Subramaniam et al., "Frailty Status, Timely Goals of Care Documentation and Clinical Outcomes in Older Hospitalised Medical Patients.," *Internal Medicine Journal* 51, no. 12 (December 2021): 2078–2086, https://doi.org/10.1111/imj.15032.
32 Ruth S. Martin et al., "Healthcare Providers' Experiences with Advance Care Planning and Goals of Patient Care Medical Treatment Orders in Residential Aged Care Facilities: An Explanatory Descriptive Study.," *Internal Medicine Journal* 52, no. 5 (May 2022): 776–784, https://doi.org/10.1111/imj.15374.
33 Andrew S. Epstein et al., "Goals of Care Documentation by Medical Oncologists and Oncology Patient End-of-Life Care Outcomes.," *Cancer* 128, no. 18 (September 15, 2022): 3400–3407, https://doi.org/10.1002/cncr.34400.
34 Andrew S. Epstein et al., "Goals of Care Documentation by Medical Oncologists and Oncology Patient End-of-Life Care Outcomes.," *Cancer* 128, no. 18 (September 15, 2022): 3400–3407, https://doi.org/10.1002/cncr.34400.
35 Diane E. Meier, Stephen L. Isaacs, and Robert Hughes, *Palliative Care: Transforming the Care of Serious Illness*, first edition, Robert Wood Johnson Foundation Series on Health Policy (San Francisco, CA: Jossey-Bass, 2010), page 9.
36 Diane E. Meier, Stephen L. Isaacs, and Robert Hughes, *Palliative Care: Transforming the Care of Serious Illness*, first edition, Robert Wood Johnson Foundation Series on Health Policy (San Francisco, CA: Jossey-Bass, 2010), page 9.
37 R. Buckman, *Breaking Bad News: A Guide for Health Care Professionals* (Baltimore, MD: Johns Hopkins University Press, 1992).
38 W. F. Baile et al., "SPIKES—a Six-Step Protocol for Delivering Bad News: Application to the Patient with Cancer.," *Oncologist* 5, no. 4 (July 2000): 302–311.
39 W. F. Baile et al., "SPIKES—a Six-Step Protocol for Delivering Bad News: Application to the Patient with Cancer.," *Oncologist* 5, no. 4 (July 2000): 302–311.
40 David Dickson et al., "Health Professionals' Perceptions of Breaking Bad News," *International Journal of Health Care Quality Assurance* 15, no. 7 (December 1, 2002): 324–336, https://doi.org/10.1108/09526860210448492.
41 W. F. Baile et al., "SPIKES—a Six-Step Protocol for Delivering Bad News: Application to the Patient with Cancer.," *Oncologist* 5, no. 4 (July 2000): 302–311.
42 M. Jawad Hashim, "Patient-Centered Communication: Basic Skills," *American Family Physician* 95, no. 1 (January 1, 2017): 29–34.
43 Nancy Berlinger, Bruce Jennings, and Susan M. Wolf, *The Hastings Center Guidelines for Decisions on Life-Sustaining Treatment and Care Near the End of Life*, revised and expanded second edition (Oxford: Oxford University Press, 2013), page 203.

44 Daniel P. Sulmasy and Lois Snyder, "Substituted Interests and Best Judgments: An Integrated Model of Surrogate Decision Making," *JAMA* 304, no. 17 (November 3, 2010): 1946, https://doi.org/10.1001/jama.2010.1595.
45 Daniel P. Sulmasy and Lois Snyder, "Substituted Interests and Best Judgments: An Integrated Model of Surrogate Decision Making," *JAMA* 304, no. 17 (November 3, 2010): 1946, https://doi.org/10.1001/jama.2010.1595.
46 Courtenay R. Bruce et al., "A Qualitative Exploration of a Clinical Ethicist's Role and Contributions During Family Meetings," *HEC Forum* 28, no. 4 (December 2016): 283–299, https://doi.org/10.1007/s10730-015-9300-x.
47 Courtenay R. Bruce et al., "A Qualitative Exploration of a Clinical Ethicist's Role and Contributions During Family Meetings," *HEC Forum* 28, no. 4 (December 2016): 283–299, https://doi.org/10.1007/s10730-015-9300-x.

BIBLIOGRAPHY

Baile, W. F., R. Buckman, R. Lenzi, G. Glober, E. A. Beale, and A. P. Kudelka. "SPIKES—a Six-Step Protocol for Delivering Bad News: Application to the Patient with Cancer." *Oncologist* 5, no. 4 (July 2000): 302–311.

Berlinger, Nancy, Bruce Jennings, and Susan M. Wolf. *The Hastings Center Guidelines for Decisions on Life-Sustaining Treatment and Care Near the End of Life*. Revised and expanded second edition. Oxford: Oxford University Press, 2013.

Bibler, Trevor M., Myrick C. Jr. Shinall, and Devan Stahl. "Responding to Those Who Hope for a Miracle: Practices for Clinical Bioethicists." *American Journal of Bioethics* 18, no. 5 (2018): 40–51.

Boissy, Adrienne, Amy K. Windover, Dan Bokar, Matthew Karafa, Katie Neuendorf, Richard M. Frankel, James Merlino, and Michael B. Rothberg. "Communication Skills Training for Physicians Improves Patient Satisfaction." *Journal of General Internal Medicine* 31, no. 7 (July 2016): 755–761. https://doi.org/10.1007/s11606-016-3597-2.

Bolcic-Jankovic, Dragana, Brian R. Clarridge, Jessica L. LeBlanc, Rumel S. Mahmood, Anthony M. Roman, and Bradley D. Freeman. "Exploring Determinants of Surrogate Decision-Maker Confidence : An Example From the ICU." *Journal of Empirical Research on Human Research Ethics: An International Journal* 9, no. 4 (2014): 76.

Bowman, Brynn, and Diane E. Meier. "Palliative Care for Respiratory Disease: An Education Model of Care." *Chronic Respiratory Disease* 15, no. 1 (February 2018): 36–40. https://doi.org/10.1177/1479972317721562.

Bruce, Courtenay R., Trevor M. Bibler, Adam M. Pena, and Betsy Kusin. "A Qualitative Exploration of a Clinical Ethicist's Role and Contributions During Family Meetings." *HEC Forum* 28, no. 4 (December 2016): 283–299. https://doi.org/10.1007/s10730-015-9300-x.

Buckman, R. *Breaking Bad News: A Guide for Health Care Professionals.* Baltimore, MD: Johns Hopkins University Press, 1992.

Cooper, Zara, Andrew Courtwright, Ami Karlage, Atul Gawande, and Susan Block. "Pitfalls in Communication That Lead to Nonbeneficial Emergency Surgery in Elderly Patients with Serious Illness: Description of the Problem and Elements of a Solution." *Annals of Surgery* 260, no. 6 (December 2014): 949–957. https://doi.org/10.1097/SLA.0000000000000721.

Czernik, Zuzanna, and C. T. Lin. "Time at the Bedside (Computing)." *JAMA* 315, no. 22 (June 14, 2016): 2399. https://doi.org/10.1001/jama.2016.1722.

Dickson, David, Owen Hargie, Karen Brunger, and Karyn Stapleton. "Health Professionals' Perceptions of Breaking Bad News." *International Journal of Health Care Quality Assurance* 15, no. 7 (December 1, 2002): 324–336. https://doi.org/10.1108/09526860210448492.

Dufault, Karin, and Benita C. Martocchio. "Hope: Its Spheres and Dimensions." *Nursing Clinics of North America* 20, no. 2 (June 1985): 379–391. https://doi.org/10.1016/S0029-6465(22)00328-0.

Epstein, Andrew S, Michael Riley, Judith E Nelson, Camila Bernal, Steven Martin, and Han Xiao. "Goals of Care Documentation by Medical Oncologists and Oncology Patient End-of-Life Care Outcomes." *Cancer* 128, no. 18 (September 15, 2022): 3400–3407. https://doi.org/10.1002/cncr.34400.

Hashim, M. Jawad. "Patient-Centered Communication: Basic Skills." *American Family Physician* 95, no. 1 (January 1, 2017): 29–34.

Hui, David, Maria Agustina Cerana, Minjeong Park, Kenneth Hess, and Eduardo Bruera. "Impact of Oncologists' Attitudes Toward End-of-Life Care on Patients' Access to Palliative Care." *The Oncologist* 21, no. 9 (September 2016): 1149–1155. https://doi.org/10.1634/theoncologist.2016-0090.

Institute of Medicine Committee on Approaching Death. *Addressing Key End-of-Life Issues, Dying in America: Improving Quality and Honoring Individual Preferences Near the End of Life*. Washington, DC: The National Academies Press, 2015.

Johnson, Kevin B., Michael J. Neuss, and Don Eugene Detmer. "Electronic Health Records and Clinician Burnout: A Story of Three Eras." *Journal of the American Medical Informatics Association* 28, no. 5 (April 23, 2021): 967–973. https://doi.org/10.1093/jamia/ocaa274.

Martin, Ruth S., Barbara J. Hayes, Anastasia Hutchinson, Paul Yates, and Wen Kwang Lim. "Healthcare Providers' Experiences with Advance Care Planning and Goals of Patient Care Medical Treatment Orders in Residential Aged Care Facilities: An Explanatory Descriptive Study." *Internal Medicine Journal* 52, no. 5 (May 2022): 776–784. https://doi.org/10.1111/imj.15374.

Meier, Diane E., Stephen L. Isaacs, and Robert Hughes. *Palliative Care: Transforming the Care of Serious Illness*. First edition. Robert Wood Johnson Foundation Series on Health Policy. San Francisco: Jossey-Bass, 2010.

Melnick, Edward R., Elizabeth Harry, Christine A. Sinsky, Liselotte N. Dyrbye, Hanhan Wang, Mickey Todd Trockel, Colin P. West, and Tait Shanafelt. "Perceived Electronic Health Record Usability as a Predictor of Task Load and Burnout Among US Physicians: Mediation Analysis." *Journal of Medical Internet Research* 22, no. 12 (December 2020).

Musschenga, Bert. "Is There a Problem With False Hope?" *The Journal of Medicine and Philosophy* 44, no. 4 (July 29, 2019): 423–441. https://doi.org/10.1093/jmp/jhz010.

Roberts, Linda, Charles Cornell, Mathias Bostrom, Sandra Goldsmith, Titilayo Ologhobo, Timothy Roberts, and Laura Robbins. "Communication Skills Training for Surgical Residents: Learning to Relate to the Needs of Older Adults." *Journal of Surgical Education* 75, no. 5 (September 1, 2018): 1180–1187.

Rosenbaum, Lisa. "Transitional Chaos or Enduring Harm? The EHR and the Disruption of Medicine." *New England Journal of Medicine* 373, no. 17 (October 22, 2015): 1585–1588. https://doi.org/10.1056/NEJMp1509961.

Salimi, Hamed, Haniyeh Bashi Zadeh Fakhar, Mohammad Hadizadeh, MohammadEsmaeil Akbari, Neda Izadi, Reza MohamadiRad, Hosna Akbari, and Ramtin Hoseini. "Hope Therapy in Cancer Patients: A Systematic Review." *Supportive Care in Cancer* 30, no. 6 (June 2022): 4675–4685. https://doi.org/10.1007/s00520-022-06831-y.

Subramaniam, Ashwin, Ravindranath Tiruvoipati, Cameron Green, Velandai Srikanth, Lionel Soh, Aun Chian Yeoh, Faisal Hussain, Michael Bailey, and David Pilcher. "Frailty Status, Timely Goals of Care Documentation and Clinical Outcomes in Older Hospitalised Medical Patients." *Internal Medicine Journal* 51, no. 12 (December 2021): 2078–2086. https://doi.org/10.1111/imj.15032.

Sulmasy, Daniel P., and Lois Snyder. "Substituted Interests and Best Judgments: An Integrated Model of Surrogate Decision Making." *JAMA* 304, no. 17 (November 3, 2010): 1946. https://doi.org/10.1001/jama.2010.1595.

Tavares, Nuno, Nikki Jarrett, Tom Wilkinson, and Katherine Hunt. "Clinician Perspectives on How to Hold Earlier Discussions About Palliative and End-of-Life Care With Chronic Obstructive Pulmonary Disease Patients: A Qualitative Study." *Journal of Hospice & Palliative Nursing* 24, no. 3 (June 2022): E101–E107. https://doi.org/10.1097/NJH.0000000000000858.

Thorne, Sally E., Barry D. Bultz, Walter F. Baile, and the SCRN Communication Team. "Is There a Cost to Poor Communication in Cancer Care?: A Critical Review of the Literature." *Psycho-Oncology* 14, no. 10 (October 2005): 875–884. https://doi.org/10.1002/pon.947.

Tinetti, Mary E., Aanand D. Naik, and John A. Dodson. "Moving From Disease-Centered to Patient Goals-Directed Care for Patients With Multiple Chronic Conditions: Patient Value-Based Care." *JAMA Cardiology* 1, no. 1 (April 1, 2016): 9. https://doi.org/10.1001/jamacardio.2015.0248.

Chapter 10

Developing a Healthcare Ethics Consultative Service

INTRODUCTION

Healthcare ethics programs were virtually nonexistent in the 1960s and 1970s and, as recently as the early 1980s, were present in only 1% of US hospitals. By the late 1980s, however, ethics committees grew to over 60% of US hospitals.[1] Subsequently, the presence of ethics committees increased to over 90% by the late 1990s. An ethics consultation service is available in all US hospitals with 400 beds or more, along with federal hospitals and Council of Teaching Hospitals members.[2] But why this growth?

In the 1940s, Dutch physician Willem Kolff built the first dialysis machine by modifying an automobile fuel pump to circulate blood outside the body, which was filtered through a series of tubes and then returned to the body.[3] The problem with Kolff's device was accessing an artery to deliver blood to the machine and then a vein to return the filtered blood to the body. Alas, the technology in the 40s allowed these blood vessels to be accessed only once, significantly decreasing the number of times a patient could be dialyzed. This problem was solved in the 1960s when another physician, Belding Scribner, working at the Swedish Hospital in Seattle, developed a permanent indwelling that allowed for repeated dialyzing through the same sites. Therefore, patients could receive the dialysis treatments needed to prolong their life.[4] This lifesaving medical advance, however, raised multiple ethical issues.

A key question raised was how appropriate patients should be selected for an innovative but limited procedure that could save lives. An article in the 1965 *Annals of Internal Medicine* discussed this ethical dilemma in detail.[5] The committee making these selections was infamously dubbed the "Seattle God Committee."[6] Its beginning revealed many vital features that ethics committees later emerged to address: technology-creating choices that previously seemed unlikely, value-based

DOI: 10.4324/9781003654124-11

problems that go well beyond what medical science can manage, a multicultural setting where not all the participants have the same values, and the need for quick decisions.[7] These challenges became fertile ground for creating ethical committees in the healthcare setting.

Clinical ethics committees in the United States typically perform multiple functions. The most noticeable is individual case consultations in response to requests from clinicians or occasionally from patients or their families. Furthermore, providing ethical input into hospital policies, developing guidelines, and educating health professionals within the institution is also essential. Although case consultation is often carried out by individual ethicists gradually, it is being performed by small multidisciplinary teams, including ethics committee members as part of the team.[8] The following sections of this chapter will look at the development of ethics programs based on the work of the American Society for Bioethics and Humanities (ASBH) and the Veterans Health Administration (VHA).

AMERICAN SOCIETY FOR BIOETHICS AND HUMANITIES

The American Society for Bioethics and Humanities (ASBH; https://asbh.org) was created in January 1998 by combining three existing organizations: the Society for Health and Human Values (SHHV), the Society for Bioethics Consultation (SBC), and the American Association of Bioethics (AAB). SHHV was officially founded in 1969 as a professional organization whose primary objective was to encourage and promote informed concern for human values as an essential, explicit dimension of education for health professionals. SBC was officially established in 1986, and its mission was to study ethics consultation and support those who provided it in healthcare at that time. Lastly, AAB was formed in the fall of 1994. Its purpose was to promote the exchange of ideas among bioethics scholars, enhance bioethicists' clinical activities, and encourage discussion and research in bioethics. It also urged the teaching and development of new scholars and participants in the field. Representatives of all three associations organized the consolidation. The entire membership overwhelmingly approved the merger in 1997.[9]

One of the most significant contributions by the ASBH is the second edition of the *Core Competencies for Health Care Ethics Consultation*. The 57-page monograph is divided into four sections: "The Nature and Goals of Ethics Consultation," "Core Competencies for Health Care Ethics Consultation," "Evaluating Health Care Ethics Consultation Services," and "The Ethical Dimensions of HCEC [healthcare ethics consultation] as an Emerging Professional Practice."[10] The first section defines HCEC as "a set of services an individual or group provides in response to questions from patients, families, surrogates, health care providers, or other involved parties. This committee seeks to resolve uncertainty or conflict regarding value-laden concerns that emerge in health care."[11] The report goes on to distinguish consultations in which the ethics consultant interacts with the patient and family and writes a note in the patient's health record as a category named "case consultations." Likewise, "non-case consultations" refer to HCEC's endeavors to work with institutions and other stakeholders to develop ethics-based policies.[12]

The most common challenge for healthcare ethics programs to meet ASBH practice standards is a lack of resources; however, external certification as quality improvement was the least favored solution.[13] Some survey respondents saw this as a way to reduce the time required to practice before the certification exam. However, "lowering the bar" would not likely help smaller nonacademic centers and may obstruct the growth in practice at larger academic centers. Indeed, expanding healthcare ethics programs to smaller, nonacademic hospitals is desirable, but lowering ASBH standards to accomplish this goal is not recommended.[14]

VETERANS HEALTH ADMINISTRATION

Along with ASBH, the IntegratedEthics (IE) model from the US Department of Veterans Affairs (VA) National Center for Ethics in Health Care (NCEHC) was also developed. The IE model looked to replace its traditional, siloed ethics committee approach with a single, fundamental ethics program that directs and supervises the organization's ethics services obligation across the full range of content areas.[15] Key components included a literature review, a survey study of 600 US hospitals to identify strengths and weaknesses in ethics programs, and interviews with a national sample of ethics program leaders to identify factors contributing to effective ethics programs. From 2002 through 2006, NCEHC developed and refined tools and strategies to enable facilities to implement IE.[16]

The IE project developed a system with reference materials describing the program and administrative tools to help program managers organize, document, and assess their programs. The program also included ethics education materials for multiple target audiences and communication tools to promote staff and leadership support. This process was completed with a year-long demonstration project in 25 Veterans Health Administration (VHA) facilities to test and improve the model, tools, and implementation strategy (2005–2006). The IE program was rolled out nationally in 2007, and the IE tools included in the rollout established specific quality standards for the IE model.[17]

The IE program divided its contents into four sections: "Program Management," "Ethics Consultation," "Preventive Ethics," and "Ethics Leadership." The first section, on program management, is dedicated to the person or persons tasked with developing the ethics program for their facility. It begins with an explanation of the importance of ethics. "Individuals and organizations must each respond effectively to ethical concerns. When ethical concerns are not resolved, the result can be errors or unnecessary and potentially costly decisions that are bad for patients, staff, the organization, and society. When employees perceive that they have no place to bring their ethical concerns, the result can be moral distress—a recognized factor in professional burnout—a major cause of staff turnover, especially among nurses."[18] This section also provides the reader with written materials (the "Primer"), videos, and a web-based training module.[19] In addition, this material includes instructions on developing an ethics program with sections on staff development, meetings, integration, and leadership.

The second section explores the "heart of the matter," ethics consultations. The IE model defines an ethics consultation in healthcare as "activities performed by an individual ethics consultant, a team of ethics consultants, or an ethics committee on behalf of a health care organization to help patients, providers, or other parties resolve ethical concerns in the health care setting. Ethical concerns are uncertainties or conflicts about values."[20] IE recommends using what they have called the CASES approach to complete this task, where C is Clarify, A is Assemble, S is Synthesize, E is Explain, and S is Support. Ethics consultants and their teams can effectively navigate the complex process to resolve ethical concerns. The authors of this protocol state that these steps can be used in the same way clinicians use a standard format for taking a patient's history, performing a physical exam, or writing up a clinical note. Although not all consultations require the specific application of a particular step, each step should be considered part of every ethics consultation.[21] By working methodically through each step of clarifying requests for consultation, assembling relevant information, synthesizing that information to identify ethically acceptable results, explaining the synthesis to the affected parties, and supporting the overall consultation process through follow-up and evaluation, the ethics consultation service helps to ensure that ethical concerns are addressed thoroughly within the healthcare organization.[22]

The third section of the Primer discusses preventive ethics (PE). The authors of IE define preventive ethics as "activities performed by an individual or group on behalf of a health care organization to identify, prioritize, and address systemic ethics quality gaps."[23] Further, they define an ethics issue as a "quality gap that results from poorly performing, unreliable or ill-defined systems and processes that can arise anywhere in a health care organization."[24] The ultimate goal of PE is to significantly improve quality by identifying, prioritizing, and addressing ethics quality gaps on a systems level.[25] As with the ethics consultation and the CASES approach, the IE authors used another mnemonic to remember the steps needed for PE. In this situation, the approach is named ISSUES. It refers to the following steps: Identify an issue, Study the issue, Select a strategy, Undertake a plan, Evaluate and adjust, and Sustain and spread.[26] The example given in the Primer of an issue for PE was the lack of assistance provided to patients in a cardiac rehab program for completing advance directives. By offering this innovative method and practical tools to improve ethical quality, the authors conclude that ISSUES enhances VA's experience as a leader in healthcare quality measures.[27]

The final section of the IE Primer discusses the topic of ethical leadership. The authors emphasize the importance of leaders fostering an environment and culture that supports ethical practices.[28] They underscore that leaders play a critical role in creating, sustaining, or changing all aspects of organizational culture, including ethical culture. Furthermore, where employees perceived that supervisors and executives regularly pay attention to ethics, take ethics seriously, and care about ethics and values as much as the bottom line, all outcomes were significantly more positive.[29] The authors conclude that ethical leadership promotes the importance of ethics consultation, preventive ethics, and the other core functions of an IE program. These three core functions have helped promote ethical practices through the VA's healthcare system.[30]

In this section, the efforts of ASBH and the VA system discussed the historical need for ethics programs. ASBH, with its Core Competencies, and the VA, with its IE program, provide excellent information regarding building programs. In addition, both programs detail the need for ethics in an organization that goes beyond ethics consultation. The following section will provide further details on what is needed to build an ethics program.

DEVELOPING A MATRIX FOR RESOLVING ETHICAL DILEMMAS

Learning is doing; for the healthcare ethicist, this is the challenge. Knowing ethics is vital but not enough; an ethicist must use that knowledge to help others. This mission means learning to use ethics knowledge in clinical situations and developing the skill set to complete ethics consultations. However, the mission goes beyond that; it also means creating a program that fosters ethical decisions for that institution. Fortunately, excellent information is available to help the ethicist achieve this objective. The ASBH and VA programs are two such examples.

This section will explore the material from these organizations and others to help the ethicist attain the needed expertise to accomplish this goal.

What Do You Need to Know?

Within the field of clinical ethics, organizations such as ASBH and the VA are attempting to standardize the medical ethics practice. In the past, interested health professionals, along with practitioners of philosophy, theology, and the law, essentially chose to focus their efforts in this area and became bioethicists through years of experience and individualized study.[31] However, training programs specific to bioethics have grown through fellowships, graduate degrees, and certification programs. These training programs vary widely, from week-long certificates to two-year fellowship programs. For example, while the American Society for Bioethics and Humanities (ASBH) offers a healthcare ethics consultant (HEC) certification examination, no current standardized method exists throughout their training program or the programs themselves.[32] Nevertheless, there is broad agreement that successful assessment of bioethics education requires demonstration that the student has acquired the specific skills or competencies defined by the curriculum.[33]

The *Core Competencies for Health Care Ethics Consultation* report represents a commitment by the ASBH to ensure that qualified persons provide high-quality clinical ethical consultation. The organization lists a knowledge base recommended to achieve this goal.[34] Similarly, in their IE program, the VA suggests the same proficiencies.[35] These competencies include familiarity with shared decision-making with "patients, ethical practices in end-of-life care, ethical practices at the beginning of life, patient privacy and confidentiality, professionalism in patient care, ethical practices in resource allocation, ethical practices in business and management, ethical practices in the everyday workplace, and ethical research practices."[36] The VA also adds domains relevant to the consultant's organizational setting, such as ethical practices in government service, mission integration, or military medicine.[37] Besides this knowledge base, the learner must also achieve a skillset that incorporates ethical assessment and analysis, process skills, communication, professionalism, courage, humility, and prudence.[38] Finally, proficiencies in academic research, writing, presenting, and teaching are also essential.[39]

Additional competencies are required if the healthcare professional provides ethics services for a religion-based institution. The Ethical and Religious Directives for Catholic Health Care Services (ERDs) are directives the United States Conference of Catholic Bishops promulgated to govern Catholic health facilities.[40] First published over 70 years ago, moral theologians created the ERDs and healthcare professionals from the United States and Canada based on natural law understood in the light of revelation. In 1971, the National Conference of Catholic Bishops (now called the United States Conference of Catholic Bishops) revised and approved a new set of ERDs that was more universally adopted. In 1994, a significant revision occurred, focusing on the importance of human dignity. Unlike earlier versions, the document prohibited certain practices. It positively explained the Church's moral doctrine with more social justice issues and clinical conditions.[41] Compared to the elements listed by ASHB, for the most part, there is agreement. Nevertheless, these directives could conflict with the core competencies set forth by the ASHB and need to be examined.[42]

Catholic hospitals are duty-bound to follow ERDs. ERD Number 5 reads:

> *Catholic health care services must adopt these Directives as policy, require adherence to them within the institution as a condition for medical privileges and employment, and provide appropriate instruction regarding the Directives for administration, medical and nursing staff, and other personnel.*[43]

This directive is not optional and could be problematic for ethics committee members unfamiliar with ERDs or who are not even Catholics themselves. For Catholic hospitals, several procedures are forbidden. Examples of intrinsically evil acts include abortion, euthanasia, suicide (both assisted and unassisted), sterilization, and contraception.[44] These procedures may be legal and available at other local health centers not affiliated with the Catholic Church, and it is essential to inform patients about these restrictions and their options if relevant.

Contemporary HCECs are looking away from a single ethicist to a more team approach. This approach should include someone with religious expertise, especially in a Catholic setting. The following section will look at recommendations for building a healthcare ethics team.

Who Do You Need to Recruit?

ASBH has attempted to standardize the knowledge base for healthcare ethicists by establishing Core Competencies. The society has also published guidelines for establishing a healthcare ethics consultative (HCE) service. These widely accepted practice standards are frequently used to measure quality. They are recognized as authoritative sources of practice standards for ethics consultation as defined in the second edition of the ASBH's *Core Competencies* report.[45] Their report describes three models for healthcare ethics programs: a single individual, a small team (a physician, a nurse, and a third person who is neither a physician nor a nurse), and a full ethics committee. While the *Core Competencies* report establishes that using all three models is "ideal," it also acknowledges that "local resources and contextual realities influence which EC model(s) are most practical for a given organization." Indeed, it seems impractical to expect hospitals to perform HCEs using all three different models when the median number of case consultations conducted annually in US hospitals is only three. While the wording of the current *Core Competencies* report's standards suggests that using all three models is ideal, future standards will look to define situations where it is essential to either use or not use each model.[46] That said, there is evidence that a small team may have advantages.

Although three people may be ideal for an HCE consultation, it is recommended that more people be involved in a healthcare ethics committee. For example, the VA writes about what they refer to as an IE model and recommends certain professionals for committee membership. This list includes facility leaders and senior staff who regularly encounter ethical concerns and are engaged in improving ethics quality at the facility, such as executive leadership team members or equivalent, quality management, patient safety, compliance, clinical services, chaplaincy, and human resources, fiscal, learning, research.[47] An IE program can be created by gathering these people into one program. So, what constitutes an IE program?

IE programs organize and streamline existing programs in three ways. First, in many institutions, ethics consultations are performed by parties and programs such as ethics committees, leadership, and institutional review boards in relative isolation from each other. IE programs have an integrative "umbrella" structure that combines these programs into a single organization. Second, whereas traditional ethics support services focus on specific content areas, such as clinical or research ethics, IE programs are comprehensive and may include many ethical issues facing the organization. Third, whereas traditional ethics support services may concentrate on a limited amount of tasks (e.g., ethics consultation, staff education, and policy review), IE programs can accomplish tasks these goals by cooperating with other programs and individuals throughout the organization.[48]

What Do You Need to Do?

In this section, two functions of ethics programs, other than consultations, will be examined: preventive ethics and ethics education. Preventive describes preventive ethics (PE) is one of the three core functions of the VA's (IE) program.[49]

The term preventive ethics was first introduced in the bioethics literature in 1993. It was used to describe "explicit, critical reflection on the institutional factors that influence patient care." PE is used in various contexts to highlight how organizational factors influence ethical practices.[50] In addition, PE aims to improve ethics quality on a systems level by identifying, prioritizing, and addressing ethics quality gaps.[51]

For example, unlike an ethics consult that looks to determine the ethically appropriate action in a particular case, PE addresses why this action is not done consistently throughout the system. Next, PE recognizes that organizational ethical behaviors are strongly influenced by the organization's systems, practices, and processes. Therefore, ethical errors occur not only because of the shortcomings of humans but also because of flawed organizational systems, practices, and processes. PE aims to improve systems and processes so that effective, ethical practices become automatic. Finally, PE recognizes that ethical practices in healthcare can be operationalized, measured, and improved. Doing metrics differentiates PE from other ethics program activities within healthcare organizations. For these items to occur, leadership support is essential.[52] In the end, leaders are accountable for the viability of all programs, and PE is no exception. High-level administration priorities can allocate resources to support these goals.[53]

Developing a PE program in a hospital should first involve looking for patterns that occur with the type of consultation received. For example, an active ethics consultation service will likely know their institution's ethical challenges.[54] Once this evaluation is completed, some experts have suggested using a web-based electronic tracking tool (ECWeb).[55] This program categorizes all completed ethics consultations by healthcare ethics domain (for example, shared decision making) and topic (for example, advance care planning) and therefore promotes the efficient identification of common challenges associated with ethics quality gaps.[56] Identifying these issues on an organizational level allows ethics committees to develop practical strategies to narrow the gap. PE can then wrap up with a systematic application, evaluation, and follow-up to ensure any ethics gaps can be tightened or eliminated.[57]

These findings suggested that providing general ethics education around resolving some common dilemmas may align more closely with the needs of acute care settings. In addition, 64% of the respondents wanted more ethics education sessions in more accessible languages, at more convenient times/locations, and tailored to different audiences. This training included frontline worker education and sessions to capture better the true scope of ethical dilemmas healthcare workers experience. They concluded that a culture of ethics could be created only through comprehensive education, and preventive ethics can only occur in this setting.[58]

CONCLUSION

Bioethics is a relatively young field that is rapidly developing as technology moves forward. As stated earlier in this chapter, dialysis introduced medicine to the need for decision-making regarding limited supplies of life-preserving treatments. Questions about whether these brilliant but expensive therapies should be used, withheld, or withdrawn will continue to trouble patients, caregivers, healthcare professionals, and administrators at an accelerated pace as new treatments emerge and new challenges arise. This undertaking requires the professional to learn multiple skills. First, what is intellectually known must be translated into knowledge that can be used clinically. Next, the clinician must also develop a program that includes a means to provide consultative services and fill other institutional ethical needs. These demands include program development, education, preventive ethics, and research.

TAKE-HOME POINTS

- An ethics consultation service is available in all US hospitals with 400 beds or more, along with federal hospitals and Council of Teaching Hospitals members.
- The American Society for Bioethics and Humanities (ASBH) was created in January 1998 to set standards and guidelines for healthcare ethics consultative services.
- Along with ASBH, the IntegratedEthics (IE) model from the US Department of Veterans Affairs National Center for Ethics in Health Care (NCEHC) was also developed. The IE model looked to replace its traditional, siloed ethics committee approach with a single, fundamental ethics program that directs and supervises the organization's ethics services obligation across the full range of content areas.
- For healthcare ethics consultations, the IE recommends using the CASES approach to complete this task, where C is Clarify, A is Assemble, S is Synthesize, E is Explain, and S is Support.
- IE defines preventive ethics (PE) as activities performed by an individual or group on behalf of a healthcare organization to identify, prioritize, and address systemic ethics quality gaps.
- Identifying problematic issues on an organizational level allows ethics committees to develop practical strategies to narrow the ethics gap. PE can then discover a systematic approach to tighten or eliminate these gaps.

- The *Core Competencies* report represents a commitment by the ASBH to ensure that qualified persons provide high-quality clinical ethical consultation.
- The Ethical and Religious Directives for Catholic Health Care Services (ERDs) are directives the United States Conference of Catholic Bishops promulgated to govern Catholic health facilities.
- Ethics committees are committed to fulfilling institutions' needs: consultative services, program development, education, preventive ethics, and research.

NOTES

1 Mark P. Auslisio, "Why Did Hospital Ethics Committees Emerge in the US?," *AMA Journal of Ethics* 18, no. 5 (May 1, 2016): 546–553, https://doi.org/10.1001/journalofethics.2016.18.5.mhst1-1605, page 546.
2 Mark P. Auslisio, "Why Did Hospital Ethics Committees Emerge in the US?," *AMA Journal of Ethics* 18, no. 5 (May 1, 2016): 546–553, https://doi.org/10.1001/journalofethics.2016.18.5.mhst1-1605, page 546.
3 Mark P. Auslisio, "Why Did Hospital Ethics Committees Emerge in the US?," *AMA Journal of Ethics* 18, no. 5 (May 1, 2016): 546–553, https://doi.org/10.1001/journalofethics.2016.18.5.mhst1-1605, page 546.
4 Mark P. Auslisio, "Why Did Hospital Ethics Committees Emerge in the US?," *AMA Journal of Ethics* 18, no. 5 (May 1, 2016): 546–553, https://doi.org/10.1001/journalofethics.2016.18.5.mhst1-1605, page 546.
5 George E. Schreiner, "Hemodialysis for Chronic Renal Failure: III. Medical, Moral and Ethical, and Socio-Economic Problems," *Annals of Internal Medicine* 62, no. 3 (March 1, 1965): 551, https://doi.org/10.7326/0003-4819-62-3-551.
6 Mark P. Auslisio, "Why Did Hospital Ethics Committees Emerge in the US?," *AMA Journal of Ethics* 18, no. 5 (May 1, 2016): 546–553, https://doi.org/10.1001/journalofethics.2016.18.5.mhst1-1605, page 547.
7 Mark P. Auslisio, "Why Did Hospital Ethics Committees Emerge in the US?," *AMA Journal of Ethics* 18, no. 5 (May 1, 2016): 546–553, https://doi.org/10.1001/journalofethics.2016.18.5.mhst1-1605, page 547.
8 A.-M. Slowther, "Clinical Ethics Committees," *BMJ* 321, no. 7262 (September 16, 2000): 649–650, https://doi.org/10.1136/bmj.321.7262.649.
9 See the ASBH website at https://asbh.org for more details about their history.
10 American Society for Bioethics and Humanities, *Core Competencies for Health Care Ethics Consultation* (Glenview, IL: American Society for Bioethics and Humanities, 2013).
11 American Society for Bioethics and Humanities, *Core Competencies for Health Care Ethics Consultation* (Glenview, IL: American Society for Bioethics and Humanities, 2013).
12 Anita J. Tarzian and ASBH Core Competencies Update Task, "Health Care Ethics Consultation: An Update on Core Competencies and Emerging Standards from the American Society for Bioethics and Humanities' Core Competencies Update Task Force," *The American Journal of Bioethics* 13, no. 2 (February 2013): 3–13, https://doi.org/10.1080/15265161.2012.750388, page 5.
13 Ellen Fox et al., *Ethical Leadership: Fostering an Ethical Environment & Culture* (Washington, DC: National Center for Ethics in Health Care, US Department of Veterans Affairs, 2020), page 13.
14 Lynn Sipsey and Joan Henriksen, "Ethics Consultant Training Standards: Don't Lower the Bar Without Benefit," *The American Journal of Bioethics* 22, no. 4 (April 3, 2022): 67–69, https://doi.org/10.1080/15265161.2022.2044561, page 67.

15 Marion Danis et al., "Health Care Ethics Programs in U.S. Hospitals: Results from a National Survey," *BMC Medical Ethics* 22, no. 1 (December 2021): 107, https://doi.org/10.1186/s12910-021-00673-9. Page 2
16 Melissa M. Bottrell, Robert A. Pearlman, Mary Beth Foglia, and Ellen Fox, "The IntegratedEthics Facility Workbook: An Evaluation Tool to Support Health Care Ethics Program Implementation and Quality Management," *AJOB Primary Research* 4, no. 1 (January 2013): 59–70, page 60.
17 Melissa M. Bottrell, Robert A. Pearlman, Mary Beth Foglia, and Ellen Fox, "The IntegratedEthics Facility Workbook: An Evaluation Tool to Support Health Care Ethics Program Implementation and Quality Management," *AJOB Primary Research* 4, no. 1 (January 2013): 59–70, page 60.
18 National Center for Ethics in Health Care, *Ethics Consultation: Responding to Ethics Questions in Health Care* (Washington, DC: National Center for Ethics in Health Care, 2006), www.bioethics.pitt.edu/sites/default/files/CEP/Dober%2C%20VHA%20Integrated%20Ethics.pdf.
19 National Center for Ethics in Health Care, *Ethics Consultation: Responding to Ethics Questions in Health Care* (Washington, DC: National Center for Ethics in Health Care, 2006), www.bioethics.pitt.edu/sites/default/files/CEP/Dober%2C%20VHA%20Integrated%20 Ethics.pdf.
20 Kenneth Berkowitz, et al. *Ethics Consultation: Responding to Ethics Questions in Health Care*, second edition (Washington, DC: National Center for Ethics in Health Care, US Department of Veterans Affairs, 2015), page vi.
21 Kenneth Berkowitz, et al. *Ethics Consultation: Responding to Ethics Questions in Health Care*, second edition (Washington, DC: National Center for Ethics in Health Care, US Department of Veterans Affairs, 2015), page viii.
22 Kenneth Berkowitz, et al. *Ethics Consultation: Responding to Ethics Questions in Health Care*, second edition (Washington, DC: National Center for Ethics in Health Care, US Department of Veterans Affairs, 2015), page 49.
23 National Center for Ethics in Health Care, *Ethics Consultation: Responding to Ethics Questions in Health Care* (Washington, DC: National Center for Ethics in Health Care, 2006), www.bioethics.pitt.edu/sites/default/files/CEP/Dober%2C%20VHA%20Integrated%20Ethics.pdf.
24 National Center for Ethics in Health Care, *Ethics Consultation: Responding to Ethics Questions in Health Care* (Washington, DC: National Center for Ethics in Health Care, 2006), www.bioethics.pitt.edu/sites/default/files/CEP/Dober%2C%20VHA%20Integrated%20Ethics.pdf.
25 National Center for Ethics in Health Care, *Ethics Consultation: Responding to Ethics Questions in Health Care* (Washington, DC: National Center for Ethics in Health Care, 2006), www.bioethics.pitt.edu/sites/default/files/CEP/Dober%2C%20VHA%20Integrated%20 Ethics.pdf.
26 Mary Beth Foglia et al., "Preventive Ethics: Addressing Ethics Quality Gaps on a Systems Level," *The Joint Commission Journal on Quality and Patient Safety* 38, no. 3 (March 2012): 103–111, AP1–AP7, https://doi.org/10.1016/S1553–7250(12)38014-8, page 103.
27 National Center for Ethics in Health Care, *Ethics Consultation: Responding to Ethics Questions in Health Care* (Washington, DC: National Center for Ethics in Health Care, 2006), www.bioethics.pitt.edu/sites/default/files/CEP/Dober%2C%20VHA%20Integrated %20Ethics.pdf.
28 National Center for Ethics in Health Care, *Ethics Consultation: Responding to Ethics Questions in Health Care* (Washington, DC: National Center for Ethics in Health Care, 2006), www.bioethics.pitt.edu/sites/default/files/CEP/Dober%2C%20VHA%20Integrated%20Ethics.pdf.
29 National Center for Ethics in Health Care, *Ethics Consultation: Responding to Ethics Questions in Health Care* (Washington, DC: National Center for Ethics in Health Care, 2006), www.bioethics.pitt.edu/sites/default/files/CEP/Dober%2C%20VHA%20Integrated %20Ethics.pdf.
30 National Center for Ethics in Health Care, *Ethics Consultation: Responding to Ethics Questions in Health Care* (Washington, DC: National Center for Ethics in Health Care, 2006), www.bioethics.pitt.edu/sites/default/files/CEP/Dober%2C%20VHA%20Integrated%20Ethics.pdf.
31 Kimberly E. Sawyer et al., "Competencies and Milestones for Bioethics Trainees," *The Journal of Clinical Ethics* 32, no. 2 (2021): 127–148, page 127.

32 Kimberly E. Sawyer et al., "Competencies and Milestones for Bioethics Trainees," *The Journal of Clinical Ethics* 32, no. 2 (2021): 127–148, pages 127–128.
33 Denise M. Dudzinski, Rosamond Rhodes, and Autumn Fiester, "Pedagogical Goals for Academic Bioethics Programs," *Cambridge Quarterly of Healthcare Ethics* 22, no. 3 (July 2013): 284–296, https://doi.org/10.1017/S0963180113000108. Page 286.
34 Anita J. Tarzian and ASBH Core Competencies Update Task, "Health Care Ethics Consultation: An Update on Core Competencies and Emerging Standards from the American Society for Bioethics and Humanities' Core Competencies Update Task Force," *The American Journal of Bioethics* 13, no. 2 (February 2013): 3–13, https://doi.org/10.1080/15265161.2012.750388, page 4.
35 National Center for Ethics in Health Care, *Ethics Consultation: Responding to Ethics Questions in Health Care* (Washington, DC: National Center for Ethics in Health Care, 2006), www.bioethics.pitt.edu/sites/default/files/CEP/Dober%2C%20VHA%20Integrated%20Ethics.pdf.
36 Anita J. Tarzian and ASBH Core Competencies Update Task, "Health Care Ethics Consultation: An Update on Core Competencies and Emerging Standards from the American Society for Bioethics and Humanities' Core Competencies Update Task Force," *The American Journal of Bioethics* 13, no. 2 (February 2013): 3–13, https://doi.org/10.1080/15265161.2012.750388.
37 National Center for Ethics in Health Care, *Ethics Consultation: Responding to Ethics Questions in Health Care* (Washington, DC: National Center for Ethics in Health Care, 2006), www.bioethics.pitt.edu/sites/default/files/CEP/Dober%2C%20VHA%20Integrated%20Ethics.pdf.
38 Kimberly E. Sawyer et al., "Competencies and Milestones for Bioethics Trainees," *The Journal of Clinical Ethics* 32, no. 2 (2021): 127–148, page 129.
39 Kimberly E. Sawyer et al., "Competencies and Milestones for Bioethics Trainees," *The Journal of Clinical Ethics* 32, no. 2 (2021): 127–148, page 129.
40 David F. Kelly, Gerard Magill, and H. ten Have, *Contemporary Catholic Health Care Ethics*, 2nd ed (Washington, DC: Georgetown University Press, 2013), page 197.
41 Sybert, Christine, "The ERDs: Part One—The Social Mission of Catholic Health Care Services," *The Linacre Quarterly* 88, no. 4 (2021), page 348.
42 Elliott Louis Bedford, "The Core Competencies: A Roman Catholic Critique," *HEC Forum* 23, no. 3 (September 2011): 147–169, https://doi.org/10.1007/s10730-011-9169-2, page 147.
43 Catholic Church et al., *Ethical and Religious Directives for Catholic Health Care Services.* (Washington, DC: United States Conference of Catholic Bishops, 2001).
44 Elliott Louis Bedford, "The Core Competencies: A Roman Catholic Critique," *HEC Forum* 23, no. 3 (September 2011): 147–169, https://doi.org/10.1007/s10730-011-9169-2, page 162.
45 Anita Tarzian et al., "Ethics Consultation in US Hospitals: Adherence to National Practice Standards," *AJOB Empirical Bioethics* 13, no. 1 (January 2, 2022): 10–21, https://doi.org/10.1080/23294515.2021.1996118, page 10.
46 Anita Tarzian et al., "Ethics Consultation in US Hospitals: Adherence to National Practice Standards," *AJOB Empirical Bioethics* 13, no. 1 (January 2, 2022): 10–21, https://doi.org/10.1080/23294515.2021.1996118, pages 10–21.
47 National Center for Ethics in Health Care, *Ethics Consultation: Responding to Ethics Questions in Health Care* (Washington, DC: National Center for Ethics in Health Care, 2006), www.bioethics.pitt.edu/sites/default/files/CEP/Dober%2C%20VHA%20Integrated%20Ethics.pdf.
48 Marion Danis et al., "Health Care Ethics Programs in US Hospitals: Results from a National Survey," *BMC Medical Ethics* 22, no. 1 (December 2021): 107, https://doi.org/10.1186/s12910-021-00673-9, page 2.
49 National Center for Ethics in Health Care, *Ethics Consultation: Responding to Ethics Questions in Health Care* (Washington, DC: National Center for Ethics in Health Care, 2006), www.bioethics.pitt.edu/sites/default/files/CEP/Dober%2C%20VHA%20Integrated%20Ethics.pdf.
50 Mary Beth Foglia et al., "Preventive Ethics: Addressing Ethics Quality Gaps on a Systems Level," *The Joint Commission Journal on Quality and Patient Safety* 38, no. 3 (March 2012): 103–111, AP1–AP7, https://doi.org/10.1016/S1553-7250(12)38014-8, page 104.

51 National Center for Ethics in Health Care, *Ethics Consultation: Responding to Ethics Questions in Health Care* (Washington, DC: National Center for Ethics in Health Care, 2006), www.bioethics.pitt.edu/sites/default/files/CEP/Dober%2C%20VHA%20Integrated%20Ethics.pdf.

52 Mary Beth Foglia et al., "Preventive Ethics: Addressing Ethics Quality Gaps on a Systems Level," *The Joint Commission Journal on Quality and Patient Safety* 38, no. 3 (March 2012): 103–111, AP1–AP7, https://doi.org/10.1016/S1553–7250(12)38014-8, page 106.

53 National Center for Ethics in Health Care, *Ethics Consultation: Responding to Ethics Questions in Health Care* (Washington, DC: National Center for Ethics in Health Care, 2006), www.bioethics.pitt.edu/sites/default/files/CEP/Dober%2C%20VHA%20Integrated%20Ethics.pdf.

54 Mary Beth Foglia et al., "Preventive Ethics: Addressing Ethics Quality Gaps on a Systems Level," *The Joint Commission Journal on Quality and Patient Safety* 38, no. 3 (March 2012): 103–111, AP1–AP7, https://doi.org/10.1016/S1553–7250(12)38014-8, page 110.

55 ECWeb Online Learning Module, "About This Module," accessed May 6, 2022, www.ethics.va.gov/ecweb/content/ecweb_html_about.htm.

56 Mary Beth Foglia et al., "Preventive Ethics: Addressing Ethics Quality Gaps on a Systems Level," *The Joint Commission Journal on Quality and Patient Safety* 38, no. 3 (March 2012): 103–111, AP1–AP7, https://doi.org/10.1016/S1553–7250(12)38014-8, page 110.

57 National Center for Ethics in Health Care, *Ethics Consultation: Responding to Ethics Questions in Health Care* (Washington, DC: National Center for Ethics in Health Care, 2006), www.bioethics.pitt.edu/sites/default/files/CEP/Dober%2C%20VHA%20Integrated%20Ethics.pdf.

58 Anita Ho, Lisa Mei-Hwa MacDonald, and David Unger, "Preventive Ethics Through Expanding Education," *HEC Forum* 28, no. 1 (March 2016): 69–74, https://doi.org/10.1007/s10730-015-9273–9, page 73.

BIBLIOGRAPHY

American Society for Bioethics and Humanities, *Core Competencies for Health Care Ethics Consultation*. Glenview, IL: American Society for Bioethics and Humanities, 2013.

Auslisio, Mark P. "Why Did Hospital Ethics Committees Emerge in the US?" *AMA Journal of Ethics* 18, no. 5 (May 1, 2016): 546–553. https://doi.org/10.1001/journalofethics.2016.18.5.mhst1-1605.

Bedford, Elliott Louis. "The Core Competencies: A Roman Catholic Critique." *HEC Forum* 23, no. 3 (September 2011). 147–169. https://doi.org/10.1007/s10730-011-9169-2.

Berkowitz, Kenneth, et al. *Ethics Consultation: Responding to Ethics Questions in Health Care*, second edition. Washington, DC: National Center for Ethics in Health Care, US Department of Veterans Affairs, 2015.

Bottrell, Melissa M., Robert A. Pearlman, Mary Beth Foglia, and Ellen Fox. "The IntegratedEthics Facility Workbook: An Evaluation Tool to Support Health Care Ethics Program Implementation and Quality Management." *AJOB Primary Research* 4, no. 1 (January 2013): 59–70.

Catholic Church, National Conference of Catholic Bishops, Committee on Doctrine, Catholic Church, and United States Conference of Catholic Bishops. *Ethical and Religious Directives for Catholic Health Care Services*. Washington, DC: United States Conference of Catholic Bishops, 2001.

Danis, Marion, Ellen Fox, Anita Tarzian, and Christopher C. Duke. "Health Care Ethics Programs in U.S. Hospitals: Results from a National Survey." *BMC Medical Ethics* 22, no. 1 (December 2021): 107. https://doi.org/10.1186/s12910-021-00673-9.

Dudzinski, Denise M., Rosamond Rhodes, and Autumn Fiester. "Pedagogical Goals for Academic Bioethics Programs." *Cambridge Quarterly of Healthcare Ethics* 22, no. 3 (July 2013): 284–296. https://doi.org/10.1017/S0963180113000108.

Foglia, Mary Beth, Ellen Fox, Barbara Chanko, and Melissa M. Bottrell. "Preventive Ethics: Addressing Ethics Quality Gaps on a Systems Level." *The Joint Commission Journal on Quality and Patient Safety* 38, no. 3 (March 2012): 103–111, AP1–AP7. https://doi.org/10.1016/S1553-7250(12)38014-8.

Fox, Ellen, et al. *Ethical Leadership: Fostering an Ethical Environment & Culture*. Washington, DC: National Center for Ethics in Health Care, US Department of Veterans Affairs, 2020.

Ho, Anita, Lisa Mei-Hwa MacDonald, and David Unger. "Preventive Ethics Through Expanding Education." *HEC Forum* 28, no. 1 (March 2016): 69–74. https://doi.org/10.1007/s10730-015-9273-9.

Kelly, David F., Gerard Magill, and H. ten Have. *Contemporary Catholic Health Care Ethics*. 2nd edition. Washington, DC: Georgetown University Press, 2013.

National Center for Ethics in Health Care. *Ethics Consultation: Responding to Ethics Questions in Health Care*. Washington, DC: National Center for Ethics in Health Care, 2006. www.bioethics.pitt.edu/sites/default/files/CEP/Dober%2C%20VHA%20Integrated%20Ethics.pdf.

Sawyer, Kimberly E., Nicolas Dundas, Anna Snyder, and Douglas S. Diekema. "Competencies and Milestones for Bioethics Trainees." *The Journal of Clinical Ethics* 32, no. 2 (2021): 127–148.

Schreiner, George E. "Hemodialysis for Chronic Renal Failure: III. Medical, Moral and Ethical, and Socio-Economic Problems." *Annals of Internal Medicine* 62, no. 3 (March 1, 1965): 551. https://doi.org/10.7326/0003-4819-62-3-551.

Sipsey, Lynn, and Joan Henriksen. "Ethics Consultant Training Standards: Don't Lower the Bar Without Benefit." *The American Journal of Bioethics* 22, no. 4 (April 3, 2022): 67–69. https://doi.org/10.1080/15265161.2022.2044561.

Slowther, A.-M. "Clinical Ethics Committees." *BMJ* 321, no. 7262 (September 16, 2000): 649–650. https://doi.org/10.1136/bmj.321.7262.649.

Sybert, Christine. "The ERDs: Part One—The Social Mission of Catholic Health Care Services." *The Linacre Quarterly* 88, no. 4 (2021).

Tarzian, Anita, Ellen Fox, Marion Danis, and Christopher C. Duke. "Ethics Consultation in U.S. Hospitals: Adherence to National Practice Standards." *AJOB Empirical Bioethics* 13, no. 1 (January 2, 2022): 10–21. https://doi.org/10.1080/23294515.2021.1996118.

Tarzian, Anita J. and ASBH Core Competencies Update Task. "Health Care Ethics Consultation: An Update on Core Competencies and Emerging Standards from the American Society for Bioethics and Humanities' Core Competencies Update Task Force." *The American Journal of Bioethics* 13, no. 2 (February 2013): 3–13. https://doi.org/10.1080/15265161.2012.750388.

Epilogue

An inane statement sometimes describes ethics consultations: "If you have seen one ethics case, you have seen one ethics case." With apologies to people who follow casuistry, each ethics case is unique. This reality is because the people involved are unique, and their problems are deeply personal. No ethics book can solve all the ethical issues that occur in healthcare. At best, a book can provide some of the tools needed to resolve healthcare dilemmas. After that, the individual must use that knowledge to make moral decisions.

Being proficient at resolving healthcare dilemmas requires multiple skills, often best provided by several rather than a single individual. The talents of healthcare professionals such as physicians, nurses, social workers, and chaplains offer the clinical and practical knowledge needed to dissect the root cause of the problem. This knowledge must be coupled with an understanding of the ethical principles involved. Challenging cases involving ethics can be both mind-numbing and heart wrenching for clinicians. Of course, let us not forget that it is also difficult for the patients and their families. Often, these cases represent the worst problem they have ever faced on the worst day of their lives. So, along with the clinical and ethical know-how needed by the professionals involved, compassion should also be added to that skill set.

Ethical principles are pretty straightforward. Autonomy is allowing people to be free to make their own decisions. Beneficence and nonmaleficence instruct healthcare professionals to do good and not bad to their patients. Finally, justice asks us to be fair when we make decisions that affect others. Knowledge of local laws and religious directives can be helpful when solving ethical issues, and it is useful to have attorneys and religious people as resources. Communication skills are needed not only for information gathering but also for conveying why specific decisions were made. Ultimately, when a decision is made, not everyone involved will agree with it. Still, everyone should understand how the decision was made and that it was made fairly.

As I said in the Introduction, this book was not written for ethicists or philosophers but for those who frequently face ethical dilemmas as part of their occupation. I doubt that I broke any new ground regarding the principles set forth by Beacham and Childress. Nevertheless, there was an attempt to explain the four principles in a way that would be more approachable to healthcare professionals. I have tried to use case histories that would be thought-provoking to the reader. Some of the stories presented are based on people I have met as a hospice and palliative care physician. Others were taken out of the headlines.

The COVID pandemic happened while I was writing this book. It provided a new scenario for applying old ethical principles. This application illustrated the principles' flexibility to new and unforeseen problems. So what is next, and what will the next healthcare crisis be? To quote Thomas Aquinas, "I would rather feel compassion than know the meaning of it. I would hope to act with compassion without thinking of personal gain."

Index

For Product Safety Concerns and Information please contact our EU representative GPSR@taylorandfrancis.com Taylor & Francis Verlag GmbH, Kaufingerstraße 24, 80331 München, Germany